Further Praise for *Green Medicine*

"*Green Medicine* is a courageous, profound, and rich journey through philosophy, culture, history, and healing practice that should be read by all who practice medicine and all who seek healing. Dr. Malerba provides the insight, wisdom, clinical expertise, and grand vision needed to recreate our health care philosophy, practices, and delivery system in ways that bring true healing and genuine holistic response to all who ail."

—Edward Tick, PhD, author of *War and the Soul* and *The Practice of Dream Healing*

"*Green Medicine* is a bold and comprehensive approach to harnessing one's life force to heal body, mind, and spirit, akin to the ancient wisdom teachings found in many cultures the world over. This book will create much-needed changes in the way we think about illness, medicine, and what it means to be truly healthy in the twenty-first century."

—Tom Cowan, author of *Fire in the Head: Shamanism and the Celtic Spirit* and *Yearning for the Wind: Celtic Reflections on Nature and the Soul*

"I wholeheartedly believe this book is needed because it shows why the materialistic/mechanistic approach of modern medicine does not work, and because it points to the critical factor left out in modern medicine: the role that a person's life force plays in healing."

—Carol K. Anthony, co-founder of the I Ching Institute, author of *A Guide to the I Ching*, and co-author of *Healing Yourself the Cosmic Way*

Green
Medicine

CHALLENGING THE ASSUMPTIONS
OF CONVENTIONAL HEALTH CARE

Larry Malerba, D.O.

North Atlantic Books
Berkeley, California

Published by   and
North Atlantic Books   Homeopathic Educational Services
P.O. Box 12327   2124 Kittredge Street #2
Berkeley, California 94712   Berkeley, California 94704

Cover and book design © Ayelet Maida, A/M Studios
Cover source images © geopaul (earth), © cteconsulting (caduceus)/iStockphoto.com
Printed in the United States of America

"I Want a New Drug (Called Love)," by Chris Hayes and Huey Lewis, © 1983 WB Music Corp., Huey Lewis Music and Kinda Blue Music. All rights administered by WB Music Corp. Used by permission of Alfred Publishing. "Unbroken Chain" and "The Wheel," Grateful Dead lyrics, © Ice Nine Publishing Company. Used with permission.

Green Medicine: Challenging the Assumptions of Conventional Health Care is sponsored by the Society for the Study of Native Arts and Sciences, a nonprofit educational corporation whose goals are to develop an educational and cross-cultural perspective linking various scientific, social, and artistic fields; to nurture a holistic view of arts, sciences, humanities, and healing; and to publish and distribute literature on the relationship of mind, body, and nature.

North Atlantic Books' publications are available through most bookstores. For further information, visit our Web site at www.northatlanticbooks.com or call 800-733-3000.

MEDICAL DISCLAIMER: The following information is intended for general information purposes only. Individuals should always see their health care provider before trying any therapies mentioned in this book. Any application of the material set forth in the following pages is at the reader's discretion and is his or her sole responsibility.

Library of Congress Cataloging-in-Publication Data
   Malerba, Larry, 1958–
Green medicine : challenging the assumptions of conventional health care / Larry Malerba.
   p. ; cm.
Includes bibliographical references and index. Summary: "Blends a philosophy of healing, ecological consciousness, and spirituality with a critique of conventional medicine and provides a new vision of health care that includes the best of orthodox medical and holistic healing methods"—Provided by publisher.
   ISBN 978-1-55643-902-5
   1. Integrative medicine. 2. Green movement. I. Title.
   [DNLM: 1. Complementary Therapies—trends—United States. 2. Clinical Medicine —history—United States. 3. Environmental Health—trends—United States. 4. Philosophy, Medical—United States. WB 890 M245g 2010]
   R733.M358 2010
   610.1—dc22   2009048215

1 2 3 4 5 6 7 8 9 SHERIDAN 15 14 13 12 11 10

Dedicated in loving memory of my grandfather
Lawrence A. Downes

My father
Robert Fortune Malerba

My good friend
Christopher Ellithorp

And to all of the ancestors and those who have come before me

Acknowledgments

To my wife, Mary, who read seemingly endless drafts and offered her wise counsel and kind criticism with patience and love: Thank you from the bottom of my heart.

Many thanks to my editor, Emily Boyd, for her professionalism, patience, and guidance through the publishing process; to Dana Ullman for his tireless advocacy, brainstorming, and belief in the project; to Greg "Captain Squeeze" Speck for his enthusiasm and for teaching me some of the finer points of writing; to Heidi Liscomb for her generosity and editing assistance; to Ed Tick for his wisdom and for introducing me to the fundamentals of publishing; to Emery Forest and Julie Purdy for helping me find the spiritual courage to complete the task; to Ed Brown for encouraging me to personalize my story; to Elaine Merrill for her painstaking copyediting; to my son Joel Malerba for his graphic art assistance; to Paul Winkeller for nudging me to write the book; to Ayelet Maida for her design expertise; and to everyone at North Atlantic for helping make this dream come true.

A debt of gratitude is also owed to those who have provided their friendship, have served as sources of inspiration, and taught me many lessons along the way: Bill Sullivan, Heinz Dill, Salvatore Ambrosino, Kirby Hotchner, Phil Robbins, Pearl Mindell, Tim Owens, and Mike Glass.

I would especially like to thank all of my patients for the many lessons they have taught me and for entrusting me with their care.

Table of Contents

Introduction

When people notice the new medicine movement now and are surprised at its swift rise and sudden popularity, they must not overlook that it is the fruition of much that was going on for a long time. It is a single common rallying point now. But its potential is barely yet realized. It is dynamite, for it challenges the principles of government and the principles of science too, and it holds the seeds of new values that might actually not be the old values in new clothing. It is not simply another tyrant awaiting the convenient overthrow of the present regime.

—Richard Grossinger, *Planet Medicine*

For all the many diseases that plague humankind, it seems that there are relatively few genuinely effective medical cures. Given all the money, effort, and research aimed at developing new treatments, real breakthroughs that help ease our struggles with human illness are rare. The very few so-called cures that are available tend to be accompanied by many nasty side effects. Not infrequently, it causes one to stop and wonder if the so-called cure is not worse than the disease. Yet the cost of quality health care continues to rise year after year, faster than all other expenses of daily living, and health industry bureaucrats and medical professionals continue to earn a healthy living as a result of those rising costs.

We know that something is very wrong and yet we cannot quite put a finger on it. People seem blinded to the realities of what is actually taking place. In fact, the medical system receives mostly praise for all the good that it does in spite of the problems that it poses for many of its patients. Glowing reports and feel-good stories appear regularly in newspapers and on the nightly news, while the side effects, casualties, and treatments gone wrong barely receive a mention.

In actuality, our nation is becoming sicker and sicker. Skyrocketing rates of allergies, asthma, autism, attention deficit disorder, depression, diabetes, fibromyalgia, heart disease, sleep disorders, and more all slip by with little explanation as to why they are increasing. Likewise, the widespread prevalence of violence, greed, and factionalism are indicators of our collectively deteriorating mental and spiritual health. The experts are at a loss and, I suspect, do not really want to look too closely because they might have to admit what they already intuitively know. And the promise of the modern pharmacological panacea is perhaps the single greatest contributor to the overwhelming degradation of an environment upon which we depend for our very survival. The unavoidable truth is that the medical system is sick and it is making its patients sick. The nation with the "most advanced health care system in the world" cannot see that its Medical Emperor is wearing no clothes.

The purpose of this book is to explore the root causes of this unsettling trend in medicine and to propose some philosophical adjustments and practical solutions. We will discover that erroneous assumptions regarding health and illness lead to inappropriate methods of treatment, which, in turn, lead to more illness and human suffering. Doctor shopping and pill popping are fast becoming recognized for the shams that they are. Conversely, a clear and unflinching awareness of the true nature of health, illness, and cure can lead to methods that promote real and effective healing. It is not too late to reverse the trend but it will require some serious thought and consideration.

A more astute understanding of the principles of genuine healing is forming the basis of a new green medicine that many are already beginning to embrace. It is incumbent upon all of us to educate ourselves regarding these issues so that we can make better health care choices. This book is designed to provide a direct and comprehensible appreciation of the flaws in medical thought and their potential remedies. An effective course correction will become possible when we shed some light on this largely unexamined subject.

The present status of medicine in twenty-first-century America parallels that of society in general. While all appears to be well on the surface, with clinics, labs, and other modern cathedrals of medicine springing up all around us, a closer look reveals a system that is failing to provide the fundamental services necessary to heal the sick. The tremendous wealth that underwrites the medical-industrial complex provides a meager return on our collective cultural investment. As with other sectors of society, the relatively well off tend to be the primary beneficiaries of the health care system while the rest of the population gets left behind.

However, this is not a book about redistribution of resources and the necessity of economic medical reform. Commonly proposed political solutions, such as single payer insurance to cover all members of society, only scratch the surface of a problem that runs significantly deeper. The real problem lies not in the financing of the system as much as with the actual practice of a form of medicine that we have proudly come to accept as state-of-the-art. Strangely though, the standard medical strategies employed by physicians remain virtually immune to scrutiny. We tend to blindly accept that doctors are maintaining the highest standards of care, given the current scientific knowledge at their disposal. But the truth is that there are a multitude of powerful and effective health care options available to us that respect the wisdom of the human body and its innate capacity to heal. Unfortunately, due to the peculiar prejudices of orthodox medicine, they are rarely given serious consideration. This book will examine the sources of this narrow-mindedness and offer an alternative perspective that is fundamentally inclusive and respectful of the diversity of healing methods.

More to the point, as I will be arguing at length, the practice of conventional medicine actually generates more illness than health. Its methods rarely result in cures and are more likely to only temporarily alleviate or worse, to suppress illness. This is a function of a quick-fix culture that has little patience for actual methods of healing that could produce long-term well-being. When disease is suppressed it may appear to be resolved, but it often smolders silently under the surface until it re-emerges, usually in more problematic form. This, too, parallels our societal proclivity to bury our truest needs and issues as we instead give paramount attention to matters of image and the pursuit of the material dream of wealth and security.

Dissatisfaction with the practice of modern medicine is fast becoming a commonplace experience. Most people have a favorite medical horror story that they can recount with little urging. We tend to dismiss or excuse these events, chalking them up to the trials and errors of medical science as it slowly gropes its way toward greater mastery over disease and illness. Quite to the contrary, I believe these adverse medical events to be an inevitability that results from an anachronistic understanding of human health and its connection to the web of life. The materialistic orientation of modern medicine compels it to spend its energy becoming proficient at treating and repairing the physical body as if it were an automobile. The consequence of such a single-minded approach is an escalating harm to the mental, emotional, and spiritual ecology of human health.

This harm is not simply a question of the neglect of these other dimensions of health but an actual unavoidable effect of the toxic and suppressive methods employed by modern medicine. The rise of chronic disease is not, contrary to common medical opinion, due to the fact that we are living longer. It is a direct consequence of our superficial and symptomatic approach to health care. The shortsightedness of a medical science that never stops to examine its own philosophical underpinnings dooms it to failure when measured against the yardstick of quality of life. Yes, it can stop most symptoms, temporarily, but this strategy rarely leads to greater health, vitality, or well-being.

The hubris and economic parasitism of orthodox medicine allows for patients to be exploited as sources of income while all other therapeutic possibilities are viewed as unwanted competition. Thus the accumulated wisdom of thousands of years of human medical experience is casually tossed aside in favor of the latest money-making "breakthrough." The consumer is programmed to respond to image and advertising and discouraged from asking too many questions. When the occasional thoughtful person naïvely attempts to bring a fresh perspective to the arena, the full force of scientific authority may be brought to bear upon such misinformed idealism. He or she may be branded a quack or simply dismissed as unscientific and ignorant. Thus the corporate medical machine, comprised largely of the pharmaceutical industry and health insurance companies, is allowed to roll on, crushing anything that gets in its path.

The entire misguided enterprise stems from one simple, basic, and very important detail: its own faulty perspective regarding the way the universe works and the way human health fits into that scheme. Not to say that there are not some valuable contributions that technological medicine has made to the betterment of mankind, but they are relatively few, highly overestimated, and grossly over-utilized. And so this present work aims to deconstruct the largely unexamined philosophical assumptions of Western medicine and their therapeutic ramifications. Concurrently, it will provide a more workable philosophical framework that accounts for the complex web of interrelationships between body, heart, mind, and soul to be incorporated into the actual practice of medicine so that health may be improved rather than death just delayed. It will take a little time to develop my argument and to provide a satisfactory explanation for these concepts but I hope that it will become clearer as you work your way through this book. I do not make these claims lightly, as they are the conclusions that I have drawn from twenty-five years of medical practice and soul searching.

The newly emerging green medical revolution is a reflection of similar changes beginning to take shape in all aspects of contemporary society. Even if the long-term implications are not yet completely clear, most people understand, at least intellectually, that all things are related, that body, heart, mind, and soul cannot be separated, that our cultural institutions must begin to reflect this fundamental truth, and that we are all in this cosmic journey together. The entrenched materialistic orientation of the medical power structure is a dead-end strategy that cannot serve the greater purposes of human health, growth, and healing. This book is my contribution toward a new understanding of these issues that will hopefully provide a sound basis for the restructuring of medical thought and practice.

SOME PERSONAL BACKGROUND

I have intended for a number of years to write this book but until this point had been unable to sit down and wrestle it onto paper. I kept waiting for a fuller perspective to emerge, only to eventually realize that the story is always being written and that this is the way it should be. Understanding the influences that lead an author to choose his or her subject matter can be illuminating, and it is in that spirit that I offer the following personal background.

I have always tended to focus my attention on the big picture. It seems to be the way my mind works. I became aware of this early on, when I met my now good friend Ed Brown after we both had recently graduated from college. Ed would regale me with the many insights he had gleaned while earning his master's degree in comparative religion. I was impressed with the breadth of his knowledge and the way he would weave this information into the concrete activities of his job as a counselor for emotionally troubled teenagers. I was reminded of an ecology class that I had taken in undergrad school. Ecology, I had come to understand, is a science that attempts to weave together many other branches of science into a cohesive whole.

After Ed and I became friends, I would occasionally tease him about his ever-evolving spiritual, philosophical, and psychological worldview, referring to it as the "Edwardian Synthesis." This was a reference to Teilhard de Chardin, one of our favorite philosophers, whose work has been collectively referred to as the "Teilhardian Synthesis." Ed has been a true source of inspiration and has given me the courage to pursue and honor my own synthesis.

Around the same time that I met Ed, an angel named Bill Sullivan entered into my life. While we were wandering around a bookstore at Harvard Square, unbeknownst to me, Bill had purchased a shopping bag full of books by Thomas Merton, the prolific Cistercian monk. As we exited the store he promptly handed the bag of books over to me as a gift. Naturally I felt obligated to read at least a few of them, starting with *The Seven Storey Mountain*,[1] and I will be forever indebted to Bill for his generosity. This divine intervention helped point me in the right direction at the beginning of my lifelong spiritual journey.

In spite of my spiritual and intellectual leanings, I nevertheless succumbed to the pervasive generational family pressure to become a "respectable" professional. I had not the courage to stand up to the powerful personality of my father, and there was little support for my own thoughts of becoming an academician. I buckled down, studied for the entrance exam, and ultimately enrolled in osteopathic medical school. After all, what was the big deal? I knew that I could at least find some common ground within the field of psychiatry.

My first day of medical school at Des Moines University arrived in 1984, just weeks after I'd read Richard Grossinger's *Planet Medicine*,[2] a remarkable volume covering the history of medicine and healing as viewed through a unique anthropological and philosophical lens. It contains several fascinating chapters on homeopathy, a system of medicine that was unfamiliar to me at the time. A week later I discovered that an instructor from the family medicine department was teaching an elective course on homeopathy during lunch hours. I promptly signed on—and became his virtual shadow for the next few years. For his patience and willingness to teach me I am deeply indebted to Dr. Kirby Hotchner, as he allowed me first to learn and then to help him practice homeopathy on many occasions in the university family practice clinic.

Just two weeks after I met Dr. Hotchner, while my wife, Mary, and I were looking for items for our first apartment together as a married couple we purchased a diploma at a yard sale. Across the top it read "Societas Medica Hahnemannia, Universitatis Iowaensis, Similia Similibus Curantur." It was the diploma of Gardner Appleton Huntoon, MD, from the University of Iowa Homeopathic Medical School, dated 1896. Much to my surprise, the medical school at U. of I. had been homeopathic (as was the case with many of our earliest medical schools) before it had transitioned into an institution for conventional allopathic medical training. In retrospect, this strange confluence of events, which I have since come to understand as a powerful synchronicity, changed the course of my life.

There was now another field of endeavor competing for my attention, but I proceeded according to the game plan. After completing a year of residency training in psychiatry and passing my medical boards, I stood at the crossroads. The subject matter of psychiatry was fascinating, but I found myself at odds with the emphasis upon disease labeling and drug therapy. The clinical results I had witnessed in Dr. Hotchner's office were far more compelling.

I took the leap and opened a private practice in homeopathic medicine. While building my practice, I worked on the side in a psychiatric emergency room that serviced a nine-county area across Upstate New York.

The many challenging and hair-raising experiences I had during my tenure there ultimately gave me the confidence to believe that I could persevere and succeed in the unusual profession that I had chosen. It also allowed me to develop a deep understanding of, and compassion for, human suffering in its many manifestations.

Now, medical school had been no piece of cake. It was tough enough for the average bright-eyed medical student but for someone like me, who had entered with a healthy dose of skepticism, it was like being thrown into the belly of the beast. Far from being a place of learning, medical school felt to me more like a boot camp designed to indoctrinate. Our minds were relentlessly stuffed with a dizzying array of seemingly unrelated tidbits and facts. Very little thought process was necessary, as everything had been carefully laid out in advance. We had no deep and heavy discussions about the purpose and meaning of illness, or even the philosophical underpinnings of medical practice. No time for that. Just go to class, study all night, and spit it back out on the multiple-choice exam the next day. I had gone into medicine looking for answers but what I found was deeply disturbing and dissatisfying. I had wanted to become a healer, not an encyclopedia of medical minutiae.

The generations of my parents and their parents tend to revere most professionals with unquestioning faith, especially doctors and the clergy. In fact, my current medical practice, which places strong emphasis upon patient participation so clients can help me to help them, can be a foreign and even frightening experience to many of the older generation. They are used to submitting to the authority of the physician. If I were to ask, for example, why an older patient continues to take a medication that is clearly making that patient sick, I might get the response that the doctor ordered it. The patient's life experience says to submit to, and obey the doctor, who is the ultimate authority in matters of health and illness, life and death. To question the decisions of the doctor is, to some, virtually unthinkable.

We live in a unique time, when the traditional structures of societal authority are freely and routinely questioned. The seeds sown by the generation brought up in the 1960s have now blossomed into an everyday recognition of our rights and responsibilities as citizens to challenge issues that we find oppressive and contrary to our basic democratic principles.

All around us we glimpse the signs of a greedy and callous medical empire that increasingly fails to fulfill its mission of service to the public. In a country with perhaps the greatest abundance of resources in the world, we have a government that refuses to provide for the most fundamental human need of protection in time of illness, and a medical-industrial complex that functions primarily to sustain its own existence. The time has come to challenge the basic assumptions of medical thought that justify the perpetuation of this monster run amok.

On a brighter note, we know that within the failed forms of the old resides the possibility of the new. If you haven't had your head buried in the sand for the past ten to fifteen years, it's been hard not to notice the enormous explosion of alternative forms of medicine and healing slowly creeping into the cracks and crevices around the edges of the allopathic establishment. The creep is so pervasive that it is often clandestinely sustained by many of the medical professionals employed by that very same health care establishment. It is not unusual for a patient to tell me that he or she was referred by a doctor but had also been advised not to reveal the source of the referral. Over the years, many professionals have confided to me their misgivings about the dysfunctional nature of the health care system that employs them.

This being said, before I go any further I would like to state with sincerity that I have enormous respect for the many dedicated doctors, nurses, physician assistants, EMTs, technicians, and paraprofessionals who have dedicated their careers to their art and to helping the sick. There are many aspects of the medical system that are valuable and indispensable, but that does not exempt it from the critique that is forthcoming in this book. Moreover, it is not the motives of the individual caretakers that I question as much as the very nature of medical education, its underlying philosophical assumptions, the system that delivers these health care services, and the attitudes of a society that embraces contemporary medicine. To some, my assessment of the state of modern medicine may seem a little harsh, but please be assured that it is offered in the spirit of constructive criticism. Ultimately, the many admirable achievements of Western medicine must be integrated, along with a variety of unconventional therapies, into a comprehensive system of care that will genuinely address the needs of the sick.

Although this may at times sound like an anti-science essay, I assure you that it is not. I love my iPod just as much as the next guy and I do not know how I could possibly have completed this project without the magic of word processing. But I *will* be questioning the extent to which we have accepted science and its worldview at the expense of a more well-rounded ecological perspective. Science, in and of itself, is fine. It is the elevated all-knowing status of medical science with which I take issue.

One result of the vacuum created by conventional medicine and its inability to accept new ideas has been a phenomenal growth of alternative practitioners and healers, which has served to fill the many gaps. Chiropractic, acupuncture, homeopathy, osteopathy, naturopathy, herbalism, nutrition, Chinese medicine, Ayurveda, Reiki, Rolfing, spiritual healing, shamanism, yoga, meditation, and tai chi are just some of the numerous forms of green medicine, healing, and self-help that have been embraced by millions of Americans. To recognize the reality of this trend and then consider the fact that standard medical practice continues to consist almost exclusively of pharmaceutical and surgical options must make any thoughtful person take pause.

At no point in the known history of our planet has there been a society that has placed greater value and trust in science than in twenty-first-century America. To understand the dysfunction of the medical system, it is useful to examine the basic assumptions that we make regarding science itself and the way that it is reflexively embraced by American culture. I will explore this in depth as well as the intimately related, corresponding American trends in consumerism and materialism. In the 1970s, Alvin Toffler warned us in his best selling book *Future Shock*[3] of the exponentially spiraling growth of technology and the compartmentalization, fragmentation, and alienation that would result. Well, that time has arrived. We are it, it is us, and it is profoundly affecting our conception of health care and the method of its delivery.

Further back in time, before the modern age, there were no doctors as we know them today. Living evidence of this exists in indigenous cultures that have been insulated from modern "civilization." There, the role of doctor is replaced by the shaman, who serves more as an organic synthesis of priest/elder/healer/doctor/teacher. We will examine the historical origins of this holistic unity and its subsequent split into distinct and separate entities, and the profound consequences of a dichotomy that has rendered the priest keeper of the soul and the doctor mechanic of the body. In today's medical environment, it would constitute scientific sacrilege to imply that soul and body have anything to do with each other. The scientist would call it silly superstition, and a doctor suggesting that your soul had anything to do with your health could be ostracized by colleagues for being unscientific and unprofessional.

Before endeavoring to critique various aspects of conventional medicine, I will need to lay some conceptual groundwork so that there is a point of reference from which to understand these criticisms. This groundwork will challenge the prevailing, and usually unconscious, assumptions that we make regarding the nature of health, illness, and cure. Of course, these widely accepted assumptions are largely generated by the steady stream of medical ideas and propaganda that we receive through the media and our interactions with the medical system. After all, who has the time to independently formulate a personal conceptual framework for understanding health and illness? Naturally, we leave that up to the doctors, scientists, and professionals whose job it should be to do that.

Unfortunately, I do not believe that health professionals are busy playing creative roles involving the conceptual development of health care. Rather, the system overwhelms its students and workers with endless details, facts and figures, and rules and regulations, leaving them little time to think outside of the box. Most importantly, it demands conformity, not free thinking. There is little incentive to be an innovator. As such it is crucial that the general public be educated regarding these issues because the medical world is too busy, for a variety of reasons, maintaining the status quo. This leaves alternative practitioners and their clients to do the pioneering work out on the fringes. Many practitioners seek a better standard of care because it is the right thing to do. In doing so, they often risk missing out on the financial rewards, social benefits, and professional perks that so readily come to mainstream practitioners.

In addition to laying a foundation and leveling my critique, I will also examine how we can retrieve what has been lost from our rich past in the hope of reconstructing a green health care philosophy that truly promotes healing, meets the needs of the sick, and recognizes the complex relationship between the internal environment and the external environment of the patient. Translating this philosophy into reality will require the medical establishment to adopt an attitude of genuine, non-competitive receptivity and a willingness to relinquish its need for absolute control. The focus must be the patient's well-being, not the doctor's ego. If this focus were the norm, under ideal circumstances the sufferer of chronic back pain, for example, might be instructed to visit a chiropractor, learn some yoga techniques, and see the appropriate therapist to deal with anger issues. Or the person whose back pain was just too far gone might be recommended for surgical intervention, followed by rehabilitation that included physical therapy, homeopathy, and yoga. Solutions such as these, which take into account the whole person, are preferable to the predictable triad of muscle relaxants, painkillers, and surgery.

You may think that this fundamental shift of medical perspective is too much to ask, that it can never happen. In response, I say that it is already happening. The inadequacies of the conventional medical paradigm have become obvious and, as a result, many patients are actively choosing other forms of care in spite of what their doctors are telling them. We can sit back and let market forces determine the character of the impending changes, thereby allowing the latest popular medical fads to become the standard of care. We can continue to allow Big Pharma and Wall Street to determine the hottest new drugs on the scene until the casualties are counted, the benefits are discredited, and we are forced to start the search all over again. Or we can educate ourselves and thoughtfully contribute to the debate, recognizing that we as patients are an integral part of the equation, and that doctors do not know everything. In fact, since physicians are the least likely to be receptive to innovation, the duty falls upon the general public to exert pressure on the profession to change. The only "reform" that we ever hear about involves the ongoing debate over how financial resources should be allocated within the existing medical structure. We rarely hear discussions about reforming the actual substance of medical practice. In any event, continued resistance to change may someday lead to the marginalization of such a narrowly focused, dysfunctional health care system.

The blueprint proposed here is not just pie-in-the-sky philosophical speculation, but a practical necessity, since the system in question is badly broken and in urgent need of change. Serious reevaluation and implementation of concrete measures that reorient medicine toward the patient and healing could have a profound and practical impact upon the quality, cost, and effectiveness of health care. Implicit in the design of a new green health care paradigm is that it effectively address the physical, mental, emotional, spiritual, and environmental needs of the individual and the community. Given that the present model really only addresses the physical and offers just lip service to the mental-emotional, it becomes clear that any meaningful reform has a long way to go. Not only does the medical profession need to reassess its thinking when it comes to the powerful connection that thought and emotion have to physical health, but it has not even scratched the surface of how religion, spirituality, purpose, and meaning fit into the equation. The healers and shamans of our distant ancestors took it for granted that the well-being of body and soul were inextricably woven together. The newly evolving paradigm will require that physicians significantly expand the scope of their understanding or else risk becoming mere technicians of the body.

We will explore some of the fundamental beliefs and concepts that are now emerging as the basis of the new medicine. While contemporary science views the human organism as a physical body with a brain at the helm, almost all religious traditions hold in common the notion that we are, at bottom, spiritual beings. If we neglect the soul and fail to incorporate matters of spirit into our everyday concepts of health and illness, we will continue to tread the naïve and nihilistic path of mechanistic medicine. The body bone is connected to the brain bone, is connected to the heart bone, is connected to the soul bone. Every person is connected to a family, is connected to the community, is connected to the nation, is connected to the planet, and is connected to the cosmos. We cannot, therefore, simply continue to repair the physical body while ignoring the unprecedented levels of environmental pollution and the social and psychic toxicity that surrounds it. Human health cannot be isolated like a specimen in a sterile lab. When we come to perceive with certainty the unity and interconnectedness of all things, we will have a starting point from which a true system of green healing can evolve. I hope that you will join me on this journey to consider some of the possibilities that I offer for your contemplation.

A note before we proceed: In order to avoid confusion, I have taken the liberty throughout to freely interchange several terms in reference to regular conventional medicine as we know it. Therefore, the words *modern, contemporary, conventional, orthodox, regular, Western, materialistic, allopathic, mechanistic,* and *rational,* while they all may carry slightly different connotations, will be used to refer to the same mainstream system of medicine to which most of us are accustomed. *Modern* and *contemporary* convey similar meanings, as do *conventional, orthodox,* and *regular. Western* refers to the primary geographical origins of our medical system. *Materialistic* refers to its almost exclusive concern with the physical body and to that which can be seen, touched, and measured. *Allopathic* indicates regular medicine's method of treatment by contraries or opposites. In other words, painkillers are used to treat pain, anti-inflammatory drugs to stop inflammation, and antidepressants to treat depression. *Mechanistic* alludes to the overly simplistic notion of the human body as a collection of parts that can be treated in the same way a mechanic fixes an automobile. And *rational* highlights medicine's use of logic and abstraction while neglecting the role of intuition and the heart in its approach to illness. In some places the more precise meanings of these words apply, and in others the words are randomly chosen so as to avoid repetition and monotony.

The Unifying Life Force

It is a fact beyond question that deep within ourselves we can discern, as though through a rent, an 'interior' at the heart of things; and this glimpse is sufficient to force upon us the conviction that in one degree or another this 'interior' exists and has always existed everywhere in nature.... In all things there is a Within, co-extensive with their Without.

—Teilhard de Chardin, *Hymn of the Universe*

CONNECTING THE DOTS

The determination of whether one possesses or lacks good health is quite arbitrary and largely in the eye of the beholder. This is partly because it is a rarely discussed and poorly defined subject—a rather strange thing to ponder, considering that Americans have been raised to believe the propagandistic proclamation that they have the "greatest health care system in the world." To my dismay, not once during medical school do I recall the subject being discussed in any class that I attended. Perhaps the only reference that I remember was the facile bromide that health is the absence of "dis-ease." In a certain sense this may be true, but it falls woefully short of what is really needed—a thorough and serious inquiry into the nature of illness, disease, health, and healing.

As a result of our cultural conditioning we are neither taught nor encouraged to look beyond the surface of things. It is not uncommon for a child who is not acting sick to be diagnosed with an ear infection after being examined by a pediatrician at a well-baby visit. This usually sets into motion a routine pattern of actions and underlying assumptions over which we feel we have little control. The doctor often prescribes antibiotics, and as long as the supposed infection has resolved by the time the pediatrician rechecks the child's ear after seven or ten days, there is no further attempt to understand how or why it happened. The problem is over—until the next discrete health care-related moment in time arises.

That may be six months later when asthma develops for the first time, or one month later when another ear infection flares up, or one week later when the child begins to have nightmares. In any event, no attempt to connect these events is made. It is assumed that they are unrelated. Since many people believe that modern medicine provides the most advanced, state-of-the-art health care in human history, we tend not to question our medical providers. We are too willing to sidestep our roles and responsibilities in such situations and instead concede control to medical authority figures. We assimilate the subconscious message that there is no point in thinking too hard about a possible relationship among symptoms. After all, if there really were a connection, medicine would have figured that out by now. Right? Wrong.

There are many questions that can be asked about the child with the ear infection. Was that really an ear infection to begin with? If the child was not acting sick in any other way, was the antibiotic really necessary? If we believe that it is an ear infection, we assume that a microbe caused it. And if a microbe caused it, we readily accept the medical mandate that the microbe must be killed. Is it correct to assume that an antibiotic has worked if the ear has improved one week later? Is it possible that the child would have recovered without an antibiotic? If the infection recurs one month later, we are discouraged from making a connection between it and the previous infection, and even if we come to the conclusion that they are related, the doctor is unlikely to change the course of treatment. Since we are not educated about other options, we assume that there is no point in putting further thought into them.

Since I have spent many years contemplating scenarios like the one depicted above, it has become second nature for me to question conventional medical attitudes and protocols. Still, I am frequently surprised at the degree to which people are seduced into suspending their own judgment regarding medical events that can have a direct and significant impact upon their lives.

The problem is that a variety of factors come into play to prevent us from trusting and believing in our own observations, intuitions, and judgments. One factor is the intimidating nature of medical jargon, which creates a convenient divide between doctor and patient, and makes the average intelligent person feel inadequate and unqualified to participate in the decision-making process. A doctor may simply rebuff the patient's statements of concern by asserting that the doctor is the authority and that the patient should not worry about things that he or she does not understand. Commonly, the fear card may be played to induce compliance. It is not unusual for parents to tell me that their pediatrician either directly stated or suggested that if the child did not take an antibiotic for an ear infection, the child could contract meningitis and possibly die. This constitutes an unwarranted form of coercion when considered in light of the most recent medical thinking, which encourages doctors to wait a few days to see if an ear infection will resolve on its own and to reserve antibiotics for more persistent and severe cases. This thinking represents a drastic and arbitrary shift in medical philosophy, thus morphing "the child could die" into "the child may possibly get over it on his or her own."

Another factor that discourages us from connecting the dots is the fragmented and compartmentalized nature of medical specialties. The physician is trained to think only in terms of his or her area of expertise, thereby making it easy to justify that accountability for a given condition lies with another specialist who deals with that other part of the body. The underlying assumption here is that our physical bodies are constructed like erector sets, each part capable of being detached and sent off to the shop as if it were not connected to the rest of our anatomy. The conscience of a physician can rest easy as long as the roles and responsibilities as defined by his or her specialty meet the specifications of current standards. Even if the physician were inspired to connect the dots, such a doctor would likely be deterred from doing so because that would include territory that fell outside of his or her medical domain. It can be a daunting task to educate oneself regarding these issues, but it is an absolute necessity if we are going to articulate what is wrong with medicine and what reforms need to be implemented in order to create truly holistic health care that serves the needs of the sick.

The science of ecology is an unusual example of generalization, in contradistinction to the prevailing medical trend of specialization. A new green perspective that seeks to transcend the current notion of medical ecology as a science that connects the *physical* body to the *physical* environment must broaden its scope to also include the relationships between body, heart, mind, soul, family, society, and environment.

Perhaps the first and most important principle to appreciate regarding the health status of any individual is that it cannot be ascertained from the viewpoint of a snapshot at a given moment in time—it must more accurately be understood using the analogy of a movie. A person's health can be improving, declining, or fluctuating over time, and is always an ongoing, unfolding story. It has turning points, climaxes, and moments of resolution. The individual frames of the film are meaningless unless run as a whole through a projector. It is not a static phenomenon but rather a process with a past, present, and future. This process cannot be appreciated unless changes over time are taken into account. The human organism is a dynamic entity possessing the ability to react, not react, adapt, or not adapt to a variety of factors that can change the direction of health at any given moment.

A thorough summertime examination of a patient with a history of recurrent winter bronchitis might reveal a snapshot of perfect health by conventional standards, but a movie of this person's life would indicate, even to the medically untrained observer, that something is amiss. It is this sort of common sense that is systematically undermined by the fragmented worldview of medical science, which teaches us to mistrust our own valid perceptions and to accept the unspoken assumption that last winter's bronchitis has nothing to do with the patient's present health status.

It is the same mindset that allows us to believe that a child's high fever and vomiting have nothing to do with the vaccination that was administered the day before. Such a mindset serves the purposes of the medical establishment in a variety of ways, most obviously in terms of responsibility and liability. Those who draw connections between medical events are advised to leave the hard thinking up to the experts. The ultimate trump card can be employed if an insolent patient insists upon believing his or her own judgment—the patient will be told that there is just no scientific proof to support such an argument. The more specialized the physician, the easier to intimidate the insubordinate troublemaker into submission by making the troublemaker believe that he or she lacks the requisite medical knowledge to make such important decisions.

The same dynamic plays itself out daily in doctors' offices across the land. The patient who had a fainting spell is told that a physical exam a week later reveals nothing of significance. All tests have come back normal and the patient is told not to worry because there is nothing wrong. Brief spells reminiscent of the faint may then occasionally recur, and subsequent return visits to the doctor continue to reveal no apparent problem. If the determined patient refuses to believe that nothing is wrong, he or she may come up against yet another tactic frequently employed when the physician has run out of options and is pressed to provide answers and solutions. The patient may be told to seek a second opinion, or the patient's mental health may be called into question when a visit to a psychiatrist is suggested. The obvious assumption here is that the problem is not in the body of the patient but in the mind, as if the two are separate and unrelated entities.

Just as health cannot be measured as a static phenomenon, it also cannot be judged by the simple presence or absence of physical signs and symptoms. Any complete assessment of health must include the emotional, mental, and spiritual symptoms, problems, and issues of the individual. While the medical profession pays lip service to these factors, those who embrace a holistic perspective must give them the real and serious consideration that they deserve.

A busy company executive may, by conventional medical standards, be the beneficiary of excellent physical health but may secretly be harboring a deep sense of purposelessness in life. A health-oriented society will someday come to view this not as some flaw that the executive is compelled to hide for fear of public shaming. It will instead embrace a medical view that this person deserves compassion, and that appropriate care should be available to address his or her wounded spirit. In the broadest sense, this calls into question the very nature and structure of corporate culture and whether in its current configuration it is compatible with the health of the individual.

Likewise, the physically healthy adolescent who is too shy to engage socially needs the proper health care resources to assist in building self-confidence before the problem leads to increasingly unhealthy life choices. While our current system tends to emphasize the physical aspects of health, it is clear that disorders of the mind or soul can have a real and profound impact upon overall well-being and, ultimately, physical health.

The next point to consider is the underlying reality that all things are related. Body, mind, emotions, and spirit are inextricably united with the physical and social environment as one whole and cannot be divided except as an exercise of the mind. This exercise is precisely what conventional medicine does and exactly where it commits its gravest error. Physical medicine rarely takes into account the deeper nature of the human being. Even when it does, it lacks an adequate framework to understand how these connections create a whole and, consequently, how to deal with them.

If a child develops frequent headaches and begins to do poorly in school, and it is discovered that the home environment is a battleground for two unhappy parents, is it sufficient or even ethical for the doctor to simply prescribe a painkiller and send the family on its way? Can the physical headaches be artificially disassociated from the emotional suffering of the child? If a prescribed medication successfully blots out the headaches, will the child's wounded spirit go unnoticed, thereby contributing to more profound health issues in the future? This is not mere philosophical fancy. It is a crucial point of conceptual orientation that determines how medical treatment and healing methods are practically applied.

Health, therefore, is not a quantity that can be measured. It is a quality that is complex, multi-factorial, and changeable. It is a dynamic process that shifts, moves, and has directionality. Considered in this way, we may conclude that ideal health is not a static state of symptomlessness. In fact, I believe that stasis is emblematic of chronic illness, whereby a person's ongoing symptoms represent a type of "stuckness" from which the person cannot extricate him- or herself. The person with chronic disease is stuck in an inflexible state, a negative feedback loop that is no longer changing, ebbing, or flowing.

The ideal is more akin to a resilient and flexible state of adaptability that can roll with the punches as it encounters life's various physical, emotional, and situational stressors. Health viewed in this way is a function of a person's resilience and susceptibility as the person interfaces with the environment. Stressful events can bounce off of an individual, leaving the person unscathed, can be absorbed and transmuted into energy for growth and change, or can penetrate into the mind-body, causing difficulties and illness.

Four children experiencing the death of a close grandparent may respond in different ways, according to their own uniqueness and the status of their overall health. One cries daily for a week, expresses emotion and discusses feelings with his or her parents, ultimately rebounding nicely, having learned valuable life lessons. Another feels the emotional impact more profoundly and becomes insecure about taking the bus to school in the mornings. The third does not cry, does not want to talk about it, and develops headaches that recur for weeks. The fourth also does not process the emotional impact of the event and, one month later, develops pneumonia for the first time ever. In each case the resulting impact can be seen as a function of the uniqueness of the child's constitutional state of resiliency or susceptibility. The first child clearly represents the ideal, while the others do not, and the fourth child is perhaps the weakest and most susceptible to this particular stressor.

If we accept the feasibility of this example, it is not a stretch to grasp that these different aspects of a living, breathing human being—mind, body, heart, and soul—respond to events as a whole, and if one is impacted then all are impacted. Any dividing line is drawn out of convenience and is purely artificial. Science, medicine, and the contemporary mind are seduced into believing in the dividing line to such an extent that they make it a fundamental principle that informs the perceived and experienced reality of those who embrace it. Such a worldview allows the physician to believe that the removal of a gallbladder is a strictly physical event that if performed with technical accuracy will have no impact upon anything except the physical body of the human being whose organ was removed.

Consequently, if this surgical patient starts having panic attacks one month later, the physician may confidently rely upon a compartmentalized worldview when he or she informs the patient that there is no connection between these two events that have occurred at different moments in time. The surgeon believes no further consideration is necessary and sees his or her role as completed once the proper referral to the psychiatrist has been made. If, on the other hand, we believe in the mind-body connection, then we see the two events as profoundly related, and the medical system that provides care for this person should be required to acknowledge and address the chain of events that has transpired.

Psychosomatics, the study of the effects of thought and emotion upon the physical body, is, for some reason, accepted by the medical establishment as plausible in a curiously limited way. Thus we are accustomed to the classic examples of job stress causing an ulcer, or a school phobia causing stomachaches and headaches. Psychosomatics acknowledges these types of connections, and medical authorities concede the role of emotional triggers for physical illnesses, but beyond this, many mind-body connections are simply dismissed or denied in the real-life clinical setting. Why is it not conceivable that a divorce can trigger the onset of arthritis? How likely is it that a man's jealousy can cause him to have back spasms? Do we allow ourselves to believe that the businessperson's fear of financial failure could precipitate an episode of acute hepatitis? Is it possible that there is a connection in the case of a woman who after being raped in the workplace parking lot develops a paralytic leg, which prevents her from returning to her job?

In addition to these psychosomatic examples of illness, causal relationships can be further differentiated into somato-somatic, psycho-psychic, and somato-psychic. In other words, an emotional trigger can lead to a physical illness, a physical trigger can precipitate a physical illness, an emotional trigger can cause an emotional illness, and a physical trigger can cause an emotional illness.

Instances of somato-somatic illness are a chronic headache caused by a concussion, arthritis precipitated by a broken bone, or even a seizure disorder induced by vaccination. Psycho-psychic illness can be exemplified by the death of a loved one causing depression, a frightening experience leading to panic attacks (as is often the case in post-traumatic stress disorder), or abusive treatment leading to chronic guilt and shame. The somato-psychic type is a little harder to fathom but is nevertheless very common. A head injury can cause depression, a bad reaction to anesthesia can be followed by out-of-body experiences, or heat stroke can be a trigger for rage attacks. The bottom line here is that virtually anything can cause anything else. There are no set rules that predetermine the possibilities, which are virtually infinite. The medical profession, therefore, must begin to develop an open-minded receptivity to each individual situation, rather than clinging to a neat arrangement of disease entities into predetermined categories.

Because its discomfort with the non-physical aspects of life is so great, conventional medicine prefers to limit its scope almost exclusively to the physical and because of this often ignores emotional triggers, psychological factors, and relationships. The blinders of medical science impose conceptual and perceptual limitations that result in a tendency for the profession to squeeze the round pegs of psychological and spiritual factors into the preconceived square holes of physical medicine. Since medicine does not acknowledge the not-so-subtle differences among the various permutations of human illness, it winds up treating all things as is if they were the same, employing tunnel vision to justify its one-size-fits-all therapeutic approach.

In deconstructing the biases of medicine's materialistic perspective and in constructing a model of how things really are, the next step is to recognize that the physical, emotional, mental, spiritual, and environmental aspects of human life exert much more than just an occasional influence upon one another. They are, by definition, one entity. One cannot be manipulated without simultaneously affecting all others. One could just as easily distinguish these different aspects as the physical, etheric, astral, mental, and spiritual planes. The distinctions are arbitrary because in the final analysis they are not separate, and together they comprise a seamless whole.

The human organic-energetic-spiritual whole is a unified system and the most complex life form that evolution has produced to date—although there is credible evidence to support the theory that the earth and all of its organic and inorganic inhabitants together comprise a vast organism of extraordinary complexity. Just like the proverbial pebble tossed into the pond whose ripples spread out endlessly thereby affecting the entire universe, any factor, no matter how small, that interfaces with any aspect of a human life ultimately leaves its mark on the whole unified system of that individual person. If we accept the truth of this, we come to see that the sprained ankle is not just a physical event, the hurt feeling is not just an emotional event, and the religious epiphany is not just a spiritual event.

Consider the following example of a child's first encounter with a medical intervention. It plunges the family into a series of events beyond their control, beginning in the clinic, where the doctor examines the child and announces that hernia surgery must be performed. Anxieties and questions are greeted with a casual "don't worry," as the gears of the medical machine are set into motion. Pre-operative routine dictates that the patient is poked with needles as blood is drawn and intravenous lines are set up. This usually occurs in a gleaming white, impersonal environment, where all personnel wear similar uniforms. It is understood and accepted that the child will be separated from his loved ones, who are made to stay out of the way in the waiting room. An artificial coma-like state is then induced with anesthesia in preparation for the surgeon, who then cuts into a body cavity to perform the "routine" procedure. The child then awakens in a disoriented fog in the recovery room to an array of unfamiliar faces, as the parents may still be discouraged from being present. Finally, providing that no complications like infection or hemorrhaging have occurred, the normal activities of the child may be severely restricted for a period of several weeks during convalescence.

If you would like to believe that hernia surgery is just a casual physical procedure, having no appreciable impact upon mind, emotion, spirit, and family, then think again. Nevertheless, the scientific medical community easily compartmentalizes and minimizes instances like this by focusing solely on the task at hand, in this case the actual hernia, thereby convincing themselves and society in general that there is nothing else to be concerned about.

Mind you, I am not suggesting that we eliminate hernia surgeries. However, I do wish to point out that in our highly technological and medically oriented society, we have come to accept many serious medical interventions as routine events having only inconsequential and temporary effects upon our physical bodies.

CROSS-CULTURAL CONCEPTIONS OF LIFE ENERGY

In the coming chapters, I will begin to define concepts like spirit and soul, explain how they are connected to the physical body, and how the conventional medical world-construct neglects these interrelationships. Along the way we shall also explore how spirit and soul may be elevated back to equal status alongside the concerns of the physical body so that balance can be restored in the quest for health and healing. For the moment though, let us next examine some ideas and beliefs regarding the driving force behind human health and illness, and how we can come to understand that force so that we can work with it rather than against it.

If we are to believe that a human being is more than a collection of body parts, more than just a bag of bones, muscles, and organs, then it is reasonable to assume the existence of some organizing force that coordinates the whole. The materialists of modern medicine posit this to be the brain, failing to grasp the implication that this still places a physical entity in control of body, mind, emotions, and soul. The popular media enthusiastically report the findings of each new imaging technique designed to visualize the brain, as if we will, one day, come to determine the exact location of where God resides in our heads.

Many cultures, mostly Eastern, believe the essence of humanity resides in the heart. The medical mind with its unique form of tunnel vision balks at this notion, unable to see beyond the physical and unable to realize that this is not meant literally. I prefer this metaphor of the heart because it counters the absurd notion that we will ever find an actual physical location wherein lies the life-giving force of a human being. This concept of a life force as a non-material entity is fundamentally incompatible with the prevailing materialism of conventional medical thought. The Western brain and the Eastern heart are very powerful images, which provide insight into the overall orientations of each respective culture. Each represents only an incomplete fraction of the whole, and a mutually respectful synthesis of the two is a prerequisite for a true revolution in the way that green medicine and healing will be viewed and practiced in the future.

Throughout history there have been many attempts to name, describe, and understand this life force that animates each living person. Naturally, this type of organizing energetic intelligence is not exclusive to humanity; it can be attributed to every living thing, whether human, plant, or animal. Many cultures and great thinkers assume all of physical existence to be imbued with a life force. A cursory glance at North, Central, and South American indigenous cultures reveals a universal belief that all animals, plants, stones, waters, and winds have spirits that animate them, which are to be respected. While the modern mind may judge this to be superstition, indigenous peoples would tend to believe that contemporary humanity's lack of soul renders it unable to see.

One of my favorite proponents of this latter worldview is the visionary Jesuit priest, paleontologist, and philosopher Pierre Teilhard de Chardin. His pioneering work, *The Phenomenon of Man,* proposes a universe where all things animate and inanimate are permeated with varying degrees of energy or consciousness in accordance with their level of complexity. The energy, or consciousness, of the Teilhardian Synthesis is purpose-driven, as all of existence strives upward from stone to plant to animal up to humans and, ultimately, to the Omega point in which the evolution of life culminates in Christ-like perfection.

Most religious traditions include the concept of an individual soul that lives on after death. Some believe that the soul goes to heaven or to hell, and some believe that it will reincarnate again in order to continue learning its lessons in the classroom of life that we call planet Earth. Some Christian denominations celebrate All Souls Day when the souls of departed ancestors are remembered and honored. In Mexico, this has become popularly known as the Day of the Dead.

Egyptian mythology contains one of the earliest recorded attempts to portray a life-giving vital energy. The creator god, Khnum, fashions two models of each person at birth, one from clay on his potter's wheel representing the physical body, and another representing the vital essence or "ka." The two are then united in the creation of each new individual. At the moment of death, the departing soul is often depicted as a human-headed bird fluttering from the mouth of the deceased. The spiritual ka continues to exist even after its mortal double has expired.

Likewise, Ayurvedic medicine from India, whose origins date back thousands of years, rests upon the premise of the vital life energy of "prana," the

Sanskrit term for breath. Prana manifests itself in countless forms, from atoms all the way up to and including all living beings. This unifying life-principle, or "breath of life," enters the body at birth, holds body, mind, and spirit together as one, and eventually leaves the body at the moment of death. Additionally, Ayurveda holds that the heart is where our true sense of who we are resides, and is the seat of human emotion and consciousness.

In the similarly ancient philosophy of Chinese medicine, Chi is the term that most closely corresponds to our concept of life force. It is the Chi (also called Qi) that drives all organs and bodily processes. Chinese medicine employs methods that restore depleted Chi and ensure the smooth flow and balance of Chi in a person who is ill. In Ted Kaptchuk's classic book, *The Web That Has No Weaver*, a groundbreaking rendering of Chinese medical thought for the Western mind, he describes the difficulty in grasping the true nature of Qi:

> We can say that everything in the universe, organic and inorganic, is composed of and defined by its Qi. But Qi is not some primordial, immutable material, nor is it merely vital energy, although the word is occasionally so translated. Chinese thought does not distinguish between matter and energy, but we can perhaps think of Qi as matter on the verge of becoming energy, or energy at the point of materializing.[4]

Here, the distinction between matter and energy begins to blur, challenging our dualistic mode of perceiving the world around us. Some gifted persons have the ability to sense or visualize the human bioenergetic field. This electromagnetic field has been referred to as the "aura" and is seen by some as colored light or radiations of energy surrounding the body. Kirlian photography is an actual method of photographing images of the auras of living creatures that was developed by a husband and wife team of Russian scientists in the late twentieth century. Beautiful and complex patterns of colored light are obtained through the use of this technique.

That such similar beliefs are to be found in so many diverse cultural settings and historical epochs is striking and lends significant credence to the notion of a life-directing force. The presumptuousness of Western science, which cannot locate, measure, or dissect this life force, tends to prejudice the physician into viewing these age-old representations as cute and quaint. I believe, however, that the emerging general consensus and consciousness of the green medical movement is beginning to debunk conventional medicine's primitive and unsophisticated emphasis upon the singularity of the physical body.

The closest likeness to the concept of a life force that science does acknowledge are the properties of energy and the laws of physics. In most educational institutions, including pre-medical curricula, the basic sciences are usually taught in a three-tiered sequence of biology first, then chemistry, and finally, physics. The trend here leads from the commonly recognizable material substance to the more abstract—from the gross anatomical or biological structure of the brain, for example, to the neurochemical transmitters that comprise brain chemistry, to the electrophysiology that measures the brain's electrical activity and the nerve impulses that travel along neurons—from the actual organ to its chemical composition to its energetic properties.

Furthermore, the basic sciences teach that biology depends upon the laws of chemistry. Without the complex biochemical pathways that drive a multitude of physiologic functions, all organisms would simply be lifeless blobs of protoplasm. But basic science also teaches that chemistry depends upon the laws of physics. Without thermodynamics and the laws of energy that drive all chemical reactions, atoms would not bond together and the chemical building blocks of nature could not be arranged to create life. Simply put, biology cannot function without chemistry and chemistry cannot function without physics.

Modern-day conventional medicine operates almost exclusively on the first two levels. The vast majority of medical treatments involve drug therapies, representing the chemical approach, and surgeries, which manipulate the biological structure and anatomy of the organism. There is a peculiarly striking poverty of thought when it comes to the therapeutic application of energy, in spite of the education of all scientists regarding its nature and properties as formulated by physics. Science acknowledges the vital role of energy in the functioning of all life but medicine acts as if it would constitute hocus-pocus to use energy as a healing modality.

Strangely, there is no lack of imagination when it comes to utilizing energy in diagnostic testing. There is an increasing abundance of technologies designed to visualize the internal anatomy of the human body. An ultrasound device can bounce sound waves off of its intended subject, X-rays use electromagnetic radiation as a beam of high energy electrons to produce an image, CAT (computerized axial tomography) scans operate much like X-rays, and MRI (magnetic resonance imaging) machines use a combination of radio waves and a magnetic field generated by a powerful magnet to produce its images.

Although these technologies are extremely effective in detecting physical anomalies, most, nevertheless, pose real dangers to human health. One of the more bizarre medical rituals is the regular application of concentrated radiation in the form of mammography directed to the breast, one of the most radiation-sensitive parts of the body. In order to detect cancers that we know can be related to radiation exposure, we repeatedly expose the body to diagnostic X-rays. In spite of the sheer power of magnetic resonance imaging, and aside from the danger it poses when in the presence of metallic iron, the MRI is currently believed to be safe, but every intuitive fiber of my being tells me that this technology will someday be recognized as a significant source of medically induced illness.

Perhaps some acknowledgement should be given to the crude therapeutic employment of energy when radiation is used to treat cancers, or when a radioactive isotope of iodine is used to destroy the thyroid gland in cases of hyperthyroidism or thyroid cancer. Some credit may be granted for the use of energy in these treatments, but the net effects are also very destructive and often dangerous. These modalities are representative of the "war on disease" mentality. As we shall see, in lieu of waging a war that tends to combat a person's vital energy, energy has many potential uses that can work in harmony with the innate intelligence of the life force. Unfortunately, with a world of promising methods of employing energy in health and healing at its doorstep, the medical establishment tends to view these potential opportunities as competitors in an "us versus them" turf battle.

MAY THE VITAL FORCE BE WITH YOU

Early medical history, on the other hand, represents a rich reserve of ideas and philosophies that had not yet been sterilized by twenty-first-century materialism. Most of these ideas have been expunged from medical education and replaced by the myriad of "facts" that contemporary science so prides itself on. Nevertheless, there have been many free thinkers who made a variety of important observations regarding health and disease, and this information is still available to those willing to do a little digging.

Perhaps the most intriguing and potentially valuable concept that conventional medicine has long declared outdated and obsolete is that of vitalism. This is the belief in an underlying force of nature, a force beyond the understanding of the laws of chemistry and physics, which nevertheless guides and informs the essence and nature of life itself. Since the life-directing force of vitalism lies at the perimeter of the sciences, it is ultimately unknowable in the manner that science would wish to know it. As such, an esoteric, metaphysical, or even religious perspective may be needed to comprehend the life force. A form of knowledge and perception different from our conventional mode of rational scientific thinking is required to become familiar with the essence and dynamics of this vital force. As we shall see, an equally viable, empirical, more direct, and experiential mode of perception may be the key to revealing its seemingly mysterious properties and secrets.

At various points in the history of scientific discovery, the theory of vitalism was repeatedly pronounced dead because it was believed that life could now finally be explained in other than mystical or metaphysical terms. William Harvey's anatomical discovery of the function of the heart suggested that this organ was the pump that drove life. With the invention of the microscope, it was believed that the secrets of life would soon become clear. Tiny microbes became the basis of Louis Pasteur's germ theory and were thus claimed to be the ultimate cause of many diseases. When chemists discovered the atomic and molecular building blocks of organic matter, the explanation for all things was thought near at hand. The visualization of subatomic particles through electron microscopy and the formulation of field theories in physics seemed to bring us even closer to the conceptual foundation of all life. James Watson and Francis Crick began to unravel the secrets of DNA (deoxyribonucleic acid), and humankind was drawn along by this proverbial carrot held before the scientific horse's nose, as popular culture anticipated that the answers to our health problems would be found when the code of the double helix was finally broken. Nanotechnology has extended the reach of technology into the realm of contemporary physics, where the latest discoveries continue to lead us to believe that the key to longer life and greater health are contained within this tiny universe. This unwavering faith in reductionistic solutions remains the dominant driving force behind modern technological culture.

One particularly persuasive refutation of the vitalistic concept accompanied the emergence of Darwin's theory of evolution. Natural selection and the science of genetics were now thought to explain life's tendency to change and evolve in certain directions, once again reducing the idea of an intelligence or guiding force to a mechanistic interplay of genes and environmental factors. Regardless of how hard science tries to reduce life to a logical system of predictable laws, there will always continue to be a variety of phenomena that remain anomalous, stubbornly refusing to conform to the prevailing theory. As we shall see, a more holistic perspective can allow for evolutionary forces and cosmic order to peacefully coexist without contradiction.

In the annals of Western medicine, various proponents of vitalism have attempted to ascertain the more specific role that the life force played in terms of health, illness, and cure. Perhaps the most well-known historical figure to advocate for a vitalistic perspective was Paracelsus, the sixteenth-century alchemist, physician, and astrologer considered by some to be the father of toxicology. Paracelsus used the term *archeus* to mean the innate vital principle that maintains and directs the life energy of all living beings. The archeus was a spiritual principle that was responsible for the health and illness of an individual.

Paracelsus's body of work effectively bridged the two worlds of science and the more esoteric. Although largely forgotten by science, he has had an enormous influence upon the modern practice of alternative medicine. Clearly, Paracelsus found it important to have knowledge of all that science had made available but he also knew that an understanding of the metaphysical was an invaluable asset.

The ideas of Paracelsus were subsequently taken up by Jan Baptista van Helmont, a Flemish physician of the seventeenth century. As a vitalist, van Helmont believed that illness took hold first upon the inner spiritual aspect of a person before it became manifest on the outer physical body. He based his medicine upon observation and experiment, placing greater value upon firsthand experience than on the logic of practitioners of the Rationalist form of medicine of the time.

Van Helmont and Paracelsus had both broken with the predominant thinking of the time, which had its roots all the way back in the second century with the ideas of Galen, an early Greek physician who practiced medicine using the Hippocratic concept of the four humors. This contentious split between Rationalist and Empiricist factions throughout medical history is a theme that will be developed in this book. The views of Galen dominated medicine for more than a thousand years and were based upon rational thought, that is, ideas about health and illness as constructed by the mind. Paracelsus, on the other hand, believed in the empirical view that experience, rather than abstract thought, was the path to true understanding.

We will see how modern medicine, which prides itself on being "scientific," is in reality largely driven by ideas that often contradict clinical experience, thereby reflecting more of a Galenist influence. I would contend that much of the empirical evidence demonstrated through modern experimental methods is frequently discarded because it conflicts with the prevailing logic and beliefs of the medical establishment. The prejudice of the rational perspective can be strong enough to blind the observer to the obvious reality sitting before his or her very nose. Something may be seen with one's own eyes and felt in the heart, but it cannot be believed because it does not jibe with the world as constructed by the rational mind.

Another prominent vitalist was the seventeenth-century physician George Ernst Stahl, who proposed that the *anima*, or "soul," was a life force centered in the stomach. This anima possessed its own intelligence, independent from the body, and was the source of a curative power that could heal illness. His theories, which influenced European medical thought for quite some time, were precursors to the establishment of the use of the terms "vitalism" and "vital force" in the early medical lexicon.

The German physician Samuel Hahnemann subsequently developed extensive theories about the vital force, which he often referred to as the *dynamis*. This body of knowledge, derived from many years of empirical observation and experimentation, came to form the underpinnings of his system of medicine, called homeopathy. Multiple revisions he made in the early 1800s of his monumental work, the *Organon of the Medical Art*, contained specific and detailed descriptions regarding the action of the vital force in relation to illness and its cure. He described how the energy of the dynamis became discernable as symptoms as it ebbed and flowed in the human organism. Thus symptoms were viewed not only as physical entities but also as evidence of the underlying life force. Hahnemann anticipated the false duality of body and mind, matter and energy, to which modern medical science so thoroughly subscribes. In his work, again, we see that the human body and energizing vital force are one, and can be divided only as an exercise of the rational mind.

The influence of vitalistic thinking is even evident in Sigmund Freud's use of the term "libido," which can be seen as an equivalent of the life force, and in Carl Jung's "objective psyche" or "collective unconscious," which he postulated as the substratum of all mental activity. Sadly, psychiatry, a field so rich in history and ideas, with such eminent thinkers as Alfred Adler, Elisabeth Kübler-Ross, Karen Horney, and Thomas Szasz, has been virtually eclipsed by the prevailing tunnel vision of psychopharmacology and the mechanistic belief in brain chemistry as the foundation of human behavior.

The psychopharmacological perspective of biological psychiatry is further reinforced by the insurance industry, which gives little respect to the role of psychotherapy and reimburses mostly for brief visits that involve the management of patients' medications. The reduction of such a potentially powerful healing profession as psychiatry to the role of gatekeeper for a specific class of drugs that primary care physicians are (rightly) reluctant to prescribe is a sad and terrible waste of medical talent.

I recall having to go to extraordinary measures when in training as a psychiatry resident, attempting to get the administration to allot funding for personal psychotherapy. I argued that it made perfect sense that all psychiatrists in training should have to undergo some form of psychotherapy. What better way to learn than to experience the psychotherapeutic relationship first-hand from the perspective of the patient? Although my request was ultimately rebuffed I remained undaunted and nevertheless funded my own analysis with a Jungian therapist from my paltry resident's stipend. Although I found this to be an invaluable experience, it ultimately became too much of a hardship both in cost and in time taken away from my resident's duties, so I had to cut it short sooner than I would have liked.

The persistence of a life-giving vital force as a notion to be reckoned with is undeniable, and its usefulness as a cardinal concept in the emerging holistic paradigm of healing is inestimable. It is only in our most modern times that the sway of the materialistic perspective in science and medicine has resulted in the virtual abolition of any consideration for the forces that lie beyond the physical boundaries of the human body. Denying the existence of a life force, or in the very least, ignoring its reality, has had a profound impact upon contemporary medicine's misguided attempts to heal the sick. The single-minded and unique success of physical medicine's divorce from mind, emotion, and spirit has already generated grave consequences for our collective cultural health, which is showing increasing signs of strain and dysfunction in almost all aspects.

Because we have the compelling proposition of the existence of a unifying and life-directing vital force, even though its existence cannot be proven because it lies outside the boundaries of conventional scientific inquiry, it must now be placed within the new model of green medicine that we are attempting to construct. The current medical model will, of necessity, be compelled to expand its boundaries into the intangible, immeasurable, immaterial universe if it is to embrace the whole of human existence so that it may successfully wrap its arms around the mystery and complexity of human health and illness.

2

Innate Healing Intelligence

Nature is the healer of disease. It is an expression of life and not a special power; it prevails over physiologic processes; it heals diseases; it is unconscious or instinct-like; it is frequently incomplete and must be assisted by the physician. It works purposefully but is based on elemental laws.

—Linn J. Boyd, MD, *A Study of the Simile in Medicine*

A CASE OF MIDLIFE SCIATICA

A very successful middle-aged man who worked as an educational administrator consulted me one day regarding the sciatic pain that he had developed. He explained that he had hurt his back from doing so much driving in his car over the past few weeks. There was pain and stiffness on the left side of his low back that felt better when he was standing and moving, and worse while he was sitting for long periods, as he had been doing while driving. At times the pain would travel down the left leg as far as the ankle, and his leg sometimes felt numb. He was also experiencing pain in the left side of his neck. The sciatica had made it difficult to sleep, requiring him to be up and walking, sometimes for several hours per night. He remarked that he'd had a similar episode years ago while attending college and he described that period as a "time of transition."

I asked if anything unusual had been happening in his life lately. He shook his head in the negative, paused for a while, and then volunteered that he had been dreaming about snakes, and had three months ago dreamed that a snake jumped into his mouth. "It woke me and startled me," he said. This experience compelled him to go out and do research about the meaning and symbolism of dreams. I asked him if he had come to any conclusion. He said he had read that dreaming of snakes symbolizes overcoming your fears. "I'm going to be fifty years old—midlife, transition," he added. "I'd like to retire at fifty-five. One of my career goals was to be superintendent of schools, and occasionally it presents itself to me. Sometimes you do things due to someone else's expectations."

I asked him if he was sure he didn't want to pursue this goal and said that perhaps he was denying himself one of his life's ambitions. He tried to assure me that this was not the case, saying, "I'm very content with what I'm doing." I remained skeptical about his response and considered the possibility that he was in denial. I was also concerned about the potential connection between his recent pain, his dreams, and his attitude toward his career and looming retirement. We had a productive session, and I prescribed a homeopathic medication at the conclusion of our discussion.

When I saw him again he told me that he had felt better almost immediately after our last visit. There was still occasional pain, but it was much less intense and less frequent. He had resumed his normal walks, which he had done for years but had given up due to the sciatic pain. When I asked him how he felt about his career he responded, "I'm much clearer that a career move is something I don't want to do." But then, to my surprise, he related an insight that he had gained after our discussion. A while back he had written a book, which had been another long-held ambition. He submitted it to publishers only to have his manuscript returned. He had intended to rework it and submit it again but had become discouraged and had just about given up on the idea of publication. This attitude of resignation had curiously occurred right around the time his sciatica had developed. "I couldn't sit at home at the computer that had the book project on it, but I could sit at the computer at work," he said. As his pain lifted he found that he was able to sit back down at his home computer, which gave him renewed enthusiasm for his book![5]

Perhaps the sciatica was the result of his inability to overcome the discouragement he had experienced, thereby preventing him from fulfilling a life's ambition. And perhaps the point wasn't that the book had to be published in order for him to feel fulfilled, but that if he had never gotten around to putting his full effort into the project he might always feel regret and be left to wonder about what might have been.

The standard conventional approach to this man's sciatica would have been a physical exam, followed by perhaps X-rays or an MRI, along with a prescription for an anti-inflammatory medication. The imaging tests would likely have been normal, thereby reassuring doctor and patient that nothing "serious" was wrong. If the pain had persisted, a muscle relaxant or stronger narcotic painkiller might have been prescribed. A more enlightened physician might have recommended physical therapy, and a more adventurous one might suggest massage therapy, osteopathic manipulation, or chiropractic. In the unfortunate event that the imaging tests had shown something suspicious, this man's pain would then have been attributed to these structural findings. Naturally, the next step would have been to consult a surgeon who might or might not have recommended the knife.

The powerful connections among this patient's physical pain, his sense of meaning and purpose, and his subconscious needs expressed in his dreams are unmistakable. The field of psychotherapy recognizes the appearance of snakes in dreams as a very common manifestation, especially in times of great transition such as this man's college experience. They are often harbingers of pent-up psychic energy looking to be expressed in a creative way. They symbolize the possibility of transformation as the old ways are shed in favor of the new, just as a snake sheds its skin. An indigenous cultural perspective might view this as more than mere symbolic imagery of the psyche such as what a psychologist or psychiatrist might conclude. Rather than a product of the mind, the dream would be considered an actual energy or visitation from an animal spirit, a potentially powerful ally to be honored and consulted.

None of the above-mentioned pharmaceutical or surgical measures would have adequately addressed the underlying life issues that were being expressed through the patient's physical symptoms. In fact, it is likely that they would have temporarily blotted out his pain, making awareness of the deeper issues more inaccessible—just as taking a pill for a stress headache can override the pain, allowing one to tend to the demands of daily life, while the original source of distress is ignored. A pill can be a great tool for getting work done, but it's also a way to avoid the warning signals of the vital force. This type of strategy, if kept up, can result in serious adverse health consequences.

Obviously, not all instances of sciatic pain have some deeper meaning, but you would be surprised at how many cases are not just strictly physical in nature. More often than not, health problems cross these imaginary physical-mental-emotional-spiritual boundaries. Knowing this, it begs us to pose the question: What happens to the poor person whose pain has some deeper, non-physical source and yet has been convinced that painkillers or worse, surgical treatment are needed? If conventional medicine can manage only the physical dimension of illness, and is poorly equipped to deal with the fundamental fact of wholeness, then it behooves us to seek holistic healing in more appropriate places, where it can be provided.

BIOENERGETIC DEFENSE MECHANISM

Let us now return to our developing concepts of health and illness. Human well-being is a function of an ongoing process involving a seamless mind-body-spirit unity that can change over time. Health can change direction, improve, decline, flow freely, or become stuck, and is dependent upon the qualities of susceptibility and resiliency. Any factor or stressor that impacts any one aspect, by definition ultimately influences the whole.

Implicit in such a definition of health is that there must be some governing principle that coordinates a health mechanism of such incredible complexity. Regardless of how we specifically define it, or whether we call it chi, prana, or soul does not concern me so much because, as in most cases of differing opinions, the truth is usually some amalgamation or synthesis of all perspectives. What does count is the fundamental reality of the role played by an underlying guiding energy. An acceptance of the existence of this energy has far-reaching implications for the way in which the practice of medicine and healing are studied and conducted. If we are to ignore this energy's existence then we will most assuredly go on as before, accepting the material medical paradigm as it is currently practiced.

If, on the other hand, we take the concept of a life force seriously, then a thorough reassessment of the current priorities of Western medicine is required. Fortunately, the stage is already being set. It would be hard not to concede the phenomenal explosion of chiropractors, acupuncturists, homeopaths, herbalists, midwives, psychics, energy healers, yoga classes, and other alternative practices that dot the landscape in towns and cities across America.

Before going any further, for the sake of clarity I would like to define "life force" as I will be using it in this book. You may call it whatever you want—it doesn't really matter—but I will variously refer to it as the *life force, vital force, vital energy,* or *bioenergetic field,* even though these terms may sound like they're out of a sci-fi movie. I will use these terms to refer to the guiding energy principle and defense mechanism of each individual human being. The innate intelligence of the individual life force can be assigned many functions other than those involving health, but the specific aspects that I will be calling attention to are its functions in maintaining health and in illness and disease. Admittedly, the role of this force is a difficult and even arbitrarily defined concept that could be interchanged with terms such as spirit, soul, or even God. This usage is simply for the convenience of my line of argument and not because I am asserting the truth or correctness of my definition.

A green medical perspective recognizes and respects the innate wisdom of the life force and its capacity for self-maintenance and repair. A good, healthy vital force that has resilience and strength will meet life's stressors with equanimity, maintaining its equilibrium under difficult circumstances. It rolls with the punches and rebounds with relative ease. It keeps its balance when facing the daily mild to moderate hassles, tensions, and difficulties that most people encounter. But sooner or later, as life's vicissitudes come our way, we begin to feel the stress, which becomes manifest either through subjective mental and emotional states, or through physical symptoms. The bioenergetic life force, in meeting the stressor, begins to generate a distress signal in the form, for example, of insecurity, anger, neck tension, or a queasy stomach. Whatever the symptom, it is the life force letting us know of the disharmony that it is experiencing.

Stressors can present themselves in almost any form, and each stressor is interpreted as such through the eye of the beholder. Some people love a challenge and some shrink from the same. Some people are bored by routine and for some it provides a sense of security. Fried eggs for breakfast may be comfort food for one person while it makes another nauseous.

Lying in the sun at the beach may rejuvenate one person while another feels faint and must seek the shade. Exposure to cold air may relieve asthma in some instances, while it actually aggravates other cases. Sleeping while lying on the back may be the only comfortable position possible for some, while it induces nightmares in others. Some do their best brainwork late at night while others become drowsy during the same hours. The perception and experience of a stressor is a function of the uniqueness of each given individual.

These examples illustrate the unique nature of each individual in terms of how the bioenergetic defense mechanism can respond to various stimuli and circumstances. The expression of the vital force in each person is largely a function of who he or she is, which is dependent upon a variety of variables. Such factors include constitutional considerations, such as genetic makeup, body type, nutritional status, and physical conditioning; mental-emotional factors, such as maturity, psychological awareness, and spiritual development; and environmental factors, such as socio-economic status and the degree of emotional support received from loved ones. These are just some of the factors that, together, form the baseline from which any individual operates. Given this complex interplay of physical, genetic, environmental, emotional, and spiritual factors one can imagine the infinite potential incarnations of unique individual circumstances. The status of the life force of any one person can never be the same as another. Thus, respect for diversity and the uniqueness of the individual constitutes another fundamental principle in any green approach to health and healing.

Special mention should be made of the concept of energetic inheritance, as opposed to genetic inheritance. Just as people may inherit brown hair, green eyes, and a stocky build from their parents, so, too, they can energetically inherit an anxious disposition, fear of heights, and a predisposition toward developing migraine headaches from their parents. While most would assume that an angry child has learned these behaviors from his family environment, it is also common for a child to inherit the angry energy of an angry parent. The difference is that while genetic inheritance is mostly immutable, energetically inherited symptoms, issues, and states can often be altered and sometimes even erased.

Consider the war veteran who had one child before entering the service and another child after returning home from conflict. At a young age, the second child showed signs that the first did not. He was afraid of being left alone and would not sleep in the dark. The source of this energetically inherited state of mind becomes clear when we reveal that the father had developed these same post-traumatic stress disorder symptoms from his combat experience, prior to conception of his second child.

In another case, a woman tragically lost her mother in a car accident and became grief-stricken. She could not fully shake off the trauma and struggled with symptoms of sadness, depression, and insomnia that she'd never had before. Two years later she gave birth to her second child. Very early on, this child was irritable, cried incessantly and had a great deal of trouble sleeping at night. The first child, born before its grandmother's death, had no such trouble as an infant. It was as if the grief state of the mother was an energy that became grafted onto the vital force or constitution of the second child.

Such energetic factors, and many more, contribute to each given person's predisposition toward certain symptoms and illnesses. This inherited tendency toward certain health problems, which may ultimately become manifest or not, is an important factor to be taken into consideration by all green health care practitioners. The term "miasm" has been used by some healers to refer to this energetically inherited predisposition toward certain illnesses.

SHOOTING THE SYMPTOMATIC MESSENGER

We can see how the complex interplay of genetic, energetic, environmental, and other factors forms the terrain of each person's unique life force. Contrast this with the desire for medical science to classify illnesses into predictable diagnostic categories with the intent of simplifying therapeutic choices, i.e., each case of heartburn receives the same predetermined prescription regardless of the particular context of the problem. The inherent conflict between Western medicine's reductionistic need to group and categorize and the uniqueness of each human life and its individual circumstances is another theme that will be developed as we proceed.

If a symptom is taken, as it should be, as a distress signal of the energetic defense mechanism, then treating the symptom is akin to shooting the messenger. I can take a muscle relaxant for a stiff neck or I can take pause to investigate the possible sources of the vital force's complaint. Perhaps I have gotten myself into a situation where I needed to say "no" early on, but instead I have passively allowed myself to be swept up into it without stating my true feelings. Maybe I have been sleeping at night with a fan blowing cool air in through the window and I haven't used common sense to protect myself from the draft. Or maybe I haven't allowed the sadness over a friend's death to be expressed because I believe that it would indicate weakness on my part. By treating the symptom in this case, I shoot the messenger by blotting out the pain so that I can persist in the same situation without correcting my course until, eventually, the situation escalates into a more serious health problem.

Just imagine how many subtle daily events like this can pile up over time, resulting in increased stress and strain on the vital force, which then begins to complain with increasing displeasure. The occasional stiff neck becomes the least of my problems as I begin to develop a series of headaches that I have never had before. I visit a doctor, who examines me and orders an MRI to rule out a brain tumor, after which he or she prescribes a painkiller in addition to a muscle relaxant. But no one has asked me how I feel about my friend's passing, and I don't really want to deal with it, so I unwittingly continue the pharmaceutical war against myself. The new medication generates an unexpected side effect of depression. Neither my doctor nor I recognize the connection between the medication and the depression and so I reluctantly consent to taking an antidepressant, which helps in some ways—but it too turns out to have several unpleasant side effects.

By now you get my drift. Had I encountered a healer with a broader perspective who had encouraged me to talk about how I feel about my friend's death, perhaps the muscle relaxant, painkiller, and antidepressant would not have been necessary. This is not an unusual course of events. Rather than being the exception, it is actually the norm in a culture like ours, which favors the quick fix and denies most mental, emotional, and spiritual associations with our physical bodies. If we were to be educated about these important connections by a more holistically attuned culture, we would be enabled and encouraged to recognize them so that corrective action could be taken more quickly, before problems escalated to the point where they required the help of a psychiatrist.

Unfortunately, the American ideal of rugged individualism is a deeply ingrained conscious and subconscious message that ensures our silence about griefs of this nature and contributes significantly to the "shake it off, tough it out" mentality that condones this approach to health care. It is not unusual for a pro football player to sustain a pretty serious injury, receive a shot of cortisone in the locker room, and return to the playing field, after which the coaches and commentators praise his toughness and courageousness. In cases like this, the obvious and morally questionable priority becomes winning the game at all costs, even at the expense of a player's health and career.

INNATE CAPACITY TO HEAL

It can be confidently stated that all signs and symptoms, no matter what their character, are unique indicators of a distressed, unhappy, out-of-balance life force. They represent the surface manifestation of an underlying energetic disturbance. The pain felt from a lacerated finger should not be the main point of concern if a cook cuts him- or herself in the kitchen. The pain is just a warning signal indicating that the penetrated skin is a potentially serious breach of the body's defenses. Naturally, tending to the wound in this case would be more imperative than dulling the pain. One of the first things I was taught in medical school is that using painkillers in instances of acute abdominal pain is to be avoided until a clear diagnosis has been established. Masking the pain could give a false sense of security, and a missed diagnosis in the event of a case of appendicitis, for example, could bring about catastrophic consequences.

If symptoms were simply warnings or distress signals, we could begin to craft a new way of approaching them, but the true purpose of a symptom runs much deeper than that. The laceration causes the cook's finger to bleed, bringing a variety of much needed components of healing to bear upon the situation. Various clotting factors are transported to the site in an attempt to seal off the wound and reestablish the body's protective barrier. White blood cells, the body's natural antibiotics, gravitate to the wound as the innate intelligence of the vital force does its best to fight off infectious agents that may have broken through the barrier. As the healing mechanism works its magic, nutrients are fed by the bloodstream to the area to help promote the growth of new skin. Clearly, the totality of this process is more than just a warning signal. It is, in reality, the vital force's magnificent and miraculous attempt to rouse up and heal itself. No better design could be imagined or concocted by the wisest of sages or scholars.

In most cases, common sense would compel us to clean a wound with soap and water and place a band-aid on it, provided it isn't deep enough to require a few stitches. With the help of the exquisitely designed human body and its mysterious vital force, the wound would heal just fine and without consequence, requiring neither antibiotics nor painkillers. In some instances, the life force might overdo it a little bit by generating some scar tissue to form a keloid, just for extra protection. On the other hand, a small percentage of lacerations like this may not heal as well and the beginnings of infection may set in. The site can swell, become inflamed and more painful, and produce pus. Even the majority of these cases with the help of basic wound care would heal without any medications.

Less frequently, the life force's efforts may fall short as the infection starts to spread, involving more of the finger. If this were to occur, good judgment would warrant intervention with a conventional antibiotic or any of a variety of natural antibiotic substances, depending upon the extent of the infection. Taking it a step further, if we simply let the body do its thing, the finger might become very infected, and eventually turn ugly colors as it becomes gangrenous. Ultimately, the finger could turn black and die. In the worst-case scenario, the infection would become systemic and overwhelm the bioenergetic defense mechanism, resulting ultimately in death.

These examples, from easy recovery, to keloid formation, to local infection, to gangrene of the finger, to death, represent a spectrum of potential responses of the defense mechanism, which are conditioned upon the severity of the injury and the overall status of the bioenergetic vital force. Each step along the spectrum still represents the life force's endeavor to heal itself. Even the gangrenous finger can be seen as a thing of beauty when we realize that it serves as a sacrifice of the digit in order to preserve a human life. A strong and vital person is less likely to develop gangrene than someone with a compromised immune system. The diminished immunity of a weakened life force can arise from a multitude of factors, including chronic disease and immunosuppressive medications such as the topical, oral, and inhaled steroids that are so abundantly prescribed nowadays.

The next important principle to be gleaned from our discussion is the fundamental truth that all symptoms, no matter what their nature, constitute an effort by the defense mechanism of the life force to heal itself. More often than not it works with potent precision. Sometimes it does a less-than-perfect job, sometimes the results are undesirable, and occasionally the life force succumbs with barely a fight. An outbreak of influenza may cause one person to develop a little achiness and a runny nose, while another develops a headache and runs a fever for twenty-four hours, and still another has fever, aches, chills, and vomiting, and, unfortunately, one vomits repeatedly to the point of dehydration, requiring hospitalization. In this example, each individual has a different response even though they are all exposed to the same microbial entity.

We are all familiar with that tidbit of holistic thinking that even the medical establishment acknowledges—that a fever serves a constructive purpose to help protect a person afflicted with an infectious illness. It is understood as an activity of the immune system designed to raise the body temperature to make the environment inhospitable to the invading "bug." I will revisit this later, but for now I'll say only that this is the basic belief that most people in our culture hold. Yet strangely, in spite of this consensus, most people and almost all doctors will use an antipyretic like Tylenol at the first sign of fever. The usual justification is that it is for the comfort of the patient but I believe the true motivation is fear and a general mistrust regarding the body's ability to heal itself. This motive forms a dysfunctional complement to the physician's need to appear to be doing something to help the patient. Furthermore, fear is induced and encouraged by a medical system that thrives on the dependency and compliance of its patients. This general societal trend has led to a gradual erosion of confidence and an atrophy of the skills of self-care and self-preservation.

The lay public is taught to rely on the advice of the experts and not to trust their own instincts.

Given our understanding of illness as the life force's warning and attempt to heal itself, what can be said of a form of medicine that indiscriminately seeks to stop symptoms at every turn? An understanding of symptoms as warning signals and as manifestations of the healing mechanism should be reason enough to reconsider the prevailing mind-set that seeks to banish them without consideration for the potential consequences. But now we add yet another layer of purpose and intention to the symptomatic expression of the vital energy, and that is the role it plays in change and transformation. Just as people can go through psychological and emotional changes when responding to challenging moments in life, so too can the physical body go through similar adaptive changes.

It is not hard to understand how a crisis can act as a catalyst for change on an emotional level. The recently laid off businessperson is thrown into a dark depression, which if handled with proper care could result in a reassessment of life's priorities, a reintegration of unresolved past emotional issues, and the courage to seek a new job that brings even greater satisfaction than the prior one, which was becoming stale. This person may look back someday and acknowledge that without being forced to look deep within the self, he or she might never have found the resources to make bold life changes.

The physical body can also change as it goes through periods of transition. Did you ever notice how some people can hold up well under great strain for as long as is necessary? For example, sometimes a person nurses a dying loved one, only to finally crash and become sick when the difficult time has finally passed. It is as if the vital force had mustered all its strength to endure and to serve a higher purpose, but now that the ordeal is over, it generates symptoms as the caregiver becomes sick and is forced to go home, lie in bed, and nurse his or her own wounds. Just as we can change and adapt psychologically to trying times, so too the physical body needs to periodically reorient itself.

Anyone who has raised children may have noticed that kids' illnesses often coincide with developmental changes in their lives. Physical growth spurts are often preceded by increased appetite and weight gain followed by an increase in height as the child thins out again. It is not unusual for the child to develop an illness, like an upper respiratory infection or flu, right in the middle of these changes, as if the life force, too, is reorganizing its energies. Taller children who grow inches in a matter of months can experience leg pains or bone pains, commonly referred to as growing pains, which can be seen as a natural and necessary consequence of such drastic physical change. In a much deeper sense, these growing pains are just a surface manifestation of the mental and emotional growing pains of the maturing young person.

Chicken pox was once viewed as a normal childhood illness, which once contracted, conferred upon the patient subsequent immunity. This, too, can be viewed as a type of growth spurt, an immunologic rite of passage that sharpens the skills of a healthy bioenergetic defense mechanism. I have met more than my share of parents who, knowing that adults who get chicken pox tend to have more severe symptoms and sequelae, seek to expose their child to the illness during an outbreak. This is pursued with the belief that chicken pox serves as a normal milestone in the development of a healthy immune system. I concur with this strategy, provided the child is of general good health and is not immuno-compromised. Contracting chicken pox, especially those cases with a good strong skin eruption component, is a legitimate way for the developing immune system to flex its muscle.

A shortsighted medical mentality that views all illness as undesirable welcomes the development of a chicken pox vaccine in the misguided hope of completely eradicating the disease. This is typical of a medical-industrial complex that institutes policies simply because they can be technically achieved (and often because a new product can be marketed), and not because of some demonstrated benefit. I am concerned that rather than eliminating chicken pox, we are creating another medical monster by delaying the age at which chicken pox may be contracted, thereby potentially increasing the number of adults that it preys upon and resulting in unforeseen consequences. Even if it were to be eradicated, nature abhors a vacuum, and the normal developmental role played by chicken pox in children's health would likely be replaced by some other viral illness for the immune system to cut its teeth on.

In many instances, illnesses and their symptoms can be seen as necessary concomitants of growth and development. The old adage "No pain, no gain" takes on significant meaning when applied to health events that accompany or precede emotional and physical transformations. From this point of view, the common cold and other common viral illnesses are desirable events, which help keep the life force on its toes, honing its skills so that it will be ready to deal with more serious health threats in the future. Illness is often a manifestation of the adaptive function of the vital force to its circumstances.

THE INTANGIBLE NATURE OF DISEASE

To this point we have been talking mainly about individual symptoms. As the bioenergetic force begins to feel the stress and strain, it may begin to generate a symptom, which alerts the person to circumstances and helps the mind-body to respond, adapt, and to heal itself. At what stage can we determine whether a person has an illness? Is a symptom the same as a disease? Is a headache a disease? How about a headache and a runny nose? A headache, runny nose, and a fever? At what point does a symptom or group of symptoms become a disease? Conventional medicine would have us believe that there are discrete disease entities with very predictable symptoms, as if they are things "out there" that we can get or catch or come down with, as if these entities have a life of their own and an external existence apart from human life. And each specific disease comes with its corresponding identifying diagnostic label. The naming of a disease has been the crowning achievement of many famous physicians and scientists who have "discovered" these diseases down through the ages.

Let's return to our case of the unfulfilled administrator with sciatica. Can we safely assume that his leg pain is the same as the disease? Knowing what we now know, the pain can be interpreted as a reflection of a deeper struggle taking place within the heart and soul of this person. Would it not be more accurate to say that the deeper struggle is closer to the true nature of the problem? When he and I first discussed his condition, neither of us knew what was really going on. It was only after the fact that he became aware of a personal issue coinciding with the onset and lifting of his pain. The diagnosis that regular medicine would have given him, sciatica, is really only a convenient label chosen for his physical leg symptoms. In this case, the conventional diagnosis would reveal absolutely nothing about the greater mystery that lay beneath the surface.

What if the same administrator with the same life issues instead of developing sciatica, began to have recurrent bouts of fever, chills, and headache, which all finally resolved in a big sweat when he suddenly came to an understanding of his problem? Would it be appropriate to argue that he had simply come down with a virus? Could we with confidence apply a diagnostic label like "viral illness" to the fever, chills, and headache and be content that we knew the true nature of his difficulties? Could we with confidence blame the illness on a particular virus even if it were to be isolated using laboratory techniques? Or were these "viral" symptoms the vehicles through which the life force did its work in bringing about a resolution to a much more profound internal dilemma?

If we based our thinking on a thorough understanding of the life force, we would have to say that the symptom of pain running down the leg is just that, a symptom, and the disease is a much more complex underlying disorder whose presence can only be known, in this particular instance, by the complaint of leg pain. The vital force may be stressed until it begins to respond, at first in imperceptible ways, and eventually in a more overt way as indicated by the emergence of a symptom. The symptom, therefore, is not the disease but rather an indicator of a disturbance in the energetic balance of the defense mechanism. The symptom is the surface manifestation of an intangible process taking place beneath the physical plane. Orthodox medicine, by contrast, occupies itself almost exclusively with the physical plane. Signs and symptoms should bring to our awareness the potentiality of an underlying energetic issue. In other words, the disease itself is more closely equated with the status of the imbalanced energy of the life force, which cannot be grasped or ascertained by direct observation. It is just like my mood, which you can never know firsthand, but which you may be able to discern by my body language and facial expression.

I contend that all disease remains out of our immediate grasp and can only be assumed by the collection of signs and symptoms that indicate its presence. The implication here, and the position that I am advocating, is that the disease will always remain an unknowable, intangible state of imbalance of the bioenergetic life force, which is constantly in flux and beyond the immediate perception of conventional science. Secondhand information in the form of external signs and symptoms can provide only a glimmer of the true inner struggle taking place as the defense mechanism attempts to reestablish balance. Other forms of extrasensory perception and energy-healing techniques may be able to detect and influence an energetic imbalance more directly, but they, too, can never ascertain with certainty the true nature of the inner problem that is made known to us by its outer signs.

Alternately, we can say that the administrator has sciatic pain on the physical level, existential pain on the psychic level, and an overall energetic imbalance. While this description may ring true, it still falls short of a complete and illuminating explanation for his situation. The disease of any individual is always a mystery and will always remain a mystery. You can see why this elusive conception of illness can be intensely frustrating to the Western rational mind, which tends to balk at the notion that something may be unknowable.

Contrast this view of disease with the attitude of certainty that a conventional allopathic diagnosis conveys. Our administrator with leg pain may receive an authoritative declaration from his family doctor that he has an inflamed sciatic nerve, while the orthopedic surgeon may assert that it is a bulging lumbar disc, and a neurologist may firmly believe a that he is suffering from a peripheral neuropathy. All three are explanations typical of the mechanistic medical paradigm but none of these diagnoses begins to touch upon the inner dynamic and energetic status of the body-heart-mind-soul of this patient. Diagnoses, we see, are largely vehicles of convenience designed to satisfy the logic of the medical mind.

It remains now to hash out what really goes on when someone is saddled with multiple diagnoses. Let us say that in addition to several recent high blood pressure readings, a female patient has had sleep difficulties over the past few years, and a life-long tendency toward constipation. Her constipation is treated with stool softeners and an occasional laxative, she takes sleeping pills as needed, and a new medication is added for her hypertension. Is it fair to say that this woman has three different health problems warranting three different diagnoses, thereby justifying three different treatments, as if the problems involve different anatomical parts, each having nothing to do with the others, each tended to by an indicated specialist who prescribes a different medication that is assumed to have no appreciative impact upon the other parts?

If the body-heart-mind-soul really does constitute an interwoven and unbroken whole, then, these three conventionally categorized conditions must be connected. Are they not occurring in the same person at the same time, and should they not be seen as an indication of the overall state of the health of this woman? Indeed, each set of symptoms provides further information about the underlying unknowable disease, and they are our best clues as to the energetic condition of her distressed vital force.

Conventional diagnostic labeling is an arbitrary and artificial construct of the rational medical mind, which chooses certain criteria to include within its scope of evaluation and excludes others that it defines as irrelevant. People's stories, their meanings, and emotional significance may serve as interesting background information to the regular physician, but are usually of no value in diagnostic assessment. Diagnoses involving mental and emotional symptoms are usually cordoned off and reserved for the unique and specific domain of the psychiatrist, who in turn is careful not to tread upon the turf of the doctors who deal with the physical body. This ensures that mind and body are kept neatly in their own little boxes. While it is true that most doctors are compassionate people with a genuine interest in their patients' stories, the actual use of the bulk of this information plays little practical role within the scheme of conventional diagnosis and treatment.

Multiple symptoms and multiple diagnoses, even when spread out across seemingly unrelated and disparate areas of the human body, are nevertheless an expression of the distress and disorder of the same life-sustaining vital force. The anxiety attacks, herpes eruptions, and cramping leg muscles experienced by a single patient are all distress signals created by the same life force. Although we may not be able to see the connection, they are intimately related on an energetic level that allopathic medicine chooses not to acknowledge. I know that this concept can be hard to grasp. We do not understand how our headaches could have any relation to our warts, but the reality is that both are expressions of the same life force.

In summary, all signs and symptoms are distress signals generated by the disturbed life force and are to be understood as attempts by the imbalanced bioenergetic force to heal itself. Some symptoms may be desirable occurrences that serve a self-regulating adaptive function. All green healing practices should seek to understand the innate intelligence of the life force, and its role in growth, adaptation, and healing. In addition, a green approach to health entails a respect for diversity and the unique status of each individual's vital force. Symptoms are not to be mistaken for the actual disease because the disease itself is more accurately characterized as an energetic imbalance of the invisible life force. Furthermore, signs and symptoms are always connected in that they are produced by the same vital force, and diagnostic names are merely artificial labels that may reveal little about the true status of that life force.

We will investigate at length how treating just the symptoms without consideration for their purpose, meaning, and relationships can have serious repercussions for both the short- and long-term health of the patient. But before we can arrive at a thorough understanding of why treating only symptoms is so problematic, I'd like to offer some preliminary historical, philosophical, and sociological groundwork upon which to construct my thesis.

Historical and Spiritual Roots

During the long Dark Age, in which separatism reigned, religion itself, as it crystallised into orthodoxy, became separated from its own source. Separation also grew between spiritual belief, scientific knowledge, psychology, medicine and education. Divorced from their one root, the Ageless Wisdom with its fundamental spiritual Laws, the arts and sciences and religions became steadily more materialistic, more separatist, and more distrustful of each other.
—Vera Stanley Alder, *The Initiation of the World*

As an Indian medicine man once said, "The white man has his medicine, but he will never be able to heal because he does not know the Ancestors."
—Matthew Wood, *The Magical Staff*

Om Sri Dhanvantre Namaha
(OM SHREE DON–VON–TREY NAHM–AH–HA)
"Salutations to the being and power of the Celestial Physician."
—Thomas Ashley-Farrand, *Healing Mantras*

ORTHODOX MEDICAL HISTORY

Popular renditions of the history of Western medicine often start with the Greek physician Hippokrates around 500 to 400 years BCE. Since few of Hippokrates' ideas resemble modern medicine, the choice of his work as its historical origin (which, incidentally, is an indication of Western ethnocentricity) seems to lie with his notion that diseases could be attributed to natural as opposed to supernatural causes. His theory of the four humors is described by historians as a "scientific" explanation of illness. But this can more accurately be described as a physical, non-spiritual explanation for illness, and hence its association with the beginning of scientific Western medicine is understandable.

The implication here is that "science," rather than indicating a methodology of observation and experiment, was a value-laden term that was used to convey a distinction between itself and magic and religion. Early Greek thinkers developed theories emphasizing rational thought and logic, as opposed to "irrational," "magical," or "superstitious" thinking. So it is not that Hippokrates was the first scientific physician as much as he was one of the first to introduce elements that enabled the eventual divorce between body and spirit.

While Western medical history places emphasis upon this version of Hippokrates for its mechanistic purposes, it is interesting to note that some of his ideas had a vitalistic theme, which viewed disease as an unknowable mystery. He was far from being a materialist; we have only to look as far as the Hippokratic Oath to see what this ancient physician intended. It was a strange and surreal experience indeed when I stood many years ago in an auditorium full of newly minted medical school graduates reciting the names of Greek gods and goddesses that had not once been uttered in our four years of education:

> *I swear by Apollo the Physician and Asclepius and Hygieia and Panacea and all the gods and goddesses, making them my witnesses, that I will fulfill according to my ability and judgment this oath and this covenant ...*[6]

I am struck by a sense of irony in recalling the time I had asked the only alternatively inclined physician teaching at the medical school about the statue standing on his desk. In response to my query about the muscular figure holding a staff around which wound a serpent he replied nonchalantly, "That's Asklepios, the Greek god of healing."

Most events of particular relevance to modern medicine have taken place within the past few hundred years. Various discoveries regarding anatomy and physiology prior to this time are usually counted by historians as events pertaining to the history of medicine. In 1553 a Spanish physician named Miguel Serveto described the circulation of blood through the lungs. In 1603 Girolamo Fabrici discovered that the leg veins have valves, which were later determined to function in preventing blood from flowing backward, away from the heart. And in 1628 William Harvey chronicled how the veins and arteries together form a circuit through which blood is pumped by the heart.

Categorizing these events more appropriately under the history of biology and anatomy, it could be argued that the history of modern medicine did not really get going until the introduction of smallpox inoculation in 1701 by Giacomo Pylarini, and the smallpox vaccination in 1796 by Edward Jenner, almost one hundred years later. Another hundred years passed by before Louis Pasteur developed the anthrax and rabies vaccines. Pasteur's work, along with the contributions of Robert Koch in the late 1800s, helped to establish the seeds of our modern germ theory, which has dominated conventional medical thinking to this day.

Even though acupuncture was used for centuries to alleviate pain in the East, one of the first uses of anesthesia during surgery in Western medical history was by Crawford Williamson Long, who used ether in 1842 while removing a tumor from a patient. Although white willow bark was used for centuries to treat aches, pains, and fevers, it was not until the 1800s that scientists isolated its "active ingredient" so that it could later be marketed by the fledgling pharmaceutical industry in the form of salicylic acid. As a result, the German company, Bayer, introduced aspirin in 1915. Wilhelm Conrad Röntgen experimented with and developed the first use of X-rays in 1895. A whole slew of additional vaccines were produced in the early 1900s, and Alexander Fleming, a Scottish scientist, accidentally discovered and subsequently tried to isolate the antibiotic substance penicillin from a fungus in 1928.

The rudimentary foundations of modern medical ideas and methods can be summed up to include germ theory, vaccination, anatomy, anesthesia and surgery, and pharmaceutical drugs. If we include Hippokrates and the intervening centuries until the advent of vaccines, we could very generously tally up 2,500 years of Western medical history. If we remove the years between Hippokrates and smallpox inoculation, the modern medical era is reduced to a mere 300 years. Even within those 300 years, the vast majority of significant events that shaped industrial-technological medicine have occurred within the past two hundred years. Put another way,

150 years ago we had no germ theory, no aspirin, no antibiotics, no anesthesia, no X-rays, and only one vaccine. In light of these facts, two possible short interpretations regarding the brevity of the modern medical era might be: "Gee, we've come a long way in such a short time," or "Where do we find the temerity to ignore thousands of years of medical history?"

FORGOTTEN MEDICAL HISTORY

If we look backward across the span of time preceding the arbitrarily chosen beginning of scientific medical history marked by Hippokrates, there are still, at minimum, three thousand years of history that must be taken into account. Ancient Greece and Rome together are usually considered the seat of Western civilization, although both were heavily influenced by Egypt and Mesopotamia. Acknowledging that this still excludes all of Eastern civilization and its history, by some accounts, Imhotep is thought to be the first physician identified by recorded Western history. (See Figure

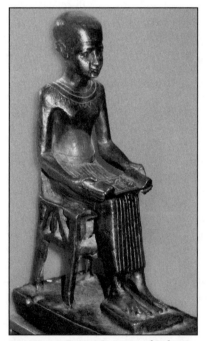

3.1.) Conventional history places him as the architect of Egypt's first pyramid, built during the reign of King Djoser, at Saqqara around 2,600 BCE. Imhotep was a multitalented vizier, architect, priest, doctor, astrologer, and scribe whose best-known writings were medical texts. He is believed to be the author of what is known as the Edwin Smith Papyrus, which lists more than ninety anatomical terms and forty-eight types of injuries. He is thought to have diagnosed and treated more than two hundred diseases, performed surgery, used plants as medicinal substances, and possibly to have founded a school of medicine named "Asklepion" in the city of Memphis.

FIGURE 3.1: *Bronze Statuette of Imhotep, Egypt (332–30 BCE), the Louvre, Paris*

In a manner similar to the canonization of Catholic saints, the Egyptians deified him after his death.

Down through the centuries, Imhotep ultimately achieved the full status of a god in the Egyptian pantheon and thus became associated with Thoth, the god of wisdom, writing, and learning. (See Figure 3.2.) A lunar god, often represented as a man with the head of an ibis, Thoth was the patron of scribes and physicians, and is thought to be the author of treatises on astrology, astronomy, philosophy, medicine, religion, and magic. He is asso-

ciated with the legendary *Book of Thoth* of esoteric lore, the contents of which remain largely a mystery to this day.

Thoth's medical knowledge was intimately related to his magical abilities, which stemmed from his command of words and the power of his use of language. The Egyptians considered magic to be closely allied with medicine and the ability to heal. We will discuss at a later point how the modern-day physician holds the magical power of life and death when words like "be-

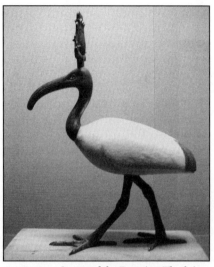

FIGURE 3.2: *Statue of the Egyptian Thoth in Ibis Form, Kunsthistorisches Museum, Vienna*

nign," "malignant," "cancerous," and "terminal" are spoken, often with stunning insensitivity and a lack of awareness of their potential effect upon vulnerable patients.

History teaches us how cultural influences over centuries can blur the lines between what we may, at first glance, perceive to be discrete civilizations. Thoth's original Egyptian name was Djehuty, or Tehuti. As Greek settlers in Egypt came to notice the similarity between their own winged messenger of the gods, Hermes, and the Egyptian Thoth, the two in time became a syncretistic meld referred to as Thoth-Hermes. When Egypt came under Greek rule in 332 BCE, the name of Khmun, the city where the cult following of Thoth was most prominent, was changed to

Hermopolis. Ultimately, the Greeks adopted him as their own, dropping Thoth from the name and then calling him Hermes Trismegistus, meaning "three times great Hermes."

Hermes, like Thoth, was a god of writing, magic, astrology and alchemy. The mythological composite of these two gods represented the ancient source of all knowledge essential to the practice of medicine and healing. Healers were seen as scientist-magicians or physician-priests, requiring experience and knowledge of both the physical world and the otherworld, or spiritual world. Both Thoth and Hermes were gods who illuminated the way safely for the dead through the perils of the underworld. This applied literally to the physically deceased or to those coming close to physical death, and even to those undergoing profound psychological and emotional crises as they experienced the transformative cycle of life, death, and rebirth.

Hermes was a great teacher who imparted his wisdom for the benefit of humanity. The creation of the large body of literature referred to as the Hermetic writings has been attributed to Hermes Trismegistus. Clement of Alexandria counted forty-two original secret books of wisdom attributed to Hermes, thirty-six of which contained the philosophical belief system of the Egyptians, with the remainder being practical essays on medicine. Here is scholar and prolific author Manly P. Hall on the inauspicious fate of these legendary volumes of ancient wisdom, which were stored in the Great Library at Alexandria in the fourth century BCE:

> One of the greatest tragedies of the philosophic world was the loss of nearly all of the forty-two books of Hermes.... These books disappeared during the burning of Alexandria, for the Romans—and later the Christians—realized that until these books were eliminated they could never bring the Egyptians into subjection. The volumes which escaped the fire were buried in the desert and their location is now known only to a few initiates of the secret schools.[7]

Hermes, one of the earliest figures associated with the caduceus, carries his magic wand, the winged rod, around which two snakes spiral upward until they meet up at the top. The medical profession has long adopted this symbol, and images of the caduceus are ubiquitous in our modern medical institutions. It is interesting to note that, just as th adopted Egyptian cultural influences, the Greek Hermes was mir the Roman god Mercury, a messenger of the gods who also carı caduceus.

ASKLEPIAN HEALING

Perhaps the best-known Greek god associated with healing is Asklepios, the son of Apollo, an Olympian god also associated with healing. There is some indication that, before he became immortalized, Asklepios was an actual historical figure. The earliest reference to his name occurs in Homer's *Iliad,* which scholars say was written around 800 BCE. An important distinction needs to be made between Hippokrates, the father of medicine, and Asklepios, the god of healing, as the contrast parallels the theme drawn out in this book. The commitment of modern scientific medicine to concrete and measurable physical health parameters has had the net effect of pulling it further and further away from real healing in the truest sense, as true healing is a holistic phenomena that transcends the physical body alone and must involve the seamless whole of body, heart, mind, and soul.

The impact of Asklepios upon healing in the ancient world is well documented with grace and beauty by Edward Tick in his book, *The Practice of Dream Healing.* All physicians in training should be required to read this remarkable accounting of an important early chapter of our Western medical heritage. Tick takes us on a tour of the ruins of several sites that were once healing sanctuaries where the sick would go to seek relief from their suffering. Archeologists have documented 320 of these temples of Asklepios, each referred to as an Asklepion, predominantly located in Greece and Asia Minor, but also found all across Europe and North Africa. The largest such center dedicated to the god of healing was in Epidauros, on the Greek Peloponnesian coast, which is estimated to have been an active site run by the physician-priests, or Asklepiads, for over 1,000 years, dating from 600 BCE.

Asklepios, according to Greek myth, was born of a divine father, Apollo, and a human mother, Koronis, and raised by Chiron, the centaur. One account of the story explains the psychic wound that Asklepios carried due to the circumstances of his birth, a wound that was necessary for his evolution into a great healing god:

> *... while Asklepios was still in the womb of his mother, a raven came to Apollo with the tidings that Koronis was unfaithful to him, whereupon Apollo straightway cursed the raven, which, in consequence, was changed forever from white to black, and hastening to Koronis, he slew her and burned her body on a pyre. Snatching the child from the midst of the flames, he took him to Chiron, who trained him in the chase and the mysteries of healing, whereby Asklepios became so skilful as a physician that he not only kept many men from death, but even raised to life some who had died ...*[8]

Chiron was half-man, half-horse, and he, like Asklepios, had suffered an accidental wound (his at the hands of Herakles) that would not heal. Any successful healing involves the reconciliation of mind and body, spirit and nature, as signified by the man-horse unity represented by Chiron, the mentor of Asklepios. We will discuss this powerful theme of the wounded healer at length later on, but for the moment, Edward Tick deftly paints the picture of this dilemma faced by Chiron and Asklepios:

> *Thus the mentor as well as the apprentice was a wounded healer. In fact, the wound that refuses to heal, and is even unjust or undeserved, is often a necessary motivation for becoming a healer. "Physician, heal thyself!" is not just a corrective cry against incompetent healers. The future healer must be driven to seek healing for him or herself. The search for healing must be successful so that the healer later knows how to conduct others down a healing path that works.*[9]

Like Thoth-Hermes, Asklepios was associated with the mythological serpent, although his staff was somewhat different from the short rod of the caduceus with its two snakes. Many archeological and historical artifacts depict Asklepios holding a long staff around which is wound only one serpent. It is instructive to note that Hermes was also considered the god of commerce and patron of merchants, and it is his caduceus that has been adopted as the modern symbol of medicine. Some have attributed this to a mistake in printing by a publisher of medical text books that unwittingly switched the two symbols, resulting in the common usage of the caduceus rather than the staff of Asklepios. Perhaps this was a mistake, or maybe a synchronistic reflection of the modern attitude toward the marketing of medicine and the commodification of health care. In addition, some historians note that when the United States Army Medical Corps chose the caduceus as its symbol in 1902, this further cemented its place in modern medical symbology. It is worth pointing out the parallel between its use by our military institutions and the role of conventional medicine in its war-like posture toward disease. It is a war often waged over the battleground of the confused and helpless patient's body.

Viewed from another perspective, the trend toward separation of body and spirit that began with Hippokrates and which has reached alarming proportions today, may be metaphorically represented by the twin snakes of Hermes' caduceus, while the single snake on the staff of Asklepios may more accurately resemble the power of true healing, which attempts to integrate the fragmented pieces of a wounded person into one whole. Some modern medical institutions have initiated a trend in recent years toward restoring the staff of Asklepios to its rightful status, but this will amount to mere window dressing if it is not accompanied by meaningful reform in the actual substance of medical practice.

In the ancient world, a person in need of medical care could seek the counsel of the gods by visiting an Asklepian temple of healing. The physician-priests would guide the seeker in preparation for his or her encounter through methods of ritual purification, such as bathing, fasting, and dressing in white robes. This is not unlike Native American vision questing, where the seeker waits in the wilderness until a message from the gods is received. The person would then be instructed to enter the abaton, a type of sleeping or incubation chamber, where he or she would wait for hours or even days to receive a healing dream from Asklepios or one of his emissaries. The supplicant's contact with the god in a dream would often achieve an outright cure, or the dream might reveal instructions for healing.

This form of healing through dreaming was far from unusual in ancient times, although it tends to be viewed as superstitious, or even dangerous by modern standards. I have encountered more than a few patients who report having had significant dreams, but sadly, often their first impulse is to dismiss them as silly, crazy, or embarrassing. A gradual process of re-education will be required for us to overcome the prevailing cultural bias in order to understand and accept that dreams can sometimes hold the key to our future well-being.

Asklepios would often visit supplicants as himself or in one of his three main animal forms: the snake, dog, or cock. The dog, as guide and protector when one visits the other side, the underworld, or dreamworld is a common motif in world mythology. And like the rooster's call at dawn, its appearance in dreams is a call to a new awakening and greater consciousness. The serpent in particular can be a powerful harbinger of change and transformation. As we have seen, the snake as cosmic messenger carries with it the multi-potentiality of light and dark, of positive and negative energies—as the shedding of its skin symbolizes the cycle of life, death, and rebirth. It is common to dream of snakes even in our modern times, and the accompanying message urging one toward change can be ignored at one's own risk, or can be heeded, with the potential for reaping great rewards.

Additional healing power and inspiration could be derived from any of Asklepios three daughters, who were also involved in the field of health and accompanied him in his work. Hygieia, Panaceia, and Iaso can be translated from the Greek as "health," "all-cure," and "healing," respectively. Hygieia enjoyed particular prominence in the ancient world and was often depicted in sculpture, in relief, and on coins side by side with her father.

Just as Thoth of the Egyptians had been embraced by the Greeks as Thoth-Hermes or Hermes Trismegistus, so, too, the Romans came to adopt Asklepios from the Greeks. How this came to be is documented in Ovid's *Metamorphosis*. The Romans, faced with a terrible plague that would not yield to the efforts of their priests, sought the counsel of the gods through divination by consulting the Sibylline books, whereupon they were advised to seek answers not from Apollo but from Apollo's son, Asklepios. A delegation was sent to Epidauros, in Greece, where one of the Roman ambassadors received a dream in which Asklepios indicated that he would return with the delegation to bring his healing influence to the new land. This chapter in mythological history is summarized succinctly in *The Mythology of All Races:*

> The outbreak of a pestilence at Rome in 292 BC turned the Romans to a consultation of the Sibylline books, where they discovered directions enjoining them to send a deputation of citizens to the healing shrine of Asklepios at Epidauros, the envoys bringing back a serpent as a living symbol of the god, and at the same time instructions for establishing the new worship. It happened that when their ship reached the city, the serpent leaped overboard and swam to the island in the Tiber, where the new shrine was built, the god's name being given the Latin form of Aesculapius.[10]

So now the Greek Asklepios had become the Roman Aesculapius. (See Figure 3.3.) The reincarnated god continued to flourish in his new surroundings for centuries until the Roman Empire eventually came into conflict with the new religion of Christianity. As the two worldviews began to collide, much religious persecution was perpetrated by Rome, but gradually the forces of Christianity began to gain the upper hand. During the reign of Constantine in the fourth century CE the old pagan gods and goddesses, including Aesculapius, came under attack. As the trend of replacing the old polytheistic beliefs with the new patriarchal monotheism took hold, many statues were destroyed and temples desecrated, and the healing god and his cohorts were ultimately demonized and banished.

SCIENCE VERSUS RELIGION

Most Westerners are well acquainted with the life of Christ, and in particular the miracles that he performed. Some of the most notable of his miracles occurred when he healed the sick, allowed the lame to walk, and restored sight to the blind; the sufferer had only to believe to be made well again. And Jesus had only to lay hands on the infirm and they would be returned to health. The similarities between the story of Asklepios and that of Christ are striking, as both were wounded healers born to a divine father and a

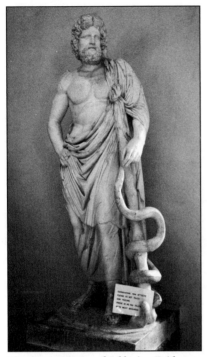

FIGURE 3.3: *Statue of Asklepios, Epidaurus Museum, Mycenae, Greece*

mortal mother. Although they existed side by side for a period, the Roman Aesculapius gradually faded as he was replaced by Christ, the new savior and healer.

While the life of Christ has powerfully and rightly inspired many millions for the past two thousand years, it is only at the hands of flawed human beings like you and me that his message of love has become mangled. And so it is—especially with institutions that become preoccupied with power, wealth, and glory—that dogma becomes enshrined, while the true meaning of the original message tends to get lost. Initially, Christ's views were deemed blasphemous. But over time, the tables were turned, and the religious beliefs of millions of pagan worshipers, which went back over centuries of time, were deemed heretical by virtue of the growing influence of an overzealous Christian power structure.

The multiplicity of male and female deities with their corresponding mythical stories and powers, whose influence had stretched back over Roman, Greek, Egyptian, and other civilizations, were now replaced by the "one true," all-encompassing, and all-powerful male god. An enormous wealth of history, culture, and knowledge was systematically and tragically wiped out as the new institutions of Christianity attempted to eradicate all traces of pagan worship. That which could not be eradicated was assimilated and given a fresh facade. Despite the claims of newness, the similarity of beliefs and practices of the pagan and Christian religions were striking and numerous. A discussion of this topic could fill multiple volumes, but that is not my purpose here.

Given the prominence of serpent symbolism when it comes to medicine, health, and healing, it is interesting to note that within the Christian Church the snake has assumed the role of representing the forces of evil. Prior to this turn of perception, throughout human history the serpent had been a ubiquitous and sacred symbol indicative of themes relating to the goddess, soul, transformation, and the cycle of life, death, and rebirth. Its persistence as the modern symbolic emblem of medicine stands in stark contrast to its popular cultural and religious depiction of all that represents darkness, evil, and even the devil himself. In the course of visiting numerous churches over the years, I have observed that many statues of Mary, the Mother of God, depict her standing with her foot pressed against and crushing the serpent on the ground below. This image derives from the story of the fall in Genesis in which Yahweh discovers that the fruit of the forbidden tree of knowledge has been eaten. Adam then promptly blames the woman, Eve, who in turn blames the serpent.

In contrast, even within the patriarchal monotheistic worldview of the Jews, the serpent is depicted as a force of deliverance and healing in the Old Testament when God punishes the impatient Israelites with a plague of poisonous snakes. After Moses looks to God for guidance, he is instructed by Yahweh to place a "brazen serpent" on a pole, and those who gaze upon the image are then healed.

This motif in which the source of an affliction holds the promise of cure for the very same affliction is a foreshadowing of Hahnemann's homeopathic system of medicinal treatment with similars. The writings of Paracelsus echo this concept, and even Hippokrates argues that illness can be treated by either method—through the use of an agent producing an effect opposite to the ailment, or with an agent that causes results similar to the condition.

Even within the Christian tradition, the view of the serpent as strictly a representative of evil cannot be justified with confidence, for it was Christ himself who warned his disciples as they set out to spread the news of his new doctrine of peace:

> *Behold, I send you forth as sheep in the midst of wolves: be ye therefore wise as serpents, and harmless as doves.*[11]

Here the message is clear: the serpent is equated with wisdom, and the disciples are enjoined to share the wisdom that they possess in an attitude of kindness and love.

The evolution of the ancient Christian world and its institutions roughly paralleled the rise of rationalism and the development of scientific thought and its many discoveries regarding the natural world. The first healers and physicians to embrace rational thought and natural causation still held to a fundamentally wholistic worldview, by which the natural world was contained within divine creation. Priest and physician were, for a time, one and the same, and later, at least respected for their respective abilities to contribute to the health and well-being of the infirm. Eventually, the two predominant influences of the time began to lay exclusive claim to their own domains.

Science, logic, and rationalism gradually became aligned with the physical world, and hence the physical body. Supernatural and spiritual causes were rejected in favor of natural and physical causes. The causes of diseases and their solutions were increasingly thought to lie in the unexplored scientific frontier, from which, it was assumed, further investigation would someday remove the veil of mystery. As an understanding of the workings of the natural world and the human body grew, the importance of the spiritual connection to the material world and to human health receded into the background.

On the flip side of the coin, the forces of Christian influence became the authorities on issues of the soul and matters of higher standing, like God, salvation, and the afterlife. The physical world and the human body became temporary, but undesirable way stations before one reached the true destination of life in heaven after death. Hardly a Catholic friend of mine who grew up in my generation would deny the prevailing attitude of guilt and sin associated with the physical body and human sexuality promulgated by the Church and its representatives. In the extreme, certain aspects of the material world and the human body became evils to be overcome only through looking upward toward the higher principles of the spiritual life.

In essence, medical science became caretaker of the body, while the Christian Church proclaimed itself keeper of the soul. This chapter of human history might be described as the seminal period when specialization stepped in to split our world in half. As science attempted to discredit religion on rational grounds, religion fought back with the weight of its moral authority. The Church's persecution of Galileo for suggesting that the earth revolves around the sun was but one of many instances of the clash between these two forces of history.

Alongside these cataclysmic changes came the rise of the masculine principle. The androgynous cosmic world of gods and goddesses was supplanted by the materialistic bias of the patriarchal culture generated by *both* science and Christianity. The authoritarian orientation of each is plainly evident—and they are the forces that have shaped our modern world over the past few thousand years. Both science and Christianity were co-conspiratorial precursors to sweeping changes in human consciousness that led to the same net effect: the dualistic split between spirit and science, between mind and body. The division was coupled with the pervasive belief that the masculine principles of logic and mind were superior to the feminine principles of intuition and soul. This divorce of medical science from its spiritual roots carries with it profound implications for contemporary culture.

LOST CONTINENTS

If we dare to step outside of the accepted bounds of conventional history and established scientific fact, we can tap into a vast field of knowledge that has been repeatedly discredited by most contemporary cultural authorities. This largely neglected field of esoteric knowledge has much to say regarding ancient medical history and the nature of health and healing. There is significant geological, historical, and literary evidence to suggest that ancient Egypt and Sumeria did not represent the first civilizations. Most scholars of esoterica would tend to trace the origins of civilization back at least to the mythological lands of Atlantis and Lemuria.

The prevailing theory is that these advanced cultures, which pioneered humankind's understanding of math, science, astronomy, spirituality, medicine, and healing, were destroyed by cataclysmic environmental events approximately ten thousand years ago, and may have dated back as far as one hundred thousand years. It is believed that Atlantis existed in the regions of the Atlantic Ocean and that its survivors settled in Egypt, where they contributed much knowledge to the development of Egypt as a technologically advanced culture. Atlantis is presumed to be the main contributor of masculine yang energy and influence on Earth. Likewise, Lemuria is supposed to have existed in the Pacific region, and it is believed that the descendents of aboriginal cultures hailed from this ancient civilization. Correspondingly, Lemuria is presumed to be the source of feminine yin energy and influence that is most closely reflected in the surviving nature-based cultures on our planet.

Various authors and students of esoteric knowledge believe that these early civilizations, far from being primitive, had acquired advanced spiritual awareness and knowledge, which afforded them powerful insights into medicine and healing. By recognizing the patterns of the natural world as understood through the study of astronomy, astrology, mathematics, geometry, herbology, and more, it is believed that these cultures had a profound awareness of the interrelatedness of all things and the energetic nature of all phenomena. The priests and healers of these cultures knew that all things material and immaterial vibrate at their own unique frequencies. They were able to use the energies of sound, color, plants, stones, and gems to treat illness, which was thought to result from disharmony with one's surrounding energetic environment. We have only to contemplate phenomena such as Stonehenge and the pyramids of Egypt and the Americas to realize that the ancients knew much more than we are willing to give them credit for.

This brief tour of the more recent development of scientific Western medicine, contrasted with the earlier spiritual history of the great gods, goddesses, and figures of ancient medicine and healing, should give one a sense of the vastness of human history and the relative immaturity of our modern medical perspective. The common refrain that the United States has "the greatest health care system in the world" is, in reality, an egocentric proclamation that only highlights the prevailing conceit and small-mindedness of the scientific medical establishment, which, in turn, serves to cover up its underlying insecurity and fear of change. This claim to medical greatness can, unfortunately, be disproven by a variety of measures including life expectancy and infant mortality rates, astronomical costs, tremendous waste, unparalleled pollution, and the ever-rising prevalence of chronic disease and mental illness.

The green medical movement is one that is cognizant of its roots and respects its history. It does not discard the old simply because it is old, or the new because it is different. It does not restrict its knowledge and understanding to the physical body and to physical causes. It embraces that which lies beyond the physical—spirit, soul, heart, and vital energy—even if it cannot quantify or examine them with its instruments of measurement. It embraces culturally and historically diverse perspectives regarding health and healing as it ads to its repertoire those methods and ideas that have been effective in relieving suffering and in furthering human growth and evolution.

4

Shamanic Journey to the Soul

Modern man does not understand how much his "rationalism" (which has destroyed his capacity to respond to numinous symbols and ideas) has put him at the mercy of the psychic "underworld."

He has freed himself from superstition (or so he believes), but in the process he has lost his spiritual values to a positively dangerous degree. His moral and spiritual tradition has disintegrated, and he is now paying the price for this break-up in worldwide disorientation and dissociation.

　　—Carl G. Jung, *Man and His Symbols*

Healing is painful because so much has become unconscious in us; the cure is a journey to the Underworld to reclaim our freedom and lucidity.

　　—Richard Grossinger, *Planet Medicine*

LEFT VERSUS RIGHT

Whether we consider the legends of Atlantis and Lemuria as mythological tales or historical fact, they nevertheless serve as useful frames of reference for viewing the history of modern medicine and its prehistory. While the Atlantean influence traces its way up through Egypt, Greece, and Rome, and then across Europe and into contemporary America, the Lemurian influence is found in the Pacific Islands and along the rim of the Pacific in Australia, China, South and North America, and across to India and Africa.

The development of rational thought and scientific thinking is decidedly Atlantean and is predominantly left-brain in its orientation. The left brain is the seat of mathematical and spatial abilities and logical thinking.

We naturally associate these characteristics with the masculine tendency to quantify and analyze. Indeed, the masculine gods of Judaism and Christianity combined with the rise of science, together form the greater part of the story of Western civilization. Modern America is the pinnacle of this trend, and I believe that our country's recent deterioration, as exemplified by its rising crime rates, rampant addictions, unchecked consumerism (in spite of increasing debt), economic inequality, and dependency upon warmaking, is a function of the excessive left-brained emphasis within our culture.

We periodically hear the cries of cultural authorities that we must produce more students with superior math and science abilities. The language that refers to children as our most valuable "resource" is a telling indictment of a culture that has depersonalized human life. We must ask ourselves if it is acceptable to treat students' lives like commodities to be molded for the benefit of the state's desire for technological dominance.

The emphasis on the masculine, along with the devaluation of the feminine, is a societal reality, and our collective cultural, mental, emotional, and physical health is reflective of our status as individuals within that culture. The road toward salvation depends upon the long and gradual process of restoring balance through embracing the feminine in our emotional, spiritual, and cultural lives. A green approach to healing also seeks to restore balance, because all illness originates from some form of imbalance.

The right-brain complementary counterpart to the Atlantean masculine is the Lemurian feminine, as illustrated by the native cultures remaining on our planet today that have not yet been "civilized." The origins and traditions of these nature-based cultures stretch back to the dawn of human history and reveal a worldview that is alien to most modern Westerners. Of prime importance to members of these societies is the fundamental belief that all things are connected and that all things have a spirit or are of spirit. The earth, the sky, the stars, stones, waters, winds, plants, and animals all have spiritual essences. Maintaining a healthy and respectful relationship with the web of life ensures ongoing prosperity for both humans and their environment. This type of Lemurian collective tribal mentality tends to be viewed as primitive and inferior by modern rational people, but overcoming this prejudice may hold the key to finding our way back to a place of balance and health.

Indigenous cultures, of necessity, are attuned to their environments in very intimate ways because their very survival depends upon it. Their belief systems, mythologies, and philosophies are a remarkable testament to the relationship of equality and interdependence between humans and nature. The cosmos and natural worlds are one, and can provide guidance and instruction; they should not be viewed as resources to be mined.

Modern culture, due to its technological advances, has become increasingly and frighteningly dissociated, enabling it to coast along under the illusion that the environment is not all that important. Nature may be viewed with outright hostility by those who feel their modern lifestyles cramped by the encroaching reality of environmental issues. Bill Plotkin, in his book *Soulcraft*, warns us about the impact of such cultural priorities:

> *All children and adolescents fashion personalities that fit within their native culture. In the West, that means a society largely materialistic, synthetic, technological, anthropocentric, ethnocentric, and egocentric. Fitting in with such a culture is difficult to accomplish without losing contact with our souls and with nature, the web of life.*[12]

SPIRITUAL REALITY

The mediator between the spirits and humans within nature-based cultures is the medicine man or woman, or shaman. The term "shaman" probably originated with the Tungus tribe of Siberia and translates as "one who sees in the dark." The shaman, often from an early age, shows a unique predilection for seeking an understanding of the mysteries of the various dimensions of the universe outside of the three-dimensional physical world. He or she has come face to face, whether through personal crisis or illness or through arduous initiation under the guidance of tribal elders, with what Michael Harner, in his groundbreaking work *The Way of the Shaman*,[13] calls "nonordinary reality" or the "shamanic state of consciousness." His work as an anthropologist with the Jivaro Indians of the Ecuadorian

Andes and the Conibo Indians of the Peruvian Amazon has given us an experiential document of the shaman's role, which has been elaborated upon by many others following in Harner's footsteps. Tom Cowan offers an alternate derivation of the word "shaman" in his book *Shamanism as a Spiritual Practice for Daily Life:*

> *Among the early root words from which shaman may have been derived are words for "knowledge" and "heat"—two ideas that capture fully the rich traditions of classic shamanism and its modern counterparts. The shaman is someone on fire with certain kinds of knowledge that come from the spirit world. In any era, the practice of shamanism puts one on the path that leads to a growing awareness of the spiritual mysteries of the universe.*[14]

This nonordinary state of consciousness is similar to the dream state that you and I can enter when we sleep. The difference is that while most people do not consciously control when and if they receive a dream, the shaman has learned how to or has the ability to travel to this space of altered consciousness at will and by choice. Although indigenous cultures have often used psychoactive substances like psilocybin mushrooms or peyote buttons to facilitate entry into the altered state, the same state can be achieved by other means, such as trance drumming or chanting. The shaman has developed a familiarity with the terrain of this otherworld of altered consciousness and utilizes this knowledge for the benefit of others. He or she moves between states of consciousness safely and with ease, and functions naturally and without difficulty at all levels. It is at these other levels of consciousness where the spirits of all things are encountered.

Again, the judgmental mind of the logical Westerner will tend to write this all off as mere fantasy, but the shaman and the shaman's fellow tribe members take this very seriously and experience nonordinary reality as no less real than conventional physical reality. Likewise, one can either dismiss a dream about one's deceased relative as a product of brain chemistry, or one can view it as a visitation from the spirit of an ancestor. More than once I have witnessed a profound transformation in mood and perspective of a patient to whom I have suggested that the dream of their deceased loved one was actually the spirit of that person. It is moving to see a person respond favorably to such an interpretation, as if he or she had simply needed permission to accept this obvious reality, which the surrounding culture has denied or rejected as nonsense.

Taken a step further, the appearance of a wolf in one's dream can be seen as a visitation by the spirit of wolf, who may have an important or helpful message to offer. Even a tree is part of the spiritual universe and may choose to speak to the shaman who travels to the other side. The academic term "animism" has been applied to this type of ancient worldview wherein all things human, animal, plant, and elemental, are possessed of intelligent and communicative life energies. This is the standard view of most indigenous peoples, who do not see themselves as individuals separated from their environment, friends, relatives, or ancestors. Such certainty as to the unbreakable bond that humanity has with the entire natural and spiritual world is highly instructive to those green practitioners who seek a model to learn from and to emulate.

A shaman is not an independent agent free to wander indiscriminately in the other worlds without guidance. (See Figure 4.1.) A shaman needs helpers and guides once reaching the other side because he or she is only

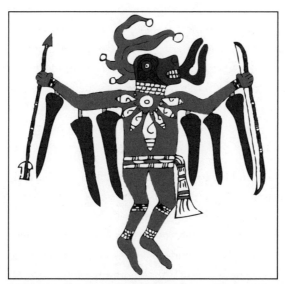

FIGURE 4.1: *Shaman Image Modeled after an Engraved Cup Found in the Craig Mound, Le Flore County, Oklahoma*

an intermediary making a visitation on behalf of someone in need of information or healing. Commonly, the shaman will have developed an intimate relationship with a spirit guide often in the form of an animal. In native cultures this helper is usually called a "power animal"—power referring in this case to spiritual power. The shaman journeys to the other side to seek the counsel of his power animal and other spirit guides and helpers.

A number of pioneers, beginning with Harner, have studied and trained with shamans and have experienced this contact with the spirit world firsthand. These techniques have been brought back to contemporary society and are being employed by some healers, therapists, and shamanic practitioners to help their patients. It is important to note that shamanism is not a formal religion and does not require belief in any particular set of rules or dogma. One simply has to open one's self up to the possibility that this life is comprised of more than just our daily physical existence. The shaman does not evangelize in favor of any particular belief system. Rather, the shaman is occupied with learning from personal experiences how to act as a guide to others. As Harner puts it:

> *The shaman is forever trying to articulate his personal revelatory experiences as though they were pieces of a great cosmic jigsaw puzzle ... A true master shaman does not challenge the validity of anybody else's experiences ... The master shaman will try to integrate even the most unusual experiences into his total cosmology, a cosmology based primarily on his own journeys ... The master shaman never says that what you experience is a fantasy. That is one of the differences between shamanism and science.*[15]

The basic technique used by shamans can vary but usually goes something like this: A steady and rapid drumbeat is used, designed to entrain the consciousness, thereby bringing the shaman's and/or patient's brainwaves into the theta frequency range, which is most conducive to producing an altered state of consciousness. This prepares the cosmic traveler as he or she approaches the portal to the otherworld of nonordinary awareness. This mental or psychic portal can vary as widely as the human mind can imagine, but is often a familiar place that in physical life leads into the ground, such as the trunk of a tree, or a cave, or a hole in the ground. The drumbeat carries the traveler along, down into the ground, and through a tunnel that leads to the other side.

Once there, the shaman meets or seeks out his spirit guide or power animal, in order to pose a question or present a problem in need of a solution. All the while the drumbeat continues in the background to keep the traveler focused on the mission. At the conclusion of the journey the drumbeat guides the subject on the return trip back through the tunnel to the portal, where the physical world of conventional consciousness is reengaged. Philip Gardiner and Gary Osborn characterize this shamanic trance state in their book *The Serpent Grail,* which seeks to understand how we may heal through reconciling the dualistic opposites of our divided consciousness:

> ... *a non-ordinary state of consciousness which has many levels to it. It is accessed via the hypnagogic state. This is the mid-point or in-between state in the waking-sleeping cycle, where one is both 'awake' and 'asleep' at the same time—a superimposition of opposites, a 'third state.' While our consciousness is balanced like a tightrope walker in this third state, we transcend the normal duality of the mind ... As such the hypnagogic state is responsible for all kinds of paranormal, psychic and mystical phenomena ...* [16]

This method of shamanic journeying can be undertaken by the healer for the benefit of a patient, or the patient may be taught to do this for him- or herself. While this may seem far-fetched to some, it is as simple as trusting the power of the imagination to kick in, in place of the ego and rational mind, which insist on maintaining control at all times. We have seen how this can work, for example, when a complete novice takes the leap and firewalks across a bed of hot coals. The novice is able to suspend any fundamental disbelief, trusts in instinct, and is ultimately rewarded with an epiphany, which changes the way he or she sees the world. No longer is it just the three dimensional physical world where one grows up, works, and then dies. It is now a world of fresh new possibilities. A bit of this "voodoo" has even crept into the modern hospital setting where cancer patients are instructed in methods of guided imagery and encouraged, for example, to visualize the cancer cells being eaten up by their chemotherapy medications.

DARKNESS AND LIGHT

The study of comparative mythologies, religions, cultural symbols, and belief systems by Carl Jung, Joseph Campbell, Mircea Eliade, and others have impressed upon their readers the striking similarities between ethnically and geographically disparate cultures. Likewise, a map of the terrain of the shaman's otherworldly travels reveals a surprising resemblance to the Christian concept of earth in between, heaven above, and hell below, although the interpretation of the significance of these regions is quite different in many respects. We are well acquainted with the Christian tendency to paint this physical life here on earth as a necessary burden. The faithful await greater rewards in heaven above if they have lived good lives, or the suffering and pains of hell below if they have been less than exemplary. Traditional Christianity portrays a black or white, up or down, right or wrong, good or bad outlook on this life, with little gray area left for reconciliation between these extremes.

An experienced shaman can travel to comparable regions in cosmic space, often designated as the upper, middle, and lower worlds. The middle world corresponds to physical life here on earth although it is not physical. It is the etheric version, or psychic double of this physical universe, through which the shaman may access a person's spiritual past coinciding with this lifetime. The shaman may go back in time and space to visit events that took place long ago and may bring back memories of those events.

The upper world is not much different from the Christian heavens. Here, things of spirit are to be found: evolved spiritual beings and entities, saints, angels, archangels, deities, divinities, and God. It is upward, beyond the physical sky, upward toward the light. It is the region of the light-giving solar Sky Father. Bill Plotkin ventures to define the upper world of spirit, toward which many of the world's great religious teachings aspire:

By spirit I mean the single, great, and eternal mystery that permeates and animates everything in the universe and yet transcends all. Ultimately, each soul exists as an agent for spirit ... the concept of spirit points to what all people, all things, have in common, our shared membership in a single cosmos, each of us a facet of the One Being that contains all. Spirit encompasses and draws us toward what is most universal and shared.[17]

These upper and middle world notions are relatively comprehensible to the Western mind; it is the lower world and its associations that give us so much trouble. Lower world journeying brings the shaman into the realm of the divine feminine, Mother Earth, the Earth Goddess. The spirits of the lower world are the spirits of nature, of trees, plants, and animals, and of humans, our predecessors and our ancestors. The lower world holds the dark womb of the earth, the cosmic yin, the mysterious forces of nature, the unconscious depths of our psyches. It is the dark night, the time when the moon becomes visible, and most importantly, it is the home of soul.

Matters of soul are deeply connected to our own sense of uniqueness and individuality. Soul is related to the true inner self or higher self, rather than the ego's constructed image of itself. One's soul is connected to one's personal sense of purpose and destiny. A personal sense of meaning that is unique to me is to be found by plumbing the depths of the darkness, and returning with bits and pieces of answers that I have found to the questions that I have asked.

The consensus of esoteric wisdom is that our soul chooses its mission in this life before birth. We also choose our parents and the circumstances under which we incarnate into physical body form so that the soul may learn new lessons as it works out its own unique destiny. Of course, most people have no recollection at birth of this chosen mission, and it becomes the task of the soul to gradually recollect its calling during this lifetime, which it can then choose to heed or to ignore. Shamanic soul-work can facilitate this process of personal knowledge and evolution in powerful and revealing ways.

Of necessity, for the sake of healthy ego development, it is the rational mind that becomes aware of itself, and comes to see all things through the lens of dualism, which then deals the decisive blow that rends the world into pairs of opposites. In the process, the concept of the lower world has been oversimplified and stereotyped by Westerners, ultimately being equated with the Christian conception of hell and evil. As a result, most of us are precluded from receiving the potential benefit that could derive from experiencing and understanding the realm of soul. The darkness is shunned at all costs, mainly because lack of familiarity with it generates fear and mistrust.

I have learned over the years to be very cautious about how I phrase my questions when inquiring whether a patient is feeling depressed. The word "depression" itself can produce instant fear and denial, as some are quick to make it clear that they are not "clinically" depressed. Understandably, they are concerned that acknowledging feelings of depression will sentence them to the stigma of a psychiatric label and a lifelong course of antidepressants. So rather than acknowledge what most will experience sooner or later if they are honest with themselves, the walls of defense rise up, ensuring that the unprocessed emotion and its corresponding issues will continue to smolder and grow internally until they can no longer be ignored.

Medical science also tends to deny the darkness. The lopsidedness of this rational perspective would have us look only toward the light, to the exclusion of half of all human experience. Just ask any person who has seen a loved one die in a hospital setting at the hands of well-intended, but often inappropriate, "heroic" medical measures. In spite of all indications that the person may have been ready to die, all resources are focused upon the goal of keeping him or her alive at all costs. Since no professional dared to recommend the alternative of helping the person die with dignity because that would represent failure in the face of death—as if we have any control over the inevitability of death—the patient and the patient's family may have been reluctant to spoil the doctor's valiant attempts to stave off the unavoidable. What could have been a powerful and natural endpoint, bringing family together to mark another transition in the sacred cycle of life, death, and the afterlife, becomes something to be feared and avoided. The hospice movement is a step in the right direction, but hospice services are sorely underutilized and often misunderstood in the United States today.

In the end, it is not a question of either/or, because the purposes of spirit in the upper world do not have to be opposed to the soul's downward pull toward nature in the lower world. Spirit and soul are two sides of the same coin: sky and earth, light and dark, male and female, life and death. They are complements that, taken together, constitute wholeness. Excluding one or the other generates only a fractured piece of the whole, which in turn engenders more human pain and suffering. Again, Plotkin shows us the way in *Soulcraft:*

> *A man's fear of the feminine is often a fear of his own soul and his own deeper nature ... Soul shows us how we, as individuals, are different from everybody else. Spirit shows us how we are no different from anything else, how we are one with all that exists. In relation to spirit, everyone has the same lessons to learn; for example, compassion and loving-kindness toward all beings, as Buddhism teaches ... In relation to soul, we each have lessons and qualities as unique as our fingerprints.*[18]

The theme that I am developing here should not be misconstrued as meaning that men are masculine and of the spirit and women are feminine and of soul. The two are not mutually exclusive. A man has within himself the potential to be both masculine and feminine, and the ideal is to develop a balance, so that he knows when to be strong and when to be soft, when to take charge and when to lay back, when to use his mind to approach a problem and when to access his feelings and intuition to deal with the same. The same concept applies to a woman, and for that matter, to all things. The polarities of light and dark, male and female, are contained within all things.

This wisdom of balance between light and dark, creative and receptive, is nothing new under the sun, but it is sadly lacking in contemporary technological society. The Chinese philosophy of Taoism and its associated yin-yang symbolism have made some inroads into popular American culture, but a more serious evaluation of the understanding that Taoism has to offer can yield great benefits to any seeker. The *I Ching* is an ancient Chinese classical text believed to be four to five thousand years old that contains the lessons of Taoism and Confucianism. It is an oracle used for divination by those seeking assistance and insight from the gods or the greater powers of the universe. The commentary on the second hexagram (See Figure 4.2), titled "the Receptive" in the landmark translation by Richard Wilhelm and Cary F. Baynes of the *I Ching*, or *Book of Changes*, sheds light upon our topic with great eloquence:

> *This hexagram is made up of broken lines only. The broken line represents the dark, yielding, receptive primal power of yin. The attribute of the hexagram is devotion; its image is the earth. It is the perfect complement of The Creative—the complement, not the opposite, for the Receptive does not combat the Creative but completes it. It represents nature in contrast to spirit, earth in contrast to heaven, space as against time, the female-maternal as against the male-paternal.*[19]

Yin and yang are paired opposites, which when taken as a whole transcend all dualism. In contrast to the closed-minded factual certainty of conventional medicine, the green practice of medicine and healing assumes a humble attitude of respect toward the many sources of ancient wisdom available to modern humanity, just one of which is the *I Ching*.

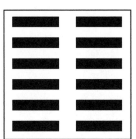

FIGURE 4.2: I Ching *Hexagram 2*

SOUL LOSS

Within tribal cultures it is taken for granted that illness arises from disharmony on the spiritual plane, and the shaman's sacred wisdom is sought in order to restore spiritual health. Emotional and even physical health issues can be resolved through making things right with the forces of nature, the spirits, and the ancestors. Health is a function of spiritual strength, which ultimately derives from right relationship with the invisible world—an invisible world that most scientific authorities would claim does not exist.

It is a spiritual world that might be entertained privately by some, but would never be acknowledged in the public arena of medical journals, institutions, and clinics.

Loss of spiritual power or, as some indigenous cultures would phrase it, "soul loss," is viewed as one of the most common causes of illness. The soul or parts of the soul of an individual may have strayed or decided to withdraw, thus leaving the vital energy or spiritual essence depleted. Tribal members are likely to attribute this to the soul's having been frightened away, or even stolen. Viewed through the lens of contemporary psychology, it becomes more acceptable if we suggest that traumatic events can lead to a condition that resembles soul loss.

The shock of a traumatic incident can leave an imprint upon the vital force, manifesting itself initially as a dazed or confused state. The classic example is the victim of a car crash, wandering around at the scene of the accident unaware of being traumatized, only to find out later from X-rays at the hospital that an arm or leg bone has been fractured. We may wonder how someone can feel no pain with a broken bone, but it is actually a common experience. It is as if the physical or emotional pain of the event is too great to bear. The vital force, in its innate wisdom, creates a buffer by partially withdrawing its energy from the location of the trauma, whether that trauma occurs on the emotional or physical level. One can surmise that this is to allow the individual to absorb the impact of such a terrible event more slowly over time rather than all at once.

This condition of shock can also be explained as a person's energy or essence beginning to leave his or her body. Out-of-body experiences are well documented and described frequently by those who have been traumatized physically or emotionally. I have had many people tell me how they had witnessed their own trauma as if they were standing nearby, or hovering above the scene in the air. The etheric body can separate from the physical body, giving the impression that there are two selves. The soul partially withdraws from the physical body, creating a floating sensation, an otherworldly, unreal feeling, or dream-like quality.

A healthy and strong spirit or vital force can rebound and return fully into the body within seconds, minutes, or even hours, but, unfortunately, this is often not the case. In many instances the body's energetic double does not fully return, and the person subsequently never feels quite the same, complaining of vague symptoms, or just not feeling normal. Symptoms of spaciness, confusion, poor concentration, or dizziness may persist. It is as if the person is still hovering out in space and has not fully gotten his or her feet back on the ground. A multiplicity of long-lasting chronic consequences may develop from having the body out of synch with its energy field or spiritual double, including irritability, depression, anxiety, fatigue, headaches, and generalized aches and pains, to name just a few. The million-dollar workup, including the latest in high-tech imaging, will be unable to detect any problem because this energetic phenomenon is not physical and does not fall within the scope of conventional medical diagnostics.

Out-of-body experiences and soul loss are pretty much the same condition as described by two different worldviews, and can be precipitated by a wide variety of circumstances. Situations of extreme duress, such as a motor vehicle accident, the death of a loved one, being held up at gunpoint, rape, or witnessing a violent crime can be so frightening or threatening as to make one's soul recoil from the body. The steady diet of pervasive and shocking levels of violence fed to Americans through television and movies is symptomatic of a populace that is already significantly numbed out in the face of such violence, and being numbed out to such a degree is already an indication of soul loss. A fascination with increasing levels of violence may represent a subconscious attempt to be shocked out of the numb state in order to feel fully alive again. People who are well attuned to the influence of their own souls would not wish to routinely expose themselves to such violence. The common usage of the term "lost soul" in popular culture reflects a deeper reality than many are probably willing to admit.

Diametrically opposed to the numbed-out souls are an increasing number of children displaying signs of hyperactivity. Young children, who are incapable of differentiating their own everyday experiences from either fantasy violence on television or real violence on the news, are particularly vulnerable to the destructive effects of media violence upon their immature psyches. We are raising a generation of children who are acquiring post-traumatic stress disorder-like traits. I believe this routine exposure to violence is one of the principal factors contributing to the rising tide of attention deficit disorder diagnoses in our overstimulated culture.

While we can easily wrap our minds around why one would leave the body under extreme conditions, it is a little harder to accept that this can happen in more subtle situations. Consider failing an exam, losing a job, contracting an illness, being punished by a parent, being laughed at by one's peers, miscarrying a pregnancy, or having a pet die. Remember how each individual's vital force is unique and reflective of different degrees of health or resilience. All it takes is a combination of the right trigger with the wrong vital force, and the consequences can be penetrating and devastating. While it may require significant force to cause some to lose their energetic balance, a relatively minor stressor can be the straw that breaks the camel's back for others.

The soullessness engendered by the industrial age, and its emphasis upon material existence, were key contributing factors to the restless discontent of the 1960s generation in the United States. Young adults knew that something important was missing and went looking for it, and the values of peace and love embraced by the antiwar movement comprise part of what their explorations found. In his book *Drumming at the Edge of Magic,* Mickey Hart, drummer of the Grateful Dead, gives an insider's honest assessment of the dangers of LSD and the role it played as catalyst to this explosion of spiritual consciousness across the nation:

> *None of my friends talked about shamans, and yet that's what we were all trying to become, without knowing it. We were climbing around in the World Tree of consciousness like adolescents, intent only on the thrill that came from playing in these dangerous spaces so far above the ground.*
>
> *And how could it have been otherwise? There was a community waiting to be healed, but there were no teachers—or very few— and there was no tradition of exploring these states. The tradition that we had inherited disavowed their existence, insisting that the tiny box of consciousness that we all inhabited was all there was. And yet 250 millionths of a gram of a powerful psychochemical suggested that when it came to the mind and its attendant powers,*

the science of the twentieth century was no closer to solving the riddle than the science of the Egyptians or ancient Greeks had been.[20]

Here we had a whole generation suspecting that their collective soul was being sucked away by the impersonal forces of a war-making machine all too willing to sacrifice the country's youth for its nefarious purposes. I fear that the current generation is so deeply anesthetized by the sensory overload of commercial culture that it may be unable to even recognize that it is being led to the slaughter all over again for the sake of oil in the Middle East. Many Vietnam veterans have spent their post-war lives grappling with the soul loss, or post-traumatic stress disorder, induced by their experiences overseas. The implications for the war-trauma victims of these different generations are staggering. A green medical perspective recognizes the collective damage wrought upon humanity by all forms of war and would support such action only as an absolute last resort.

A surprising percentage of people will respond in the affirmative when asked if they have ever had an out-of-body experience. The majority of these episodes have been the result of traumatic events or of taking psychoactive drugs. Sandra Ingerman is a therapist and shamanic practitioner who has written a book about soul loss titled *Soul Retrieval.* She poses an interesting question that arises when the psychotherapeutic process encounters the reality of soul loss:

> *In modern times, psychology has provided our primary model for addressing the painful sense of incompleteness and disconnection that many of us experience. We may spend years in therapy or self-help groups trying to uncover traumas and to become whole. I hold a master's degree in counseling psychology and have employed many of its methods, but experience has shown me that psychotherapy works only on the parts of us that are "home." If a part of our vital essence has fled, how can we bring it back?*[21]

A CASE OF NARCOLEPTIC FOG

We can't do psychotherapy with a soul part that is not there. Therapy can effectively deal with the ego and its issues here in the middle world, but it cannot access the lower world, to which the missing soul parts have likely fled. A patient that I once saw often exhibited a dreamy, distant quality. He did not speak of himself in this manner, perhaps because he was mostly unaware of it. He did explain that he was always working on being "more present" in his daily life. A carefully chosen homeopathic treatment was followed by a powerful dream experience that seemed to wake him from out of the fog. He dreamed that a friend of his, whom he had not seen in years, appeared above him while he was sleeping and tried to wake him from his slumber. The patient got up to witness the friend complaining to someone, saying that he'd had enough and could not go on anymore. The day after the dream, the patient got up with a gnawing feeling, which eventually compelled him to call his old friend. The friend's wife answered the phone and informed him that her husband had just passed away. The profound impact upon the dreamer was evident when he returned to my office to report what had happened. He seemed different, and even though I had never mentioned the word to him, he said that his lifelong "narcoleptic" tendency was starting to diminish, and that he was awakening to the desire to build better interpersonal relationships.

Now I cannot speak with absolute certainty, but it strikes me that an intervention from the other side had taken place, as the spirit of the patient's old friend lent his assistance by helping this slumbering soul to awaken once more. Perhaps this spirit had at least one more important job to do before he moved on to the next life. And the patient's first response to this deep healing event was to reprioritize the value that he placed on relationships with others. This was a beautiful and perfect conclusion, indicating to me that my client had been the recipient of a spiritual gift that was likely to lead to greater overall health. It is reasonable to assume that he will be able to derive much greater benefit from psychological counseling now that he has emerged from the fog and is more fully present, as he had originally wished to be.

PERSONAL SOUL QUEST

Now we turn our attention back to the shaman, whose role it is to travel to the other side on behalf of another to seek ways to restore spiritual power to the suffering individual. The shaman enlists the assistance of his or her power animal and spirit guides to lead the way on the journey. Remember, just as the minister is the intermediary between God and his congregants, so, too, the shaman is only an intercessor between the supplicant and the spirit world. The shaman travels back and forth across the border with news and information.

If it is suspected that a person's ailment may be due to soul loss, a shaman may undertake a journey to inquire whether there are any lost souls or soul parts. If there are, a power animal may lead the shaman into the underworld to where these souls have fled, where they may be asked or coaxed by the shaman into considering a return to their rightful home. Provided that they agree, the shaman may, through a process called "soul retrieval," bring these soul parts back to the person who needs and wants their presence in order to be whole again.

My personal healing journey once led me to a shaman's doorstep deep in the Vermont woods, where he graciously agreed to teach and assist me. After much preparation and calling upon the help of the spiritual world, with my wife providing the steady beat of a drum in the background, we lay on our backs with eyes closed side by side, with ankles and shoulders touching as he journeyed. (See Figure 4.3.) Upon returning to ordinary reality, he rose up and leaned over me, cupping his hands while blowing several times into my heart region and into the crown of my head. He

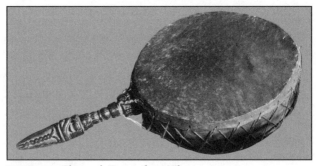

FIGURE 4.3: *Shaman's Drum, from Tibet*

informed me that he had been led by his power animal to three souls, all of whom consented to coming home, and that he had just blown them back into me. I told him that during the ceremony I had glimpsed images in my mind of my mother, my grandfather, and my father, in that order.

Being a skeptic, I was not very impressed until he offered further information regarding these long-lost souls. Without my having given him any prior information about these souls, he said that the three shared a common theme, which he struggled to put into words. He said it was as if all three had just decided to leave because they were not getting what they felt entitled to receive. The first was a vital, happy, playful eleven-month-old child crawling on hands and knees. He had been trying to engage an adult in a game of hide-and-seek, and had crawled off to hide. But when no one had come to find him, and after he'd unsuccessfully attempted to draw the adult into playing with him, he'd felt wounded and had decided to leave. The second soul was approximately six years old, but his situation was less clear. There was just a feeling that he had not been getting something he was entitled to, and so he had left in disappointment. The third was a teenager, perhaps fifteen years old, who had been at odds with a father figure. Although the teen had been standing strong under fire and holding his own, the parent just had not understood the significance of the struggle. Since he had not received the praise he had deserved for his transition into manhood, he too had decided to leave.

Upon hearing this information, I began to internally protest, "These aren't the traumas that I need healed!" But then, as I burst into tears, a dawning realization came over me. I suddenly knew what the shaman was referring to. I honestly cannot recall anything from the age of eleven months, but one of my clearest and earliest memories is from about age five or six. I had become so upset at my mother, for reasons I do not recall, that I grabbed a small suitcase, packed some stuff into it, and took off down the street, away from home. After I had gone quite a distance and was becoming concerned that no one was coming after me, my grandfather pulled up alongside me in his car, told me to get in, and took me back home.

I also remembered that one of the defining moments of my teenage years occurred when I refused to get my increasingly lengthy hair cut. I felt that in spite of my having lived up to paternal expectations of getting good grades in school and of being a very responsible young man, I was getting no slack with something that symbolized to me my budding individuality. Push came to shove and I left home, putting quite a scare into my father, even though I had only hidden myself in the upstairs bedroom at a good friend's house.

The correlation between the three souls, my three fleeting images during the journey, and the actual events in my life, was dramatic. To my further amazement, as if to confirm the profound nature of what had just happened, I received visitations in dream form from two of these souls within the next few days. First, I dreamt that I reached out and joyfully scooped up a naked and smiling baby boy who was crawling on the ground. In the second dream I was walking with a teenage boy as we looked for our class at the university. We came upon the Science class but this was not where we belonged. A little more searching brought us to the Religion and Science class, and we knew we had found the right place. I will leave speculation regarding the connection between this last dream and the current enterprise of writing this book to you, the reader.

The overwhelming disposition of Western culture is to look upward toward the light, to acknowledge only the positive, while denying the negative. To suggest that our scientific, technological, and medical advances do not necessarily make us the greatest nation on earth is considered unpatriotic by some. To suggest that we may never conquer disease is considered heretical by many who place their hope in technological innovation and wish to believe in the eventual triumph of scientific progress. As a materialistic culture that is uncomfortable with genuine spirituality, we have lost our collective soul, and we have instead placed our faith in the will of the scientific mind to triumph over the unpredictable forces of nature. It is illusion to think that we can live only in the light without integrating the dark.

Most journeys by shamans and those who seek their help seem to be to the lower world because this is where most of the healing work needs to be done. Although many do not want to go there, it is necessary to look down into the dark feminine underworld of the unconscious, where the soul resides. No one ever benefited from psychotherapy by avoiding coming to terms with the secret feelings of pain, grief, anger, hurt, inadequacy, and insecurity that are harbored inside. The courage to dive into the darkness brings with it the promise of rebirth, making it possible for one to return to the surface as a more balanced and whole individual.

This glimpse into the worldview of shamanism illustrates just one of the possibilities for healing that lies outside the domain of the left-brained materialism promulgated by the scientific establishment. Not unlike Asklepian dream healing, shamanic journeying provides a powerful method for tapping into unseen healing dynamics that physical medicine is incapable of accessing. The asymmetric tilt toward quantitative, reductionistic medicine is, by its very nature, productive of illness, since all disease issues forth from a state of imbalance within the individual and his or her surrounding culture. While medical science rightly deserves a place at the table, its inflated sense of itself will require serious reappraisal in order to restore balance and create legitimate room at the very same table for a right-brained, qualitative, green approach to health, disease, and human understanding.

5

Perceiving the Natural Order

Treating the whole person, which is now accepted on a rhetorical level by everyone, should be more than a theoretical dictum; it should be an applied reality.
    —George Vithoulkas, *A New Model for Health and Disease*

SYMPTOMATIC HIERARCHY

All symptoms are not created equal. A big toenail discolored by fungus is not on a par with arthritic knee pain, and knee pain is not as problematic as a suicidal mood. An astute evaluation of the unique health status of any given person involves careful discrimination and judgment as to the depth of pathology and consequent limitation that it places upon the suffering patient. Each individual symptom can be assigned its place in the hierarchy of the patient's complaints, just as the overall pattern of symptoms, taken together, can be used to gauge a person's health status and the condition of the underlying vital energy.

At first glance a hierarchical assessment of symptoms may seem easy enough to achieve. Obviously, we must ascribe greater significance to a person's migraines than to some itchy patches of eczema. The annoying itch of a skin condition cannot be compared to the severe pain of a migraine that lasts for hours. But is this always the case? What if the migraines are rather mild and infrequent, occurring perhaps twice per year and lasting only an hour, while the eczema is relentlessly itchy to the point of keeping the poor person awake at night, scratching until he or she is raw and bleeding?

How about the high school track star's asthmatic cough compared to the small warts on the hands of the team cheerleader? Slam dunk, no comparison, right? A little further investigation reveals that the cough occurs only in very cold air and has little, if any, impact upon the athlete's performance, and his prescribed inhaled medication is almost never used or required. The cheerleader on the other hand, when carefully questioned, reluctantly admits that she is contemplating quitting the squad because the warts make her feel disgusting and ugly. She acknowledges that the way she feels about the warts is even affecting her social relationships at school.

Now, admittedly this is a trick question regarding warts versus asthma, because the warts, in this instance, are not the limiting symptom. It is the self-image associated with the warts that has become so problematic for this girl. It may be illuminating to note that another hypothetical girl on the cheerleading squad also has had warts on her fingers for a couple of years, but she has never thought twice about them. If we are to grade these symptoms according to the threat that they pose, the warts themselves are of least concern, the asthmatic cough would place second, and the feelings of self-disgust are most troublesome.

Let's try another example. A young woman complains that she has used birth control pills for a few years, but now that she is ready to try to conceive she finds that, since discontinuing the pill, her regular menstrual cycles have not returned. In addition, she is experiencing hot flashes that she says are driving her crazy. Before all of this set in, she would have said that her biggest complaint was seasonal allergies, which manifested mainly as itchy eyes and a runny nose. When asked which of these symptoms bothers her most, she clearly indicates the hot flashes, followed by the allergies. A little surprised, I question why the lack of menses does not bother her more. She confides that although she used to feel certain about her desire to have children, she is not so sure anymore, and besides, it is rather convenient not to have to deal with a monthly period. Upon further questioning, she discloses that her libido has been diminished for some time, perhaps a year or more, and she can give no emotional or psychological reason for this since she is happy with her relationship.

This scenario is an example of a very common syndrome that results from birth control medications, which, although experienced by many thousands of women, few medical professionals seem willing to acknowledge. The altered hormonal balance that can result from using birth control pills manifests as a subtle or not so subtle ambivalence, indifference, or outright aversion toward the idea of becoming a mother. The natural emotions and attitudes regarding motherhood become distorted, and these changes can be chronic and, in some cases, permanent, even when the person may have ceased taking the pill months or even years ago. In our example, this hormonal imbalance shows itself as a suppression of the menstrual cycle, a decreased sex drive, an ambivalence toward childbearing, and hot flashes.

This woman's own assessment of the relative discomfort of her symptoms gave us a list of hot flashes, itchy eyes, and runny nose, in that order. It is common that maternal ambivalence and lack of sexual desire are not even perceived as symptoms, although some can be quite aware of such changes and may complain about them but may be unable to explain them. While this woman arranged her symptoms based upon the level of discomfort that they produced, the observant clinician may use different criteria. All green health care practitioners need to be cognizant of the big picture and should be trained to exercise their judgment as to the relative threat to well-being that each symptom poses.

A hierarchical assessment of threats to health and well-being would, in this case, produce a list of symptoms from most to least problematic as follows: cessation of monthly periods, recent development of ambivalence toward childbearing and motherhood, diminished libido, hot flashes and, last, the allergy symptoms. Some may claim that I am making a sexist judgment in this case, and assert that a woman has the right to choose whether she wants to bear children. I completely agree that a woman has the right to choose not to become a mother, as long as it is not unwittingly forced upon her by chemical means. If this propensity toward hormonal imbalance created by birth control medications were fully disclosed to prospective consumers, many would think twice about their method of prophylaxis.

The point that I am making is that all symptoms are not the same. Some represent greater dangers to health than others. If we accept this fundamental assumption, there must be some way to assess and grade symptoms so that we know where to direct our greatest attention. Mistakenly focusing on superficial symptoms and issues can inadvertently produce a medical nightmare. The average clinician of orthodox medicine might well oblige the woman complaining of hot flashes by attempting to adjust her hormonal balance, or lack thereof, by prescribing yet more hormonally active medications. Rarely have I seen a satisfactory outcome from this type of hormonal tinkering; the more common result tends to be symptomatic chaos and a variety of unpleasant side effects.

Let's return for a moment to the cheerleader who is upset by her warts. A shortsighted approach that neglects to investigate the underlying issues could similarly produce serious long-term consequences, just as such an approach fell short for the woman on birth control pills. The obvious standard of treatment here would be to have a doctor remove the warts. Quite possibly the cheerleader would feel relieved for a time, but let us assume for argument's sake that a year later she begins to lobby her parents for a nose job because she has become displeased with her appearance. Not unlike the issue raised in our discussion of hernia surgery in a previous chapter, a not-so-benign procedure is then performed by a plastic surgeon, who believes that this can help to improve this young woman's self-image. Fortunately, she comes through without complications and returns to school excited about her new look.

All the while, parents, teachers, and physicians are enabled to look the other way, thus disregarding the true nature of the illness involved. Several years pass, and college seems to be going well until this young woman calls home one day and announces that she cannot cope any longer and is thinking of dropping out. Consultation with a psychologist reveals that she is showing signs of significant anxiety and depression, and she admits that she has been severely restricting her diet. She has now become anorexic. But this should hardly come as a surprise. The original feelings of self-disgust have, sadly, remained all along, never having been adequately addressed but instead only temporarily masked by periodic superficial adjustments to the patient's physical appearance.

It turns out that the warts and imperfect nose were merely the focus for, and not the actual cause of, her internal negative assessment of herself. And yet our cultural milieu and physically focused medical system are customarily complicit in sending the distinct message that these types of internal conditions can be treated or solved by external means. The rational mind of science is unlikely to see through to the inner heart of the matter.

THE BODY-HEART-MIND-SOUL CONTINUUM

An effective healer must become proficient at reading the language of the life force, which can express itself in a variety of ways through physical, emotional, mental, and/or spiritual symptoms. Consequently, he or she must always consider the possibility of an underlying message behind any given physical symptom. Sometimes there is a clear message, sometimes it is more subtle, sometimes there is a message but it is beyond our understanding, and occasionally a physical symptom is what it is, just a physical symptom.

A framework for understanding symptoms and their import is needed. Fortunately, one need look no further than the writings of the pioneers of homeopathic medicine over the past two hundred years to find a great deal of accumulated knowledge concerning the subject. Practitioners and patients alike need to be educated regarding the natural order of symptomatology so they can make informed decisions when they face important health care issues. Much of this information has been cogently summarized for the contemporary reader by Greek homeopath George Vithoulkas, in his book *The Science of Homeopathy*. Vithoulkas identifies three levels, mental/spiritual, emotional/psychic, and physical, which, in reality, are not separate. Although I am in essence saying the same thing, for my purposes I make a distinction between mental and spiritual levels, and will refer to this natural order in terms of the following four levels of increasing importance:

1. Body (Physical, the most superficial layer)
2. Heart (Emotional)
3. Mind (Mental)
4. Soul (Spiritual, the deepest layer)

This natural hierarchy of body, heart, mind, and soul is roughly equivalent to physical, emotional, mental, and spiritual levels.

The physical plane corresponds to the domain of conventional medicine and includes physical symptoms, like headache, nausea, and joint pain, and physical signs like increased blood pressure, and elevated temperature. It also includes phenomena that orthodox medicine does not usually consider, such as food cravings, sleep positions, and sensitivities to environmental factors like heat, cold, humidity, and wind. The anatomical components of the human body and their various physiological and biochemical processes are of the physical level. The circulatory system, digestive system, endocrine system, and nervous system are examples of this.

The emotional plane encompasses the entire range of human emotional experience, including love, hate, anger, fear, anxiety, grief, joy, sadness, irritability, depression, hurt, and despair. The passions and desires that drive people to do what they do are part of the emotional lives of all individuals. Emotions can be positive or negative and can be experienced in balance, in excess or to extremes, or may be diminished or lacking.

When we speak of the mental plane, we mean the mind and its ability to think and reason. The ability to use language, to analyze, to calculate, to draw conclusions, and to make judgments fall into this category. The capacity to create, to communicate, to plan, and to imagine and envision are mental functions. Memory, concentration, attention span, and clarity or confusion of thought processes are also characteristics of the mental plane.

By its very nature the spiritual plane is a little more elusive, although arguably there is some degree of overlap with the mental plane. A sense of meaning, destiny, or purpose, and a belief or disbelief in something greater than oneself are spiritual qualities. Altruism and charity, love and respect for one's neighbor and for all humankind regardless of differences, and a sense of obligation to nurture the earth and its fragile ecosystems can all be thought of as spiritually motivated. Prayer, and communication with angels, spirits, and the ancestors are spiritual activities. A sense of oneness with the universe or conversely, a loss of faith, can both be spiritual experiences. Even atheistic and agnostic sentiments are spiritually related, as they are defined by their degree of opposition to God or a higher power.

As discussed earlier, the frontier, or bridge, between mind and spirit lies somewhere between waking and dreaming, between the conscious and the unconscious mind. The immature ego frequently attempts to erroneously assert its superiority, by declaring the "irrationality" of an activity like beseeching God's mercy or praying for a loved one's well-being. The rational function may choose to value its version of reality over what it judges to be illusion or delusion. There can be a very fine line between the conceptions of reality held by different cultures. A man who claims to have heard God speak to him may, in Western society, be evaluated by a psychiatrist to determine if he is schizophrenic, while the same man in an indigenous setting may be taken under the wing of his elders to be groomed as a shaman.

We will discuss the practical relevance of understanding the natural order of symptomatic expression at a later point but for now, perhaps, an example will suffice to illustrate. What if a person struggling with arthritis is prescribed a non-steroidal anti-inflammatory drug (NSAID) and thereafter reports significant symptomatic relief but, unfortunately, also notices the onset of emotional symptoms suggestive of depression? What if another patient with arthritis is given the same medication and experiences dramatic improvement in his or her symptoms but six months later has a heart attack? These are not hypothetical examples, as the medical community has acknowledged that the use of some NSAIDs, such as Celebrex, has been associated with numerous instances of myocardial infarction. Is this to be interpreted as a side effect of NSAIDs? Is it mere coincidence? Would these people have had heart attacks anyway? Questions of this nature and more will be explored after we have built an adequate framework of understanding upon which we can then base our answers.

We can judge the relative importance of symptoms on different levels by comparing them to each other and assessing the impact that they have upon the overall person. When choosing between a moderate degree of low back pain and a moderate degree of depression, most people would opt for back pain. Back pain is contained and affects a localized part of the body, while depression affects the whole individual in a more complete way. It is revealing to become cognizant of the way people describe each of these conditions. On the one hand we say, "*My* back hurts," and on the other, we say, "*I* feel depressed." Likewise, in comparing moderate depression to a moderate degree of memory loss, most would not choose to live with memory loss. While depression can be experienced as troublesome, memory problems can have a profound impact upon the scope of one's daily activities. Taking the comparison one step further, while one can live a purposeful life even with memory loss, a moderate degree of loss of capacity to love could cause one to question the very point of his or her existence. Recapping, we can say that back pain is preferable to depression, is preferable to memory loss, which is preferable to the inability to feel love. Given similar degrees of pathology on each level, the physical problem is less threatening than the emotional, which is less threatening than the mental, which poses less of a threat than the spiritual problem.

Within each level of our framework of spirit, mind, emotion, and body we can also describe a hierarchical division into sublevels. This is most easily seen on the physical plane, where skin issues are usually less troublesome than intestinal symptoms, which are less problematic than heart conditions, which are less threatening than central nervous system illnesses. On the emotional plane, most would agree on the order of the following, from least to most limiting: sadness, jealousy, vindictiveness, and suicidal feelings. Similarly, on the mental plane, the order from least to most undesirable would begin with a lack of aptitude for mathematics, followed by distractibility, then racing thoughts, and finally, memory loss.

In addition, we must consider qualifying factors like intensity, duration, and acuteness versus chronicity of symptoms before we can arrive at a thorough understanding of the energetic status and health of an individual. Again, a severe itch can be much more problematic than a rare migraine. And an acute viral illness with high fever, achiness all over, and sinus headache is of lesser concern in comparison to a chronic fear that someone may break into my home at night to kill me.

Through understanding the natural order of symptomatic expression, health status can be assessed by determining the locus of where the energy of the life force is most forcefully expressing itself. In other words, if I feel mildly depressed but also have asthma attacks that come on suddenly and sometimes require visits to the emergency room, then the predominant force of the illness lies on the physical plane. If I have chronically sore arthritic knees and I am concurrently experiencing significant forgetfulness such that I momentarily could not find my way home in my own neighborhood, then the force of the illness is showing itself on the mental plane. If I experience frequent mild headaches but I am also phobic about flying in a way that creates a significant impediment to fulfilling my career goals, then the imbalance is manifesting most significantly on the emotional plane. If I have moderately high blood pressure but I have also lost a sense of purpose in life and am questioning many of the things that I previously thought true, then the energetic disturbance is most apparent on the spiritual level. George Vithoulkas refers to the location of the energetic focus of an illness as the "center of gravity." Symptoms on all levels, nevertheless, remain interrelated, but tend to constellate around this center of gravity.

DIRECTIONALITY OF DISEASE

Although the scientific mind seeks absolutes, this is unrealistic in terms of human health, which is highly complex, multifactorial, and not subject to unequivocal laws. We can begin to define some fundamental guidelines, which should never be construed as written in stone. As a general rule, we can say that as the defense mechanism becomes more compromised, it manifests its distress on deeper levels. Illness deepens as it moves in the direction from physical to emotional to mental to spiritual. We can also say that this negative trend moves from the most exterior point, that being the skin, to the most interior level, that being one's spiritual essence or soul. By this standard, even a severe case of eczema that causes much discomfort is not comparable to the status of a hate-filled individual who wishes harm upon others. The center of gravity of a hateful person is much deeper, and should be considered a much more grave condition. Similarly, the center of gravity in a narcissistic person resides at a much deeper location than it does in someone with gallbladder pain or allergy symptoms.

Looks may be deceiving; a narcissistic person can be perfectly healthy in the physical sense and may never even complain to a doctor but, nevertheless, his actions can be deeply hurtful or destructive to those around him. This kind of assessment can be a little delicate because some may perceive it as being judgmental. I would contend, rather, that it involves the proper use of sound judgment. It is not a moral condemnation, in this instance, of the narcissistic individual and his or her actions or shortcomings. It is not an assignment of guilt, or rightness or wrongness, or goodness or badness. It should be a non-judgmental clinical assessment, imperfect as it may be, designed to aid the patient in the quest for healing.

A common issue that I have faced when interviewing patients is how to reassure those who may begin to feel judged by the questions that I am asking. For example, a man may want to know what my questions concerning his temper have to do with his stomach ulcer. It becomes my job then to make clear to him that I am not passing judgment on his temper but rather, like an investigator, I am sleuthing around looking for connections and patterns that may help illuminate the nature of his illness and the status of his vital energy so that proper measures may be taken to facilitate a true healing process.

A patient may not only feel judged, but may feel simple resistance to talking about certain sensitive topics. Paradoxically, these points of sensitivity often hold the key to understanding the true nature of the illness and the stuckness of the vital energy. I may, for example, find out that within weeks prior to the onset of a woman's headaches, her mother had died. When I inquire how that affected her, she may be reluctant to dredge up those painful feelings. If the headaches are to be solved, then the issues that lie on a deeper, more internal level must be addressed. Once this is accomplished, it no longer becomes necessary for the life force to generate headaches as a distress signal, since corrective measures have been taken and balance has been restored.

After losing loved ones, many are intent upon moving on and would like to believe that they have adequately grieved their loss. Unfortunately, it does not always work this way, as the vital force may demand more thorough processing and integration of the purpose and meaning of such a crucial event in a life story. Unprocessed and unresolved grief is one of the most common causes of illness. The proper handling of grief is a skill that can be learned by many and that can prevent unnecessary illness from developing.

The next rule of thumb, which we can state with confidence, is that the body-heart-mind-soul is a single, continuous entity. This unity can be visualized as a gradient along which the energy of the bioenergetic life force can move and, correspondingly, a gradient along which symptoms can move. The human organism is a fluid, dynamic, ever-changing whole that responds continuously to circumstances by adapting with either healthy resilience or dysfunctional susceptibility. Homeopath Rajan Sankaran explains how this changes our concept of disease:

> *Disease is ... not something local, not an affection of the parts, but it is the state of being of the whole person at the time, the way he feels, thinks, behaves, what he likes and dislikes, and what he tolerates and cannot tolerate on the whole ... The whole concept of disease thus changes from being something local to something general, from being a diagnostic label to being an individual's state of being. From this understanding our whole approach to treatment changes.*[22]

As examples of this fluidity, one person may describe stomach cramps that alternate with strong waves of sadness and crying, and another may report bouts of insomnia that alternate with back spasms, while they both say that their two sets of symptoms never occur simultaneously. This shifting of symptoms is, in reality, a shifting of energy from one locus to another as the defense mechanism seeks a new state of equilibrium. The modern medical mind balks at the notion that a symptom manifesting as knee pain may suddenly disappear and be shortly thereafter replaced by an attack of vertigo, which after receding is replaced again by knee pain. The mechanistic medical model leads to the assumption that the two conditions are anatomically unrelated and consequently should have nothing to do with each other. In reality, it is sufficient to assume a connection because they are energetically related. The scientific mindset may refuse to entertain the notion that an underlying energetic principle is at work, while a green perspective takes the energetic connection between all things to be a given.

The stress point in the bioenergetic field may make itself apparent anywhere along the body-heart-mind-soul gradient through the generation of symptoms. As symptoms move from one level to another there is directionality to this shift. As the energy shifts toward the spiritual plane it is moving deeper into the interior of the person, and as symptoms crop up on the physical plane they are being expressed on the more superficial or surface layer of the body. If a person who previously tended to get bladder infections has in recent months become prone to anxiety attacks, we can say that the focus of the illness has gone deeper into the system. Conversely, in a restless child who previously could not sit still and has now become calmer but, instead, has developed eczema on the arms and legs, the center of gravity of disease can be said to be moving externally toward the surface of the body as the child's health shows signs of improving.

Health status, therefore, can be assessed by determining where along the gradient an individual tends to manifest symptoms. Keeping in mind that there are sub-gradients within each level and that intensity and chronicity of symptoms must also be taken into account, we can generate a health profile that becomes very useful in gauging a person's progress or regress over time. By noting where along the gradient that symptoms tend to fall, we can discern a range of susceptibility that serves as a tool for predicting what kinds of symptoms or illnesses a person is likely to get or not to get. The range of susceptibility of a woman that has had only a couple of sinus infections, an occasional cold, and no other health problems, is skewed toward the physical level. We would not expect her to develop a deeper illness like arthritis or depression unless she were to encounter an adverse event of significant force. A different woman, one with a history of gallbladder attacks, occasional bronchitis, and a miscarried pregnancy, would be much more likely to develop arthritis or depression because her current health issues already indicate that her range of susceptibility is compatible with these additional illnesses.

Sometimes people diagnosed with cancer report that they believed they were previously quite healthy and were therefore surprised by the discovery of their disease. They commonly indicate that they hardly ever get sick and do not understand how they could have gotten cancer. The mistaken belief that the less frequently one gets sick with acute illnesses, like a cold or flu or fever, the more healthy one is, is based upon a lack of understanding of how the energy of the defense mechanism functions. Cancer represents an illness that has gone very deep into the physical body. This penetration skews the range of susceptibility away from superficial, everyday illnesses like the common cold. The defense mechanism is engaged in a battle at a deeper level and, consequently, does not tend to waste its time and energy, so to speak, with more surface matters. The big cultural lie that encourages us to pop a pill at the first sign of the slightest cold symptom can actually promote an unintentional shift of the center of gravity onto deeper levels, thus contributing to the development of more serious illnesses.

The healthiest members of a population are the ones without chronic illness who are also prone to coming down with a run-of-the-mill head cold or viral fever now and then. The immune system is functioning well when it flexes its muscle by contracting an illness, mounting a defense, and quickly recovering without subsequent complication. This is most obvious in children, the ones least likely to develop deeper and more chronic illnesses. This tendency is rapidly changing in modern industrialized societies, due to a number of factors directly related to the "advanced" type of medical care that children are receiving (more on this later). The adult members of a population, who are less likely to come down with a flu or fever, are the ones more likely to develop chronic diseases such as hypertension, arthritis, or migraine headaches.

It is no coincidence that young people tend to get acute self-limiting illnesses, while older people tend to contract chronic illnesses. As health diminishes, the previously clear and straightforward expression of the immune system as typified, for example, by a fever, chills, and sweating, becomes blunted or dulled into more low-grade, vague symptoms that no longer resemble a nice clean short-lived bout of illness. An adult who picks up the same virus as his own child may, instead of fever and chills, complain of achiness, stuffed-up head, and fatigue that can last for a week or more. While the child gets sick and recovers uneventfully, the adult may have difficulty throwing off the same illness, often experiencing low-grade symptoms for weeks or even months. Continuing along the gradient of diminishing health, the adult with high blood pressure and chronic fatigue may not even be susceptible to a viral illness because the immune system may be too busy expressing itself on a deeper level via symptoms that are ever present. And most chronic illness is unlikely to ever resolve without proper care based upon the holistic principles of green healing.

The deepest symptom that a person manifests at any given point in time represents the weakest point of the human energy field: the Achilles heel of the vital force, if you will. Any therapeutic intervention carries with it the potential of inadvertently pushing the center of gravity of the disease deeper into the organism. All the better, therefore, if we can use our knowledge and discernment to purposefully encourage the center of gravity to move in the direction of greater health.

This fluid mobility of symptomatic expression along the body-heart-mind-soul gradient is a crucial concept to understand, as it will form the foundation of my critique of the effects of most orthodox medical interventions. Since the conceptual framework of Western medicine does not account for an energy gradient along which the life force may express itself through symptomatology, its practitioners remain unable to discern the big picture and the long-term consequences of their actions. As a result, most orthodox treatments are superficial, oriented toward symptomatic relief, and likely to contribute to chronic illness.

A CASE OF CROHN'S DISEASE

The following example may help to illustrate the natural hierarchical order of expression of the bioenergetic life force. Lisa was a teenage girl who once consulted me for treatment of her Crohn's disease, a condition that involves progressive inflammation and destruction of the digestive tract, especially the intestines. Conventional treatment usually includes strong anti-inflammatory drugs, corticosteroids and, ultimately, surgical removal of the affected parts of the digestive tract. Lisa had been having severe attacks of abdominal pain and daily diarrhea for about a year and a half. These episodes of pain had continued in spite of regular medical therapy. After a year of homeopathic care under my supervision, Lisa's Crohn's disease became virtually symptom free. Her attacks of pain were gone, her appetite improved, she tolerated meals better, she gained back the weight that she had lost, and she was taking a lot less medication.

It is instructive to highlight how Lisa's progress manifested over that year. After the first homeopathic treatment, she immediately developed hives on her legs, behind the knees, similar to a bout of hives that she'd had just prior to the onset of her Crohn's disease. At the same time, she reported that her nightly attacks of abdominal pain had almost completely stopped. Most alternative healers would agree that the hives were a type of "healing crisis," a symptomatic flare-up that often precedes general improvement. After the second treatment she developed symptoms of the common cold. In spite of the runny nose and cough she found that she could eat more without getting stomachaches and she was able to gain weight as a result. Her general improvement continued, and several months later she reported a stye in one eye and a skin eruption on her hand.

Here we can see the direction of expression of Lisa's life force as she began to recover from a serious inflammatory illness. What began as abdominal pain and diarrhea became quickly transformed through several healing crises, first as hives, followed by a cough and cold, and eventually as a stye and a skin rash. This successive trade-off of symptoms was indication of the gradually increasing strength and resilience of her vital force as the threat of Crohn's disease faded into the background. An inflammatory illness of the intestines was gradually pushed toward the surface as she became healthier over the course of the year.

To summarize, the bias of physical medicine encourages a superficial understanding of symptoms, which then leads to poor therapeutic choices. A practitioner with a more thoughtful, green perspective reads between the lines to use his or her critical judgment to assess the significance of any given sign or symptom. A reliable framework for understanding the natural order of symptomatic expression can be constructed, beginning with the most external physical layer and concluding with the deepest and most internal spiritual layer. The scientific establishment tends to limit its focus to the mind and body, while often devaluing the role and significance of the emotions and spirit.

As the defense mechanism becomes more compromised it manifests symptomatology at deeper levels. Symptoms may shift within levels and from one level to another, and there need be no logical or anatomical connection between these shifting loci. The locus at which the life force expresses itself most urgently can be considered the center of gravity of a disease. The focus of an illness may shift toward deeper, more internal regions of the human organism, or toward the more exterior surface of the person. The deepest symptom and/or the center of gravity represents the weakest point of the human bioenergetic field. It must therefore be properly handled so the energy of an illness is pushed in the correct direction along the hierarchical gradient in order to facilitate healing.

An ecological perspective is one that apprehends the whole, and green healing respects the natural order of symptomatic hierarchy without losing sight of the system as a whole. An adequate understanding of this energetic framework will become the foundation for critiquing the prevailing trends in modern medical practice and for proposing an efficacious alternative approach to illness and healing. The direction taken by an illness over time, whether toward the interior or exterior, is of paramount importance.

6

Limitations of Medical Materialism

Those thinkers are absolutely mistaken ... who imagine they can prove man's nature to be purely material simply by uncovering ever deeper and more numerous roots of his being in the earth. Far from annihilating spirit, they merely show how it mingles with and acts upon the world of matter like a leaven. Let us not play their game by supposing as they do that for a being to come from heaven we must know nothing of the earthly conditions of his origin.

—Teilhard de Chardin, *Hymn of the Universe*

We have to remember that what we observe is not nature in itself but nature exposed to our method of questioning.

—Werner Heisenberg, *Physics and Philosophy*

NORMAL SCIENCE

Perhaps the most disappointing and disturbing realization that I came to after five years of medical school and residency training was that almost no one was interested in discussing the nature of health and illness, disease and cure, or the cutting edge of new developments in the quest to heal the sick. There was virtually no interest, no innovation—an intellectual vacuum. There was little desire to examine novel ideas, and sometimes even contempt for anything other than the latest state-of-the-art technological advancements within the confines of mainstream medicine.

Not a moment was spent discussing medical history or the history of scientific innovations, for that matter. It was as if to say that all that had come before was essentially irrelevant to the practice of medicine, or was only of value to the academician or the intellectually curious. Imagine if you took all photos of departed loved ones, threw them away, and resolved never to talk about them with your family and friends ever again, because it was believed to be of no practical value to the present or future. Likewise and equally disturbing was the fact that not a moment of class time was spent on the philosophical underpinnings of medical practice, or the philosophy of scientific ideas or methodologies; there was no seeking to understand what it was that we were doing or why we were doing it. Much to my dismay, even within the halls of the psychiatry department there was a remarkable lack of interest in these pertinent and essential topics.

I suppose I was naïve to expect that medical scientists would be naturally curious about the historical and philosophical origins of their profession. And yes, you can study the history of science, the history of medicine, or the philosophy of science in the rarified halls of academia, but do not be fooled into believing that these fields of knowledge inform the average doctor pumped out by the assembly line of conventional medical education. Like many successful industries, the end product is guaranteed to be of the highest quality, pre-packaged with white coats and stethoscopes, standardized and homogenized, ready to meet the needs of the demanding consumer. Independent thought is not permitted to gum up the works. And by extension, these cookie-cutter doctors are designed to serve mainstream consumers and their cookie-cutter maladies. But there is one serious glitch in the educational program. People and their ailments rarely conform to the size or shape of the cookie-cutters that medical graduates acquire by virtue of their long years of medical training.

In my initial enthusiasm as a newly enrolled medical student, I initiated the formation of an alternative medicine club. I went through the proper channels and obtained permission from the administration to use classroom space for meetings. The wheels were set in motion and flyers were made up to advertise the first meeting. But my excitement was quickly dashed when I was called to the dean's office at the last moment. I was informed that persons involved in accrediting the university would soon be visiting the campus, and that the club posed too great a potential threat to the status of the school. I remained undaunted and was given permission, ironically, by the Unitarian church directly adjacent to the university campus to hold meetings in their basement conference room. Our club was ultimately a success, and many young minds were corrupted with ideas of medical heresy that year. In fairness, that was almost twenty years ago, and I do know firsthand that the average medical student nowadays is significantly more receptive to green medical practices. However, the glacial speed with which modern medical institutions are inclined to change remains a significant impediment to progress.

Thomas Kuhn, the influential historian and philosopher of science, would have said that my frustration revolves around the nature and activities of "normal science." Normal science entails the everyday activities of scientists who are engaged in research and practicing within the framework of assumptions of the prevailing scientific paradigm. Kuhn also popularized the term "paradigm" in relation to scientific pursuits to mean the worldview, underlying assumptions, or set of rules regarding how a particular branch of science is viewed, structured, and practiced. This means that persons engaged in the activities of normal science within a given scientific paradigm are busy studying and testing phenomena that fall within the parameters of that branch of science. What they are *not* busy doing is questioning or challenging the underlying assumptions of the consensus of the scientific community and its cultural milieu.

Kuhn's most significant contribution to the field is his book *The Structure of Scientific Revolutions,* which is a staple of almost every Philosophy of Science 101 course. Some excerpts from this important work will help develop my theme:

> *Scientists work from models acquired through education and through subsequent exposure to the literature often without quite knowing or needing to know what characteristics have given these models the status of community paradigms.*[23]

They do not need to know because they are occupied with working within, and not disputing, the set of rules they have assimilated from their education and cultural environment. If an experimental outcome does not conform to preconceived expectation, then the result is commonly believed to be due to ineffective technique on the part of the investigator and not to erroneous assumptions made by the paradigm the research is conducted in. Kuhn also speaks of the peculiar colorblindness of the scientific enterprise:

Closely examined, whether historically or in the contemporary laboratory, that enterprise seems an attempt to force nature into the preformed and relatively inflexible box that the paradigm supplies. No part of the aim of normal science is to call forth new sorts of phenomena; indeed those that will not fit the box are often not seen at all. Nor do scientists normally aim to invent new theories, and they are often intolerant of those invented by others. Instead, normal-scientific research is directed to the articulation of those phenomena and theories that the paradigm already supplies.[24]

Resistance to new ideas and forcing the natural world to conform to a predetermined framework is particularly egregious in the field of orthodox medicine. Take, for example, the historical reluctance to acknowledge the existence of an illness like chronic fatigue syndrome (CFS). The rationale has been that, since CFS can not be proven through examination or testing, it can not exist. As we shall see later, the existence of all diagnostic entities can be called into question because they are artificial, predetermined constructs of modern medicine, but for now, I will frame the discussion in conventional terms. In those terms, then, once all possibilities of "real" and "legitimate" physical maladies that might account for the fatigue of the CFS sufferer, such as anemia or hypothyroidism, are ruled out, it is, by default, assumed to be a psychiatric condition. This demeaning assessment carries with it the implication that the problem is "all in the head" of the complainant.

SCIENCE AS MYTH

Popular culture tends to equate science with truth or objective fact, failing to understand that conventional science does not have a corner on the market of potential lenses for viewing the natural world. Each new pronouncement made by the scientific community is assumed to be true and tends to be accepted by the mainstream with minimal, if any, critical analysis. To recognize the extent of this wholesale yielding to scientific authority one needs only to observe how popular news programs and newspapers dutifully report the results of the latest scientific studies. Predictably, for example, each new nutritional "fact" supported by the research can trigger a cascade of food products making various health claims, which is followed by a stampede of consumers all too willing to fall for each dietary quick fix—even while the next "fact" indicated by the latest data may well contradict the previous.

A levelheaded review of these trends in medical science should make one wonder about the "scientific" nature of the science that it claims to be. Scientific flip-flopping is commonly characterized by research authorities as the price we pay for medical progress as our knowledge grows through a process of trial and error. I would propose, however, that it more closely resembles chaos, and the truth regarding its ultimate value in terms of human health is a much more difficult thing to discern. A full perspective required to make an accurate judgment is not accessible to us through truncated studies that examine only pieces of a story and parts of the human body.

There is something seriously askew in the fickle way with which the scientific community makes its authoritative claims, and the corresponding willingness of the gullible public to uncritically accept whatever they are spoon-fed. This is the very same dynamic that causes some hungering souls to accept in blind faith whatever their spiritual leaders decree as truth. Dr. Edward Whitmont, in *The Alchemy of Healing*, his powerful examination of the nature of health and illness, boldly draws little distinction between modern science and myth:

> We rarely stop to consider that any truth is multifaceted and that the postulated validity and claims of absolute truth of the current scientific ideas rest on a priori metaphysical assumptions ... these modes of belief, in their sweeping claims, have become culturally dominant modes of thinking. As a priori ideas, they are mere mythologems, the mythologems of the post-Renaissance/Enlightenment period. As mythologems, albeit contemporary ones, they have no more claim to absolute truth than any other myths.[25]

Myth here does not mean untrue, but rather denotes the stories produced by the human psyche that serve to impart meaning to humankind's existence. In this sense, the myth of the tree of knowledge in the Garden of Eden is a powerful metaphor for a psychic reality, but it is no more or less true than the story of the rise of modern technological society, whose abilities to travel to the moon and to unravel the secrets of DNA contain within them the promise of someday solving humanity's problems. Just as in the myth of Atlantis, where an advanced civilization was ultimately destroyed by greater cosmic forces because its advanced state of high technology had come at the expense of nature and soul, so too, twenty-first-century technological society flirts with self-destruction when it arrogantly presumes to be able to master and control the forces of nature. According to some, the consequences of ignoring the higher laws of the universe ultimately led to the downfall of Atlantis through a karmic correction in the form of volcanic eruptions, earthquakes, and tidal waves.

Modern humans are just now becoming aware of how their quest for control over nature may be contributing to the phenomenon of global warming. Will we heed the warning or will we plunge ahead in reckless disregard? Medical science may be able to synthesize a drug that reliably lowers a fever, but the assumption that it is desirable to lower a fever is a highly debatable question whose answer has far-reaching consequences and depends upon each individual situation. Shall we forge ahead and lower that fever anyway, simply because pharmaceutical technology makes it possible? Our lack of understanding and failure to heed the messages of nature have resulted in an unprecedented degradation of the environment and a corresponding desecration of the body-heart-mind-soul. Education of professional and layperson alike regarding green medical philosophy and its holistic/ecological worldview will be essential if we are ever to reverse this recent and rapid decline.

These materialistic and metaphysical assumptions about the nature of a universe that science aims to study are no less arbitrary than the assumptions that underpin disciplines that are not considered "scientific" by scientists, such as parapsychology, numerology, alchemy, or the study of the psycho-spiritual archetypes of Carl Jung's collective unconscious. Because scientific endeavor is usually not concerned with reflecting upon its own underlying assumptions, the vast majority of its energy is directed toward deepening what it already does know rather than expanding the breadth of knowledge into what it does not know.

This disposition toward increasing the depth of knowledge within each specialized field is often accompanied by science's tendency to overstep its bounds by making hypocritical judgments regarding areas of human endeavor over which it has no authority. It will not deign to allot scientific resources to the study of, say, astrology, which it dismisses as pseudoscience, but it nevertheless reserves the right to pass judgment upon it. The stereotype of the scientist as an egg-headed know-it-all provides a suitable image to consider here—it's akin to *Star Trek's* Mr. Spock expounding upon the irrationality and lack of utility of human emotion. Similarly, in *Planet Medicine*, Richard Grossinger points out the way in which medicine fails to recognize its own limitations:

> *We can summarily say that the thing which is wrong with orthodox medicine is not the system itself, but the way in which it presents itself as the only or most effective way to treat sickness . . . Sometimes orthodox medicine is shockingly provincial. In order to save its reputation, it gives people the illusion it is handling more than it is and that the other methods for getting things done are either primitive, untested, exotic, unscientific, or un-American.*[26]

The point of this philosophical exploration is to make clear that the conventional medical paradigm is grounded in an underlying set of assumptions that prejudice one into believing that all health problems are based in the physical body and therefore ultimately solvable through material means. Quite to the contrary, truly effective green healing will not be achievable until the left-brain of science welcomes the right-brain of emotion, intuition, the subjective, and the intangibles of human nature back into the equation of human health care. Good science knows its boundaries and acknowledges what it does not know and cannot know due to the limitations of its methodology.

A CASE OF A BROKEN HEART

The real-life impact of such a limited frame of reference is vividly illustrated by the following story. A middle-aged woman came to me one day, suffering from shortness of breath. An investigation several years earlier at the onset of symptoms had revealed that Cindy had a very mild case of hypertrophy, or thickening, of the walls of the heart muscle. Although this was the finding, her cardiologist gave no real explanation as to why this was the case. At the time, Cindy resolved to exercise regularly, which she had faithfully done for several years. The shortness of breath had been completely absent during that time until more recently when, while walking uphill, she had experienced difficulty breathing, which brought on a feeling of panic that then compounded her lack of breath.

I asked Cindy if she had gone back to the cardiologist since the return of the shortness of breath. A look of distress came across her face as she replied, "No, I don't like him. I don't want to go back to him." She explained that she had gone for periodic check ups and had liked her original cardiologist but that he had retired and she did not like the new doctor that had replaced him. I asked why not. She said that the first doctor had always said that the hypertrophy was just a mild case and was stable but, when she saw the new doctor, he had told her that it was a progressive disease and that it was going to get worse.

"So he scared you?" I queried. "Yes," she responded. I asked Cindy to be more specific about the details of her fear, whereupon she launched into a long technical explanation about progressive hypertrophy of the heart. The cardiologist had explained that, over time, her heart muscle would become thicker and thicker until one day when the heart contracted, the walls would meet as they pumped the blood out and they would stick together, at which point the heart would collapse and she would die. Whether the cardiologist had framed it in that specific way was unimportant; it was the take-home message that had been etched into Cindy's mind that I was most concerned about.

When I asked if she had any other fears, she admitted to being claustrophobic. I then encouraged her to tell me her "wildest theory" about why her heart had come to be this way. With an embarrassed look she said, "Well, I do have a very wild theory but I have no facts to back it up." I reassured her that I was not asking for scientific proof. With a good bit of certainty she related that when she was five years old, her mother had become pregnant and brought Cindy's baby sister into the world. Qualifying her statement with the fact that as an adult she obviously now knows better, she said she still feels that as a child, the diminished attention toward her that was redirected upon her sister had "broken" her heart. When I asked whether she still could get her heart broken, Cindy replied, "All the time."

Encouraged that I had taken her theory seriously, she offered, "And I can tell you where my claustrophobia comes from. When I was about eight years old I was hiding under the covers in my bedroom when my dad came in and sat on the bed." Since she always tucked the edges of her blanket in under the bed, he inadvertently left her no escape route. She felt panicked and feared she could not breathe.

Two very powerful episodes in Cindy's life, her "broken heart" and her feeling of suffocation, had set the tone, and this was compounded by the cardiologist whose explanation of material certainty was, in her mind, a very large nail in the coffin of her eventual demise. The vivid detail of this *fait accompli,* her heart's someday sticking together and collapsing, was a stunning revelation and also an example of the power that a physician's words can carry. I immediately suggested that we needed to "exorcise" the death sentence that materialistic medicine had consigned her to. I told her that her own explanation of a broken heart was not only more likely to be true, but that it left room for us to conclude that it was not an irreversible fate.

Recollecting that she had previously told me she had an unfulfilled dream of taking singing lessons, I mentioned this to her. She told me that listening to the operatic singer Pavarotti had always "made her heart sing." It was now clear that the best way to open up her heart, in order to prevent it from ever sticking together, was to find the courage to take singing lessons. I told her that one of the best ways to reverse shortness of breath was to learn breathing techniques as taught by various schools of yoga. In addition, I suggested that she might want to find a new cardiologist, one she would feel more comfortable with.

Putting the pieces of her childhood experiences together with the unfortunate prognosis of the cardiologist, along with gaining a new perspective and taking on homework assignments that offered the hope of changing what had previously seemed inevitable, left Cindy feeling quite uplifted as she left the office that day. A broader worldview that included more than just the physical possibilities was just the prescription needed. Over the ensuing months she mustered up the courage to pursue singing lessons, and she was pleasantly surprised when the first topics covered by her teacher were breathing technique and posture. Through these teachings she learned that she had been unconsciously holding a stooped posture, which had limited her breathing and contributed to her overall dilemma.

OBJECTIVITY, BIAS, AND ANOMALY

We have briefly explored some of the underlying materialistic bias built into Western medicine, and it will also serve us to examine the very nature of science itself—what it is supposed to be and what, in reality, it turns out to be when placed in human hands. The Oxford American Dictionary tells us that science is *"the systematic study of the nature of the physical and natural world through observation and experiment."* The scientific method, we are taught, involves the proposition of a problem or hypothesis, the collection of data through observation and/or experimentation, and the reaching of a conclusion regarding this information. A moment of reflection here points up the elegant simplicity and looseness of the method. Just propose a problem, gather information, and come to a conclusion. Very straightforward and very broad in its applicability, don't you think?

However, we must first deal with that pesky issue of prior assumptions that informs all scientific endeavors. If we assume that all things in the universe ultimately derive from matter, we will begin with a very different worldview and likely arrive at very different conclusions than if we assume that all things derive from spirit, or from pea soup for that matter. One may begin with the assumption, for example, that all things are made of energy, or that there is a God, or that there is no God, or that the world was created in six days, or that it evolved over vast eons of time. These beliefs affect the whole way in which we will conduct our research, and will clearly result in significant bias in our results. I believe that, in the end, it is impossible to remove the bias from what we have been conditioned to regard as objective science.

Michael Polanyi, an oft-cited philosopher of science whose ideas influenced Thomas Kuhn, questions the very possibility of an objective scientific method. His best-known work, *Personal Knowledge,*[27] defines "tacit knowledge" as innate knowledge that is possessed unconsciously by the individual and therefore very hard to identify and to transmit to others. The scientist's passions, biases, intuitions, personal inclinations, and tacit know-how are just some of the factors that influence the scientific enterprise before it even gets underway. Far from being objective, Polanyi argues, the knowledge that a scientist brings to his or her activities is "personal."

Once our prior assumptions, which are often unconscious, have been brought into the light of day, there remains the fact that a variety of preconditions are placed upon all scientific investigations, and this is necessarily done with conscious intention. This category of preconditions is virtually limitless, and is emblematic of the problem of scientific reductionism. Such preconditions may include, for example, the stipulation that only quantifiable data will be included in the analysis, or that the results must be replicable in order to have any validity, or more specifically, that no subjective statements regarding the experience of an illness will be considered, or only women from thirty-five to forty-five years of age may participate in a study.

Since the natural world in its complex enormity cannot be studied by the scientific mind as a whole, it must be broken down into parts. The minute we start to do this, we begin to stray from the reality of the world in its undisturbed state. Science requires the isolation of a very limited number of parameters that can be included in any one study; otherwise interpreting the results becomes far too complicated and open to all kinds of speculation. In this sense we can say that most of science moves in a direction opposite from the emerging green consensus. While one seeks an understanding of nature by dividing it into increasingly smaller parts, the other attempts to apprehend and appreciate it in its whole, natural state. Both perspectives have practical value and a wide array of applications, but a real problem arises when science assumes its superiority and derogatorily dismisses all other potentially valuable contributions as unscientific. Since other contributions do not come from accepted fields of scientific study or do not conform to a reductionistic methodology, science implies that they are somehow useless or deserving of contempt.

In the course of the daily activities of normal science, situations, problems, and events arise that cannot be resolved by utilizing the framework or methods of the prevailing scientific paradigm. Kuhn labeled as "scientific anomalies" these facts, bits of data, or phenomena that do not fit within the conventional way of seeing things. The Oxford American Dictionary definition of anomaly may shed some light here: "something that deviates from what is standard, normal, or expected."

When the prevailing scientific paradigm of a given historical period comes into contact with an anomaly, it tends to deal with it in one of several predictable ways. At first, the anomalous phenomenon usually goes unnoticed, as if the blinders of the particular scientific paradigm prevent its practitioners from seeing it. Once scientists notice it, they often dismiss the troublesome bit of data as if it did not occur, or tuck it into a neat little box to put on a shelf for some future date. This tendency is understandable because the scientific world cannot stop to reevaluate its fundamental assumptions every time it comes into contact with information that contradicts its expectations. Once an anomaly gets recognized, there may be attempts to force it into the scheme set up by that particular field of science. If the anomaly begins to make a sufficient nuisance of itself, sometimes the scientist who makes the community aware of it is blamed for faulty thinking or flawed research techniques. A campaign to discredit the scientist may take place, as it did when Galileo informed his contemporaries that the sun did not revolve around the earth. But sooner or later the anomaly begins to cause a ruckus and, when push comes to shove, something has to give.

CRISIS, EPIPHANY, AND REVOLUTION

We have been educated to believe that scientific progress marches on in a steady trajectory as it gradually acquires knowledge, adapts, changes, and incorporates the new information into its domain. Ever evolving, science is thought to be leading us to a greater understanding of the way the universe works. Many assume that one day we will have solved most, if not all, of our problems via the scientific method. Kuhn, however, disputes this notion of linear progress, contending instead that, as pressure builds up around and within the operational paradigm, it must eventually come to terms with the increasing volume of information that is not compatible with its preset framework of assumptions.

A sufficient threshold of anomalous information may create a crisis wherein scientists begin to question the suppositions of their own paradigm. The operational paradigm can go no further without first having to answer to the anomalous elephant now sitting in the room. At this point it is usually not a simple matter of making an adjustment here or there. Kuhn tells us that the illusion of the smooth progress of science is shattered as the need for wholesale change becomes apparent:

> *The transition from a paradigm in crisis to a new one from which a new tradition of normal science can emerge is far from a cumulative process, one achieved by an articulation or extension of the old paradigm. Rather it is a reconstruction of the field from new fundamentals, a reconstruction that changes some of the field's most elementary theoretical generalizations as well as many of its paradigm methods and applications.*[28]

The immensity of the implications and repercussions of such significant change requires much more than the usual scientific considerations to bring the change about. The mavericks, the visionaries and philosophers —those capable of thinking outside of paradigmatic boundaries—are needed for the task. Such pioneers of change are usually youthful individuals who are not irrevocably committed to the dominant paradigm.

A scientific revolution occurs when the transition from one paradigm to another has taken place. My own field of homeopathic medicine departs so radically from the conventional Western paradigm that the average physician can't be convinced of its viability by a simple explanation. Unless one is already predisposed to thinking outside of the box, as is often the case with artists, poets, and philosophers, the leap is very difficult to take. In my experience, the only way that a skeptic will change his or her mind is by experiencing the effects of a homeopathic treatment firsthand and, even then, the skeptic may employ a variety of rationalizations after the fact to deny the full impact of the changes that have taken place. The acceptance of a new paradigm does not usually take place via a logical thought process.

Kuhn refers to it as a "conversion experience"[29] more along the lines of a religious epiphany.

Evidence of anomalous information confronting our increasingly unresponsive medical system abounds. While technological medicine finds its niche most appropriately in the practice of diagnostics and emergency medicine, the majority of medical needs, especially those involving chronic illness, are poorly served by the system. The dissatisfaction of those with chronic illness comes from an increasing awareness as to the limitations and dangers of the powerful pharmaceuticals prescribed for their conditions. Well-educated modern-day patients are often unwilling to go quietly along with the prescriptions and prognoses of their doctors, who may, in turn, become rankled by such mutinous impertinence. Such factors constitute just a few of the anomalous pressures facing a medical environment that is in desperate need of change.

The coming green medical revolution will be accompanied by a paradigm shift whose colors and broad stripes are beginning to unfold and show themselves in all aspects of contemporary culture. From vegetarians to healing touch practitioners, from environmentalists to medical intuitives, from animal rights defenders to herbalists to crystal healers to dream journalers to color therapists, a certain segment of society has long been way ahead of the curve. They stand on the perimeter, observing the rise and fall of material medicine, anticipating the natural course of events that any societal institution must ultimately face when it chooses to defend its outmoded worldview instead of tending to the welfare of the citizens that it should be serving.

ABSTRACTION, FRAGMENTATION, AND DISSOCIATION

Let us return to the dilemma that contemporary medicine faces and examine the price that we pay for placing our faith in a healing method that lacks balance and perspective. When the medical experts that we look up to in times of crisis are not what the culture has projected them to be, we are often disappointed and dismayed. Although the system expends a great deal of financial, educational, and human resources to generate the illusion of medical competence, in reality, it has little to offer those whose ailments do not conform to the cookie-cutter model.

If a particular specialist cannot help you with your health problem, he or she can always refer you to another specialist. This turns out to be a serendipitous, though unconsciously constructed form of plausible deniability, which is really just a side effect of the system that it serves to protect. How many times have we heard the story of the poor person who sees multiple specialists, receives multiple opinions, but has no one doctor willing to take responsibility for the coordination of his or her health care decisions? It is often not the fault of any one doctor. It is simply the dysfunctional nature of a compartmentalized system created by the fragmented mind of medical science.

In my estimation, medical education is a smorgasbord of haphazard facts and largely uncorroborated theories that forms no cohesive whole. There is no comprehensive underlying philosophy that binds it all together. One must strain hard to see the connections between the different fields of knowledge that fall under the rubric of medical science. It has become exactly what its method of investigation will always produce—a disconnected, disembodied array of facts with no guiding principles or meaning.

Let's try to identify some of the components of this medical potpourri. One of the more obvious elements is germ theory, which tends to get stretched to the point of ridiculousness. In the search for a bug to blame for just about every human ailment, medicine reveals its lack of resourcefulness and inability to think creatively. Extrapolating from current trends we can imagine the average kid having to submit to one hundred or more different vaccines at some point in the future. Batteries of tests can tell us what we do not have, and all else can be attributed to the amorphous, generic, catch-all category of "stress," thereby blaming the patient for creating the condition by not managing his or her own stress. If you have a symptom there is almost always a drug that will at least temporarily squelch it. And if all else fails, you can have the complaining body part surgically removed. Although this may be a bit of an oversimplification, it is not very far from the truth.

The implications of such a lopsided, left-brain way of approaching life and its problems, especially health problems, are more than just theoretical and extend beyond even the traditional sciences. British physicist F. David Peat points out how the extent to which this fragmented worldview pervades all aspects of contemporary culture:

> The problem of the fragmentation of knowledge and understanding extends far beyond science into fields such as economics, sociology, psychology, practical government, human relationships, indeed to the very fabric of society. It is almost as if the twentieth century had lost its ability to perceive the larger patterns of nature and the broad contexts in which events happen.[30]

As these other fields aspire to achieve the cultural status enjoyed by science, they naturally attempt to emulate science, sometimes even achieving the status of scientific specialties on their own, thereby taking on the characteristics of harder sciences. It is truly sad to see the dry, lifeless state of some fields of modern academia—a state that has largely resulted from the selling of their collective souls in order to become more legitimate in the eyes of a culture that values hard scientific "fact" above all. The holistic perspective and more rounded judgment that these other disciplines should normally bring to the table have been traded in for a barren wasteland of quantifiable data and statistical manipulations. Yes, statistical analysis should play some role, albeit minor, in a field such as psychology. But if psychology were to proudly stand up to acknowledge and embrace the inherent messiness of the human psyche, and drop the pretense of being a hard science, what a fascinating array of inspiring subjects might be offered to students, who would then feel far more enriched by their educational experiences.

Unfortunately, even the institutions of my own background in osteopathic medicine periodically succumb to this temptation, when they show their willingness to downplay their strengths and uniqueness in order to be more like conventional allopathic MD schools. Although osteopathic medical education emphasizes generalization by encouraging young doctors to become family practitioners, it also includes training in all of the traditional medical specialties. One rotates through pediatrics, obstetrics, surgery, neurology, psychiatry, and so forth. In addition, students learn osteopathic manipulation, which is a very effective form of bodywork somewhat similar to chiropractic practices. I chose this educational direction assuming that a greater degree of receptivity to holistic thinking would be evident, but in fact, I found the reverse to be true. Osteopathic education seemed to give precedence to the need to guard its reputation and legitimacy when comparing itself to MD education. For example, one osteopathic hospital in which I trained discouraged the use of osteopathic manipulation in situations where I thought it might be beneficial to patients, and instead seemed embarrassed that such an unscientific procedure be allowed to take place within their clinical setting.

Taking this distorted need to make human health and disease predictable, quantifiable, and reproducible to its extreme, we come to what modern medicine calls the "gold standard"—the pinnacle of scientific rigor and purity—the randomized, double-blinded, controlled scientific study. A randomized controlled trial is designed to eliminate all bias on the part of the researchers and subjects involved in a study, including the biostatisticians interpreting the data. This is all well and good but it does not eliminate the bias that we have been discussing regarding fundamental assumptions made before a trial even gets under way, such as the unspoken belief that pharmaceutical drugs are the only legitimate way to treat an illness. This pre-trial bias has led to a glut of studies evaluating various pharmaceutical options, thus making it clear that medical science lives in a bubble, unaware of the myriad alternative therapeutic options available beyond conventional drugs.

This type of rigorous trial virtually guarantees a research product that is hermetically insulated from actual human beings and their actual illnesses. It preserves the purity of the fragmented perspective from which it takes its marching orders. We start with real people with real problems, place them in the sterilized clinical laboratory of research medicine, blind them and their physicians from knowing who is getting the "real" treatment, and filter it all through the abstractions of statistical analysis, until we wind up with an impersonal, sanitized database of facts, numbers, percentages, probabilities, and standard deviations. This method may be of some limited value when comparing drug A to drug B but in the process, medical science's insistence upon its own rigid methodologies neglects the all-important mission of healing the sick.

To abstract is to consider something as an idea separate from its physical or concrete existence. It entails removing something from its context in order to examine it as a theoretical construct. An abstraction is a generalized representation of something devoid of its individualizing characteristics. The process of abstraction removes the unique identifying traits from the original empirical experience of a phenomenon. The textbook description of asthma, therefore, is never the same as the actual individual suffering with asthma sitting before the physician in his or her office. It is always a step or several steps removed from experiential reality. A green perspective, on the other hand, moves in the opposite direction as it seeks to personalize each and every healing experience.

It is neither a cute slogan nor mere philosophical consideration to say that a doctor should treat *the person* with an illness rather than an idealized abstraction of the illness represented by various lab values, diagnostic test results, and book knowledge of what this patient's illness is supposed to be like. This tendency of modern medicine has more than just a passing impact upon the patient, who often feels overlooked by the doctor who studies the chart and ignores the person sitting right there in the room. A greater danger than the negative effect that disregarding the patient has upon the patient's capacity to heal is the physician who begins to believe that all cases of asthma are essentially the same. Such beliefs bring us around again to the cookie cutter model of medical treatment. Human life and illness are, once again, reduced to a predictable, quantifiable set of parameters and forced into a box constructed for the convenience of the analytical mind of medical science. The well-established tendency of medical specialists to treat the various parts of the patient as if they are not attached to other parts of the body, mind, or soul compounds the matter. The net practical effect of this dissociated form of scientific medical endeavor can be staggering.

Patients who have had to navigate the maze of medical specialties have often told me of the tendency for one doctor to be unaware of what the other is doing. This frequently results in expensive, dangerous, and redundant testing and procedures, and more drugs prescribed to treat the side effects of drugs already prescribed. You know what I mean—Joe complains to his doctor about his poison ivy, so the doctor initiates aggressive treatment with the corticosteroid prednisone. Additionally, the doctor prescribes an antihistamine like Pepcid to prevent the stomach acid problem that we know prednisone frequently causes. Joe happens to be one of a good number of individuals who are likely to suffer from the undesirable effects or side effects (more on this distinction later) of prednisone, such as swelling and chronic fluid retention. The swelling causes concern about kidney or cardiovascular disease, prompting more blood tests and diagnostics, after which Joe is prescribed a diuretic in order to drain off some of the fluid. And round and round we go, as a moderate case of poison ivy becomes a medical nightmare, with doctors responding to each mini-crisis, often seemingly unable to exercise common sense by stepping back to assess the overall situation. Regrettably, stories of this nature are legion.

This unique form of tunnel vision engendered by the exclusion of intuition, creativity, emotion, and other right-brain activities, often confuses those of us who would like to embrace a more well-rounded view of things. The possession of many facts does not guarantee an adequate understanding. In the end, only a synthesis of our higher faculties, including our personal values, intuitive hunches, and rational analysis, can produce valuable information and sound judgment. Vera Stanley Alder has written one of the most straightforward, easily comprehensible, and concise overviews of esoteric teachings in her book *The Finding of the Third Eye*. She reminds us to be neither dazzled nor intimidated by the reams of data and profusion of factual information that science produces:

> *Man realizes that "science," which has dealt so successfully with physical phenomena, has not yet succeeded in giving humanity any measure of happiness or safety ... He begins to sense the difference between knowledge and wisdom. Knowledge is the result of an accumulation of facts, and its tendency is, through specializing, to isolate subjects one from another. Wisdom is the deduction from these facts of useful laws, a process which can only take place by comparing the facts in one compartment with those in all the others, thus giving a vision of the whole.*[31]

While science and medicine claim to bring us closer to the truth, I would contend that they provide a more distorted vision of the way we, as human beings, exist in the natural world. Science may well supply us with zillions of bits of information but the common sense needed to make proper use of this data is lacking. There is no collective will to promote and develop the capacity for discernment that is so desperately needed to process this information in order to provide guidance to the scientific community. Medical science is like a monster run amok, without a moral compass. It has, in fact, historically claimed to be amoral, that is, outside the scope of morality, or, not subject to the considerations of morality. Ivan Illich, in his landmark sociological critique of industrialized medicine, *Limits to Medicine: Medical Nemesis,* explains:

> *The divorce between medicine and morality has been defended on the ground that medical categories, unlike those of law and religion, rest on scientific foundations exempt from moral evaluation ... The technical enterprise of the physician claims value-free power ... The assertion of value-free cure and care is obviously malignant nonsense, and the taboos that have shielded irresponsible medicine are beginning to weaken.*[32]

It is clear that the separation of science from morality is mere mental gymnastic, a philosophical abstraction not congruent with holistic reality and green practices. Some believe that pure science, as an objective enterprise, is amoral by its very nature. This supports the distorted and fragmented worldview held by science that allows it to maintain the delusional stance of being truly objective while operating in a vacuum, as if it has no impact upon the world or the world has no impact upon it. This, unfortunately, is the type of belief system that allowed the creation of an atom bomb, the preservation of deadly microbes for the production of agents of biological warfare, the engineering of genetically modified life forms, and the emergence of the specter of future human cloning.

My own father maintained consummate faith in the power of science and medicine to deliver him from illness and death. He was a Herculean figure who, when down to his last days, refused to relinquish his belief in his own will power and in the ability of the human mind to solve all problems—an admirable and noble sentiment but extremely painful to watch. In the end, he would broach no discussion of giving up or acknowledging a higher power. His family, dominated by the sheer force of his personality, was silenced and unable to discuss the obvious reality of the end of his physical life that was fast encroaching upon him. As a result, many things were sadly left unsaid.

This is a personal example of the way that our perceptions and assumptions about the workings of the universe can powerfully inform how we respond to critical events and issues. I suppose now you have some idea about where my issues come from—I do not deny that. I do believe that this may be part of my soul's purpose here in this lifetime, to grapple with the unavoidable issues presented by the nature of my father and his beliefs. There is no doubt that it has propelled me along my journey in search of reconciliation between soul, spirit, mind, and matter.

What science is supposed to be and how it is actually practiced are two completely different matters. Science as an objective methodology that serves humankind in the search for knowledge about the universe is a noble concept. However, in human hands, medical science becomes riddled with unconscious bias and conscious prejudice, often serving economic and political agendas that have nothing to do with health and healing. The difference between the ideal and the real forms an enormous gulf, and science alone as we know it is not sufficient to meet the needs of suffering humanity. The rigorous pursuit of, and adherence to, quantitative fact is a poor substitute for the common sense and balanced perspective of the green approach, an approach needed to produce a real impact on strategies and choices made in the everyday real-life treatment of sick individuals. The tyranny of science must not be allowed to eclipse common sense and good judgment. Am I looking to throw all of medical science out the window? Of course not. But it needs to be taken down a few pegs, and once its adherents find the ability to examine their own motives and preconceived notions, then a reasonable discussion and assessment regarding its true role and real value in the emerging green paradigm may ensue.

7

The Synchronistic Milieu

*Synchronicities are the universe whispering to us, reminding us
of our deep interconnectedness.*
   —Christian de Quincey, *Radical Knowing*

*Blessed be you, universal matter, immeasurable time, boundless
ether, triple abyss of stars and atoms and generations: you who
by overflowing and dissolving our narrow standards of measurement reveal to us the dimensions of God.*
   —Teilhard de Chardin, *Hymn of the Universe*

NUMEROLOGICAL CONSIDERATIONS

My oldest son, being rather single-minded in his academic pursuits, had his heart set on the college of his choice during his junior year of high school. That year he was chosen by the high
school for an academic award, which, much to his parent's surprise, was
sponsored by the very college of his aspirations. This prompted us to visit
the college to see the campus and talk to a professor from the field of his
interest. We came away feeling that it was a good fit for him, and we were
very pleased by everything except the hefty price tag. Over the ensuing
months, our son received a variety of standard mailings from the schools
that had accepted him for enrollment, encouraging him to choose their
programs. To complicate matters further, my wife and I were torn over the
financial implications of his preferred college and also the fact that he had
been offered a full-tuition scholarship to another reputable institution.

One day we received an ingenious mailing, a postcard that depicted the
view from behind a car rolling down the highway. Decals with the name
of my son's high school and the college of his choice were plastered onto
the rear window, while the rear license plate, instead of the usual letters

and numbers, had my son's first name on it. The car was pictured passing by a big green highway sign indicating the distance from our hometown to the college: 222 miles.

Although this amusing gimmick had caught my attention, I didn't think much more of it until I overheard my son's younger brothers talking. It turns out that they were well aware of their older brother's favorite number. I went straight to the source to confirm this and my son told me that if anyone asked him for his favorite number he would say two. If two digits were required he would say twenty-two, and if three digits were needed he would say 222. A peculiar twist to note is that if you Google the distance from our town to the school it actually turns out to be 219 miles.

Levelheaded, rational people would not normally allow such "silly" considerations to enter into their deliberations over the best place for their child to go to college, and yet it turned out to be one of the deciding factors in our final choice. We believed that the combination of his preference for this school, along with his compatibility with its programs, the award he received, and the cosmic clincher of "222" gave us significant reason to feel, in spite of the greater financial cost, that this would be the best place for his academic future. It is also interesting to note that in some esoteric belief systems the number 222 signifies the beginning of a new cycle. In coming to our decision, we did not exclude any factors—all were considered in our college choice equation.

Someone with a Western analytical mind-set might quickly dismiss the belief in the significance of 222 as superstitious, and feel that the award, while clearly desirable, was merely coincidental. These factors could be pushed aside in favor of more practical considerations, such as cost and reputation of the school in question. Just like a dream that is shrugged off as nonsense, the meaning of 222 holds no value for the left brain, which is concerned mainly with facts and figures. The limitations of this mode of perception have had far-reaching consequences for modern living and also for conventional medicine. In her very accessible groundbreaking book on synchronicity, *The Tao of Psychology,* Jean Bolen, psychiatrist and Jungian analyst, frames the issue in terms of East and West:

By our insistence that the scientific method is the only means by which anything can be known, doors of perception are closed, the wisdom of the East is denied us, and our own inner world becomes one-sided. East and West are two halves of the whole; they represent the two inner aspects of each individual man and woman. The psychological split needs healing through an inner union, allowing flow between left and right hemispheres, between scientific and spiritual, masculine and feminine, yin and yang.[33]

RECONSIDERING COINCIDENCE

It was the extraordinary Swiss psychiatrist Carl Jung who first introduced the concept of synchronicity, writing the term in the foreword of the 1949 edition of the Wilhelm-Baynes translation of the *I Ching*. There he makes the interesting observation that ancient Chinese civilization never developed science as we in the West know it—that mechanistic perspective that we have come to equate with fact and truth. Jung identifies synchronicity as the basic assumption that underlies ancient Chinese thought and is the polar opposite of the cause-and-effect thinking that science employs and most Westerners unconsciously embrace:

This assumption involves a certain curious principle that I have termed synchronicity, a concept that formulates a point of view diametrically opposed to that of causality. Since the latter is a merely statistical truth and not absolute, it is a sort of working hypothesis of how events evolve one out of another, whereas synchronicity takes the coincidence of events in space and time as meaning something more than mere chance, namely, a peculiar interdependence of objective events among themselves as well as with the subjective (psychic) states of the observer or observers.[34]

The Western mind has become increasingly familiar with the concept of synchronicity, but treats it largely as a curiosity to be amused by and doesn't take it very seriously. It represents those moments in our lives that are too uncanny to be just coincidental. Some occurrence out there in the world that would normally have no relation to us strikes us in a way that resonates, giving that event unexpected meaning—like getting a postcard from an important party with your favorite number on it. Synchronicity jars us from our everyday mode of perception because it defies the ingrained, unconscious, cause-and-effect assumptions that we make about the way the universe operates. It causes us to double-take and say to ourselves, "No, that can't be," about something we can attribute to no logical reason. Synchronicities do not lend themselves to the standard causal explanations that we so dearly need in order to believe in the things that we assume to be true.

Because synchronicities can make us uncomfortable and require that we temporarily remove the filter of rationality, many are prone to dismiss them as groundless, preposterous, or nonsensical. Those who heed synchronicities are often seen as superstitious and irrational, or as gullible, wishful thinkers. But some of our greatest minds have recognized synchronicity as the missing piece to the puzzle, the right-brained complement to the left-brained cause-and-effect societal norms to which many of us feel compelled to conform. More important, it is the key to allowing us to embrace the emerging green worldview and its anomalous precepts that challenge the reigning scientific paradigm.

A few quotes regarding synchronicity may be apropos at this juncture. Jean Bolen explains that synchronicity can be our bridge to the Tao, the central principle embodied by the *I Ching:*

> *Jung described synchronicity as an acausal connecting principle that manifests itself through meaningful coincidences. There are no rational explanations for these situations in which a person has a thought, dream, or inner psychological state that coincides with an event ... Through synchronicity the Western mind may come to know what the Tao is. As a concept, synchronicity bridges East and West, philosophy and psychology, right-brain and left. Synchronicity is the Tao of psychology, relating the individual to the totality.*[35]

Christian de Quincey's thought-provoking book *Radical Knowing* explores the nature of consciousness and the problem of mechanistic thinking. De Quincey, a professor of consciousness studies, contrasts synchronicity with causality, and here, he refers to the spiritual dimension of synchronicity when characterizing synchronistic events as:

> ... those strange "coincidences" that sometimes seem like messages from the gods ... expressions of the deep intelligence of the whole cosmos flaring up, usually at moments of personal existential crisis—"divine" clues or reminders of our profound interconnectedness and ultimate unity ... None of this involves anything "supernatural"; it just expands our notion of what is "natural."[36]

Furthermore, Robert Moss, contemporary pioneer of dreamwork for Westerners, explains, in his *Dreamways of the Iroquois*, how synchronicity is a language of the psyche:

> Navigating by synchronicity—paying close attention to coincidence, chance encounters, the play of symbols all around us— is the dreamer's way of operating in waking life ... The epiphanies of life—those numinous moments when we glimpse the deeper reality behind the manifest world and derive insight into the larger meaning of our personal existence—come with the intersection of a hidden order of events with our seemingly linear progression through space and time. The grammar of epiphany is synchronicity ...[37]

A few years ago my father called me with news that his doctor had detected an abdominal aortic aneurysm, a type of ballooning due to weakness in the wall of the body's largest blood vessel. Although not an emergency, it would require surgery sooner rather than later. As was typical of my father, he understated the seriousness of the condition, neglecting to mention that his own father had almost died from the same ailment. Sensing the urgency of the situation, I made the four-hour drive to spend an unusual day of alone time with him. After I arrived, my father drove us down to a local beach, and when I got out of the passenger side of the car I noticed that the front tire had an enormous blister, almost the size of a golf ball, sticking out of its side, looking like a thin bubble of chewing gum, ready to burst.

The obvious metaphor stared me in the face and alarmed me, but my father made no such connection, shrugged it off, and said we could stop to get it fixed on the way back. In retrospect, I understand that the synchronistic moment served to put me on notice that no matter how much my father downplayed the significance of that day, I would not be deterred from treating it as a very important occasion charged with meaning. He came through surgery successfully, but that was the first of a chain of medical interventions from which he never fully recovered. That was the last real quality time I spent with him alone and outside of a hospital room. I now hold that day close as a very fond memory of the two of us spending our time just the way it should have been, talking for hours while strolling along the shoreline together.

CAUSE AND EFFECT DEFECT

Causality is a concept that does not allow for the inclusion of chance happenings. Synchronicity, therefore, is not possible if we hold that all acceptable things must have a logical cause-and-effect explanation. Causality, after the need to reduce all things to their material origins, is perhaps the most fundamental assumption made by modern science and medicine. If a causal mechanism cannot be provided for a given phenomenon, it is often minimized or disregarded. Mechanism, especially in human medicine, presupposes that the body can be serviced like an automobile in need of a tune-up or repair. Change the oil, lube a part here, replace a part there, and you're good to go. The human body, when seen as such, is a purely logical assemblage of physical parts functioning in a predetermined way, unaffected by the mood of the driver, the phase of the moon, or the meaning of life.

My own field of medicine serves as a perfect example, and I know other alternative medical modalities can claim the same. While twenty years of clinical experience have made it clear to me that homeopathic medicine works very effectively for a wide range of health issues, even so I am unable to provide a satisfactory cause-and-effect explanation to its critics as to how it works. An entire therapeutic system thus gets summarily dismissed without a second thought because it does not make sense to those requiring a left-brain justification. Mind you, I can provide a number of very plausible theories as to how and why it works, but those theories include medical constructs that a mechanistic standpoint has predetermined to be impossible. Concepts like energy, vital force, soul, and spirit are not included in the conventional medical lexicon. Also, I can propose a number of viable experiments designed to prove that homeopathy does work, but historically there has been little interest in pursuing such research because there is no sufficient mechanistic rationale to explain how or why homeopathy works.

This is an odd scientific approach indeed that requires a mechanistic justification of *how* and *why* before investigating if something *can* be beneficial to the suffering and the sick. The proverbial cart is placed before the horse when we dismiss a viable therapy because it cannot be understood. Just imagine if I had a drug never before used by doctors, which I decided to call penicillin and which I had seen help many of my own patients. What if it were rejected when I proposed its use to the medical community, because I could not explain how or why it worked? Never mind the scientific method that, in theory, is supposed to objectively evaluate a phenomenon without prejudice before it comes to a conclusion. Instead, the method renders judgment ahead of time because the phenomenon does not conform to the preconceptions of Western medical science.

It can be illuminating to point out the unmistakable double standard evident in the daily practice of medicine. All one has to do is crack open a copy of the most ubiquitous and reliable resource used by doctors for information about prescription pharmaceuticals, the *Physicians' Desk Reference* (PDR). If you randomly flip the pages you will come to the names of specific drugs in bold print. Just under each name is the heading "Description." This section describes the chemical nature and composition of the specified drug. The next heading usually reads "Clinical Pharmacology," which details the "mechanism of action," or how the drug works. It may come as a shock that many commonly prescribed medications are listed as having "no known mechanism of action," or whose "mechanism is unclear," or whose mechanism "is believed to be," or whose "precise mechanism of action is unknown." Included in this category are drugs the public trusts and assumes to have met the standards of scientific proof, such as Naprosyn for arthritis, Thorazine for psychosis, Depakote for migraines and epilepsy, Wellbutrin for depression, and Ritalin for hyperactivity. The ugly truth is that conventional medicine arbitrarily picks and chooses which drugs, therapies, and methods it wishes to hold to its standard of proof, and which it decides to give a pass.

The intellectual foundation for the mind-matter split, the mind-body duality, was laid down in the seventeenth century by French philosopher and mathematician René Descartes, who declared, "Cogito ergo sum"—"I think, therefore I am." According to this dictum, one comes to know one's existence by virtue of the fact that one thinks. I am because I think, and by extension, my mind is primary, and my body is secondary. The mind is distinct and separate from my body and all physical matter around me. Mind and matter are two separate realms but mind reigns supreme. I am defined as my mind, not as my mind, body, heart, and soul. This conceptual split between mind and matter encouraged scientists to see the world as an array of physical parts within the machine of the universe. This mechanistic view flowed naturally from Cartesian dualism, which was to have a far-reaching and profound effect upon philosophy and science in Western civilization, the repercussions of which we are now witnessing in the dead-end materialism of modern medicine.

De Quincey's *Radical Knowing,* mentioned above, provides a concise history of ideas regarding causality and mechanism and takes us through the complex philosophical twists and turns regarding the subject. He takes as his starting point the British philosopher David Hume, who in the eighteenth century upset the scientific world when he claimed that we could never directly observe or perceive a cause. Rather, he held, we can only infer causation when the mind associates one event with a subsequent event. His claims called into question the cornerstone concept of science, the assumption that cause-and-effect is a fundamental reality. He asserted that all we can ever know are the ideas within our own minds. To the rescue came German philosopher Immanuel Kant, who proposed that causality was an intrinsic quality of the human mind. As such, causality is not something that we perceive out there in the world. Rather, it is representative of the very nature of our minds. This argument preserved the concept of causality but rendered it purely subjective. Another philosopher, Alfred North Whitehead, suggested that the world is constituted of processes. The "now" is a process of creation wherein the old is always becoming the new. As the subjective "now" recedes into the past it becomes an object, or matter, to be grasped by the next subjective moment, thus connecting mind to matter. Since we feel the objective pressure of the past exert its influence on the momentary subjective "now," we believe this to be a process of cause-and-effect.

De Quincey goes on to point out that mechanistic cause-and-effect involves the exchange of energy as per the laws of physics. As an alternate explanation for this perception of causality he proposes that the reality of what we experience as "now" is really an endless sequence of subjective moments rapidly coming in and out of existence. Since no energy is exchanged, he concludes, no cause-and-effect mechanism has been involved. This experience of "now" occurs not through a mechanistic exchange of energy but, rather, as a synchronistic exchange of meaning. From this perspective, causality is seen as a subjective experience of shared meaning.

Hume's refutation of causality as something that cannot be apprehended, Kant's claim that it is an innate quality of the subjective mind, and Whitehead's subjective now's false perception of causality all add up to a significant rebuttal of the fundamental basis of mechanistic medicine delivered by some of the giants of Western philosophy.

PHYSICS AND METAPHYSICS

In 1969, when nearly a million hippies sat in the mud for three days listening to music at Woodstock, they not only proved that they could resolve their differences peacefully but they had a good time doing it. And with the first publication of Fritjof Capra's *The Tao of Physics*, in 1975, one could almost hear the tectonic plate of the new paradigm bumping up and scraping against the old Newtonian construct. While the artists, poets, musicians, and mystics could intuitively apprehend the holistic reality of the emerging paradigm, it took physicists and philosophers to convince the scientific mainstream that something momentous was happening. Though the materialists of contemporary culture are fond of deconstructing the new message of peace, love, and unity into nothing more than sex, drugs, and rock and roll, its imprint upon society has been undeniable, and forms a significant footing upon which the new paradigm is being built.

Let me be clear, I am neither trained physicist nor philosopher—but I feel that physics and philosophy can add much to our exploration of the historical and intellectual underpinnings of a form of medicine that is proving itself inadequate in meeting the needs of the sick. My hope is to take some of the rather complex and dizzying ideas of these disciplines and render them more lucid and comprehensible to the likes of us non-specialists, and point out their relevance to our subject.

Much to his credit, Fritjof Capra does a remarkable job of translating the complexities of mathematical and theoretical physics into under-standable concepts. So fear not; I enthusiastically recommend his book to all who are interested. Capra begins by explaining how Isaac Newton's mechanical model of the universe formed the foundation of classical physics, and it is the familiar territory that we have come to know as the three-dimensional space delineated by classical geometry. This framework is a mechanistic reduction of the unknowable mysteries of the universe to a construct the rational mind can grasp:

> *All physical events are reduced, in Newtonian mechanics, to the motion of material points in space, caused by their mutual attraction, i.e., by the force of gravity ... The mechanistic view of nature is thus closely related to a rigorous determinism. The giant cosmic machine was seen as being completely causal and determinate.*[38]

Capra describes how the activities of the physicist involve the investigation of an increasingly smaller universe of particles and subatomic particles, and the discovery that, at this level of "quantum mechanics," the rules of Newtonian mechanics no longer apply. The physicist is confronted with a microcosmic world that defies cause-and-effect and throws into doubt all the previously believed laws, which are more applicable to the macrocosmic world. As physics advanced through greater knowledge accumulated from more sophisticated techniques of measurement, it had to replace the assumption of a microcosmic universe filled with zillions of tiny particles moving around in space with a model that more closely resembled a complex interactive energetic web of waves and particles connected by a field.

The mysterious and paradoxical nature of the phenomena that physicists encounter within the subatomic world, Capra believes, may force people to face philosophical issues regarding this new science. These issues will challenge Western mechanism and more accurately reflect an Eastern model of the universe, as exemplified by Buddhism, Hinduism, and Taoism. The bottom line is that modern physics, instead of seeing a universe of material particles predictably behaving in a cause-and-effect manner like a table full of billiard balls, supports the notion of a dynamic and complex unitary world of inseparable, interconnected phenomena.

In the mid-1800s, the discoveries of Michael Faraday and the research of mathematician and physicist James Clerk Maxwell led to an understanding of the basic laws of electricity and magnetism. The phenomena of electromagnetism were described in terms of fields and oscillating waves that traveled through space at the speed of light. This early discovery laid the groundwork for the later development of quantum mechanics and the theory of relativity.

In the early 1900s, Albert Einstein introduced his much-celebrated theory of relativity. According to the mass-energy equivalence formula, $E = mc^2$, that is, the amount of energy contained within a particle is equal to the mass of the particle multiplied by the square of the speed of light, establishing the fact that mass and energy are interchangeable. They are essentially the same thing, only manifesting in different forms. Capra sheds further light upon the paradigm shattering implications of this equation:

> *At the macroscopic level, this notion of substance is a useful approximation, but at the atomic level it no longer makes sense. Atoms consist of particles and these particles are not made of any material stuff. When we observe them, we never see any substance; what we observe are dynamic patterns continually changing into*

one another—a continuous dance of energy. Quantum theory has
shown that particles are not isolated grains of matter, but are prob-
ability patterns, interconnections in an inseparable cosmic web.
Relativity theory, so to speak, has made these patterns come alive
by revealing their intrinsically dynamic character.[39]

The broad applicability of the classical Newtonian worldview began to break down as physicists discovered the means to study matter at the atomic and subatomic levels. In 1927 Werner Heisenberg reported his findings regarding the measurement of electron motion around a nucleus, which have come to be known as the *Heisenberg uncertainty principle*. He determined that the precise location of an electron in space could not be ascertained with any specificity, but could ultimately be expressed only in terms of mathematical probabilities. This became one of the cornerstones of the new quantum physics and suggested that the notion of an electron as a particle of matter in space was no longer viable. A new conceptualization of subatomic particles as wave-particle dualities was required in order to accommodate this mathematical anomaly. Heisenberg's landmark work *Physics and Philosophy* profoundly influenced Fritjof Capra and inspired him to write the *Tao of Physics*.

The work of another early contributor to quantum theory, physicist Wolfgang Pauli, suggests to some that there is yet another, deeper level of ordering principle that lies beneath this world of subatomic particle waves and their fields. The *Pauli exclusion principle,* introduced in 1925, explains why particles like protons, neutrons, and electrons tend to stay away from each other and thus do not occupy the same space. It is fascinating to note that Pauli collaborated with psychiatrist Carl Jung, comparing the similarities between Jung's notion of synchronicity and the implications of the exclusion principle, which suggested that events on the quantum level are acausal or random. Pauli saw the behavior of particles not as the cause-and-effect result of forces acting upon one another, as in the notion of two negatively charged electrons repelling each other, but rather, as a function of the underlying pattern of the whole.

Adding further fuel to the fire is the concept of nonlocality, which physicists have formulated to explain how, at the subatomic level, two particles may act in concert with each other even across vast distances of space, and even though there is no mechanism to account for how this happens. For example, two quantum particles may seem to mirror each other, spinning in certain directions, with the spin on one changing instantly as the spin on the other also changes. This sort of correlated activity at a distance suggests some hidden dynamic beneath the surface of the known quantum world that throws a seriously anomalous wrench into the paradigm of causality. Larry Dossey, a pioneer in the field of mind-body medicine, has written an entire book, *Reinventing Medicine*, on the subject of nonlocality and its relationship to healing.

In the thirty-plus years since *The Tao of Physics* was written, much has happened in the world of physics. But little of it changes the book's basic premise that underlying our natural tendency to perceive the manifest world through the lens of cause-and-effect lies a deeper holistic reality based upon the unity and interconnectedness of all things. Contemporary physics continues to provide evidence in support of this cosmology, and one of its leading proponents is physicist David Bohm. Bohm developed a mathematical system that accounts for this hidden underlying order, which he called the "implicate order," and which he held directs the seemingly random events of the quantum world. The aforementioned Christian de Quincey elaborates upon the theme:

> Bohm's quantum cosmology ... made a radical break with standard physics and materialist philosophy. Bohm was saying, in effect, that below the level of the quantum lies a deeper, innate intelligence ... a metaphysical worldview that acknowledges the presence of some kind of consciousness all the way down to the deepest levels of physical reality. Consciousness, purpose, meaning, Bohm is telling us, are embedded in the very roots of what we know and experience as the manifest physical world.[40]

Taking the whole argument a step further, de Quincey proposes a cosmo-conception reminiscent of the universe as laid out by Teilhard de Chardin in his *Phenomenon of Man*, which proposes that all things in the universe, animate and otherwise, are endowed with differing degrees of consciousness. If acknowledged for what it is, this basic fact of existence eliminates the illusory dilemma of the mind-body split that we are so fond of debating. In de Quincey's words:

> *Consciousness is the innate ability of matter/energy to know and move itself purposively ... There is no dualism of mind moving body, and therefore no mysterious mind-body interaction. Our bodies move themselves—guided by our consciousness ... The whole notion of mind-body "interaction" is a hangover from Cartesian dualism ... I'm saying there really is only the one reality: sentient energy.*[41]

To summarize this foray into philosophy and physics, we can say that a superficial read of our normal, everyday three-dimensional physical world tends to engender the belief that cause-and-effect is the only mode of reality in which we operate. While the rules of mechanism do apply to the gross physical world of objects around us, the same laws are poorly suited to energetics, the subatomic realm, psychic and spiritual phenomena, and the human body and its health. Further investigation has revealed an atomic and subatomic world that *appears* to be completely random and violates all the rules of the macrocosmic world. A deeper look into contemporary theoretical physics provides information that seems to prove false the conception of the separateness of matter and energy, body and mind, and instead to point toward a unified web of existence whose primary characteristics are consciousness and meaning. By using this new information, we can reinforce our understanding of synchronicity as seemingly random events that, upon closer scrutiny, reveal an underlying pattern of meaning that seems to emanate from the depths of the cosmic order.

A HAIR-RAISING EXPERIENCE

A number of years back I was conducting an initial interview with a patient, a middle-aged woman who turned out to have a number of serious health problems. I could feel a powerful emotional intensity to her presence lying just beneath the surface, largely unexpressed, consciously or unconsciously, for reasons unknown to me. She complained of a dizzying array of physical symptoms, the sheer volume of which had my head swimming. I find when faced with a situation like this, that there is great value in trying to locate the core or essence of the story, the glue that holds it all together, the underlying energy or issue that is generating this seemingly random, chaotic assortment of symptoms. Sometimes I am successful. Sometimes it is not that simple. In this particular case, my attempts to shed light upon potential emotional contributing factors were met with a good degree of resistance.

Questions of a psychological nature caused her to respond with a nervous, rapid, tense chatter focused upon reiterating the details of her physical symptoms. In a moment of letting down her guard she did acknowledge that her cat had recently gone missing. An older and well-established house cat, it had decided to go out on a recent winter's day but, sadly, had never returned. She speculated that it had either been attacked by some other animal or had simply gone out to die alone. I could see tears well up in her eyes and, honestly, I was inclined to dismiss this as a relatively recent and superficial event, and felt that there had to be a more profound and long-standing source of distress that could be generating her health problems. Neither she nor I was inclined to dwell on the issue of the cat. But suddenly, from just outside the window of my treatment room, there rose up a long, loud, screeching howl, like one would imagine emanating from a severely wounded animal. Shocked, we sat staring at each other, eyeballs bugging out of our heads in amazement and hair standing up on the backs of our necks, as we simultaneously came to the realization that it was the cry of a cat! In the next moment this poor suffering woman erupted into a prolonged and intense explosion of gut-wrenching grief. All I could do was to sit by supportively, allowing her to cry herself out.

After the dust settled and she was able to catch her breath, we had a long discussion about what had taken place. We even laughed together at one point over the unimaginable weirdness of the moment. In the coming months, she was able to reveal and discuss a number of very painful emotional issues that had been plaguing her. A synchronistic opportunity had made possible a cathartic release that brought significant relief to this patient, and the shared moment had become the basis of a therapeutic bond of trust between us. Mere coincidence? I think not.

PSYCHIC STOREHOUSE

Complementing the conclusions drawn from our discussion of physics and philosophy is the voluminous evidence available to us from the field of psychology, especially the analytical psychology introduced and developed by Carl Jung. Jung, in addition to using the term synchronicity to mean the acausal connecting principle of meaningful events, postulated a connection between synchronicity and what he called the *collective unconscious*. Jung proposed a ground from which all manifestations of the non-conscious human psyche ultimately arise that was not unlike the unified web underlying the quantum world of physics. He divided the subconscious, or unconscious, into two fundamental layers. The first layer is the personal unconscious, which contains information derived from our personal experience that was at one time conscious but has since been forgotten or repressed or suppressed. This layer relates to personal information with which we are familiar, and is illustrated by common dreams in which, for example, we replay the previous day's events. Dreams of this nature usually do not strike us as particularly extraordinary or foreign.

It is the second, deeper layer of the psyche, the collective unconscious, that is most relevant to our discussion and which Jung connects to synchronicity. Because observers have repeatedly found that dreams can contain material that the individual dreamer could not possibly have ever consciously known, Jung concluded that this material must originate from a source greater than the individual's psyche. While the personal unconscious is unique to each individual, the collective unconscious is that which all persons have in common. Like a giant repository containing the collective experiences of human history, the collective unconscious forms a substratum that connects the individual psyche to the rest of humanity. Also referred to as the *objective* psyche (as opposed to the personal), its content is universal and inborn or inherited. Inherited here doesn't mean in the material sense of DNA inheritance, but in an energetic or psychic sense, as if each person is capable of tapping into this vast reservoir of mythic and symbolic material.

It is not uncommon for dreams to contain imagery and storylines that parallel many of the great myths of humankind, even when the individual dreamer has no prior knowledge of the given mythic story or of the information contained within the dream. Jung called these themes or stories generated by the psyche and appearing in dreams *archetypes*. They are like energetic or psychic patterns of instinctual behavior that echo through human history and still make their presence known to modern humans. Archetypes are common especially in times of crisis or change, as if to provide guideposts to those open to this form of symbolic message available to them through their dreams. The study of dreams may be particularly enriched and complemented by the study of comparative mythology and religions because dream messages and lessons have striking parallels to themes that cut across geographical regions and historical epochs, and these themes often reiterate themselves in our dreams. Or as Jean Bolen would remind us:

> We all have within us these powerful images, more varied than those provided by our parents, that reside in the collective unconscious, to which we all have access ... The ancient Greek gods and goddesses no longer live on Mount Olympus, but they are still alive and well, by whatever names we might call them, in our collective unconscious.[42]

Bits and pieces of this psychic library can surface in dreams at any time, but especially at moments of personal crisis. Dream messages often provide clues that shed light upon our dilemmas, although the messages may not be immediately comprehensible because they can appear in obscure symbolic form. Not until my wife was well into adulthood, after she had become interested in the native traditions and spirituality of the Americas, did she become cognizant of the existence of actual stepped pyramids built by the great Mayan and Incan civilizations. All the more stunning to her, when she came to realize this, because in her early teens she had dreamt of such a stepped pyramid. She had experienced a god-like presence in a dream in which she was climbing the steps of a pyramid illuminated by bright sunlight. She had long held the memory of this strange image but did not grasp its import until she had opportunity to study the cultures that produced these monumental structures. It was as if this synchronistic spiritual beacon had shone from the depths of her psyche, providing meaning and continuity connecting the many years of her spiritual journey, only to become a conscious motivating force much later in life.

Some claim they can access valuable information from this psychic library. Edgar Cayce, an American psychic well known to many in the alternative health movement, gave regular "readings" for people in search of healing while he was in a trance or semi-sleep state. He gathered his information from what some have called the Akashic records. *Akasha* is a Sanskrit word that members of the nineteenth-century theosophical movement used to denote the etheric library, which is said to contain the complete records, from the beginning of time, of all thoughts, words, and deeds, human and otherwise. Cayce channeled a vast wealth of information from the Akasha well before Jung posited the existence of the collective unconscious.

Continuing in the tradition and spirit of Fritjof Capra, Hungarian philosopher, scientist, and prolific author Ervin Laszlo brings the most up-to-date information from physics and the sciences to bear upon his theory of an Akashic field (A-field). In his celebrated book *Science and the Akashic Field,* Laszlo places his unique stamp on our understanding of the ground of all being that bridges science and spirit:

> *Thanks to in-formation conserved and conveyed by the A-field, the universe is of mind-boggling coherence, all that happens in one place happens also in other places; all that happened at one time happens also at all times after that. Nothing is "local," limited to where and when it is happening. All things are global, indeed cosmic, for all things are connected, and the memory of all things extends to all places and to all times.*
>
> *This is the concept of the in-formed universe, the view of the world that will hallmark science and society in the coming decades.*[43]

SYNCHRONICITY AND SCIENCE

Synchronistic epiphanies have been a source of inspiration for some of the greatest moments in art, literature, philosophy and, yes, even science. Or should I say, *especially* in science, since the intense focus of science upon left-brain activity almost begs the right side to assert its influence. When it does, it can often create the experience in the form of a miraculous insight. As if coming to the rescue, symbolic material from the unconscious can emerge just at the precise moment when it will be most valuable, as long as its recipient is open to the message.

One of the better-known examples of synchronistic intervention from the other side was provided by German chemist August Kekule, who was the seminal figure in the development of the theory of chemical structure in the mid-to-late 1800s and was responsible for the notion that carbon atoms could link together, thus forming a chemical bond. His discovery resulted in rapid advances in the field of organic chemistry. His most famous contribution was the discovery of the chemical structure of the benzene ring, a symmetrical six-membered ring of carbon atoms composed of alternating single and double bonds. Years later, he explained that his breakthrough had come one day while he was daydreaming and saw a snake seizing its own tail. It is notable that this message from the other side required suspension of all left-brain activity—like what happens in an altered state of consciousness such as a daydream—in order to come

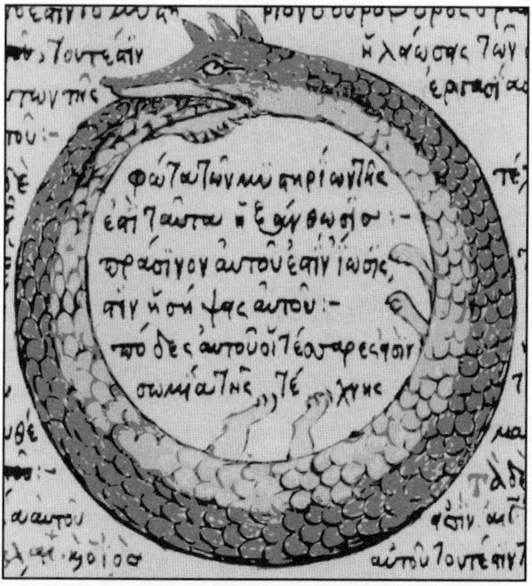

FIGURE 7.1: *Ouroboros Serpent Eating Its Tail, from Greek Alchemical Manuscript*

through to awareness. Predictably, Kekule was ridiculed by some of his contemporaries, who accused him of making this up.

The form of the snake that gave Kekule his inspiration is what is most fascinating here. It is a perfect example of one of those symbols that has been generated by the human psyche throughout the ages and across many different cultures. Known as the *ouroboros*, the serpent eating its tail, in its most basic form represents the wheel of life as depicted by a simple circle. (See Figure 7.1.) This powerful symbol was frequently used by the alchemists, the gnostics, and others to represent the primordial unity that contains within itself the beginning and the end. This life energy constantly renews and re-creates itself through the unending cycle of life and death.

What more fitting metaphor for the discovery of one of the most basic chemical building blocks of organic chemistry? This critical event in the history of chemistry does not owe itself to the labors of the rational mind but rather to an intrusion of the unconscious mind, whose symbolic gift provided the necessary change of perspective, thus making the new conceptualization possible. It is reasonable to ask if this was merely a coincidence or if there was a deeper dynamic at play that was perhaps emanating from the depths of the universe, urging Kekule on to his discovery.

Furthermore, we must acknowledge a phenomenon that has been observed many times over that begs for an explanation, and that is the occurrence of parallel discoveries. One such parallel discovery involves the English physicist and mathematician Isaac Newton and the German polymath Gottfried Leibniz, both of whom claimed to have worked out the mathematical basis of calculus. Controversy raged back in the late 1600s over who had come up with the mathematical innovation first, because the two men obviously could not have arrived at the same conclusion simultaneously in two different locations. Or could they?

This brings us back to the notion of nonlocality, in which similar phenomena occur simultaneously at a distance with no evidence of connection or cause-and-effect between the two. In recent years, biologist Rupert Sheldrake has come up with his theory of *morphic fields* to explain how all matter has a pre-existing associated field of memory that guides and "informs" the creation of the structures of molecules, minerals, plants, and animals. An example of this concept occurs when scientists attempt to synthesize a new substance. At first they often have difficulty achieving a successful synthesis, until they finally have a breakthrough, after which subsequent attempts to synthesize the same substance seem to take place with much greater ease.

Sheldrake would contend that the strength and influence of the morphic field grows with each repetition, thus playing a role in this increasing ease of synthesis of the chemical. More to our point, it has been repeatedly observed that chemists at different geographical locations, attempting to synthesize the same substance and having no communication with each other, often achieve a breakthrough at the same time. Is it possible that Sheldrake's morphic fields play a role in the simultaneous coming into being of a new substance in different locations as if by magic, thereby defying all logic?

AN EASTERN INFLUENCE

Coming full circle brings us back to Jung, who elaborated upon the nature of synchronicity in writing, for the very first time, in the foreword to the *I Ching*. This, in and of itself, is no mere coincidence and will someday be seen as one of the most important moments in intellectual history, when Western thought came face to face with Eastern philosophy. The *I Ching* is the most ancient, and perhaps most accessible and reliable, example of how synchronicity can be observed and used in our everyday lives for both practical and spiritual purposes. At first glance it is easy for the rational mind of the Westerner to dismiss the idea that throwing some coins and observing the heads and tails pattern that results can indicate a passage in an ancient Chinese oracle that will reliably provide insight to a question that is posed for its consideration. Sincerity and reverence are all that are really required when approaching the oracle with a question, after which open-mindedness and suspension of disbelief are helpful in interpreting the answer that is given. Jean Bolen confirms what many have experienced:

> *The* I Ching *is probably one of the most important books in the*
> *literature of the world, because the two branches of Chinese*

philosophy, Confucianism and Taoism, have common roots in the
I Ching. *It emphasizes eternal values in the middle of a continu-*
ally changing universe, assumes a cosmos that has a discernable
underlying pattern, and strongly advises holding to inner values
yet counsels about action and attitudes appropriate to the outer
situation. The I Ching *teaches principles through which it may*
be possible to learn to live in harmony with the Tao, the invisible
meaning-giving matrix of the universe.[44]

Obviously, this is not a matter of cause-and-effect since casting the
coins does not *cause* the *I Ching* to respond. It is hard to imagine that we
could conjure up God at our command, like a genie from a bottle, as this
presumption would violate our most fundamental spiritual principles. But
if we consider the possibility that by sincerely bringing a pressing emotional, spiritual, or practical matter to the oracle's attention we may find
that the seemingly random way the coins fall is not really random at all.
Perhaps, instead, the circumstances of one's life combined with the pattern of the fallen coins, along with the resultant reading from the oracle,
together form a synchronistic confluence of phenomena that contains
meaning and purpose. Sounds crazy, but I have repeatedly confirmed this,
as have millions of others over centuries of time.

Notice that Bolen refers to the Tao as "the invisible meaning-giving
matrix of the universe." The Tao of ancient Chinese philosophy is the natural cosmic rhythm of the universe, the yin and the yang, non-action and
action, the ever-changing negative and positive energies ebbing and flowing. One can go against the flow by imposing one's own will upon circumstances, or seek to follow the "way" or the "path" so as to be in harmony
with the prevailing tendencies. Being at one with the eternal Tao places a
person in harmony with the beneficent forces of nature. The Tao forms
the backdrop against which we consult the *I Ching* to ascertain the current status of these forces as they pertain to our personal circumstances.
Contrast this philosophy with the Western belief that the world can be
shaped and nature can be molded for human purposes and pleasures, and
the medical belief that we can manipulate and control the body and its
functions to get it to do what we wish, rather than seeking to understand

and work with its complex rhythms and innate healing capacity. A truly green perspective seeks to work with the laws and forces of nature in a spirit of cooperation, and imposes the human will against such forces in special circumstances and only when necessary.

We can teach ourselves to look beyond our cause-and-effect blinders, toward the synchronistic patterns of phenomena and events as they emerge from the invisible matrix and are perceived by the conscious mind. Is it possible that the ancient Chinese conception of the Tao, Bohm's implicate order, Sheldrake's morphic fields, Jung's collective unconscious, the Akasha, and the unified web of quantum physics are all describing a similar hidden foundation that becomes discernable to us when the acausal connecting principle of nonlocality comes into play? Physicist and author F. David Peat, whom we mentioned previously, believes so, and sees synchronicity as the complement to cause-and-effect rationality:

> These synchronicities therefore must transcend the normal laws of science, for they are the expressions of much deeper movements that originate in the ground of the universe and involve, in an inseparable way, both matter and meaning ... Synchronicity could therefore be thought of as a counterbalance to fragmentation, for it always deals in the widest context and seeks its patterns across boundaries and categories. Clearly if the scientific and analytic approach to nature could be integrated with the more holistic, pattern-seeking, and meaning-valued aspects of synchronicity, then a creative surge of considerable energy would be possible.[45]

Twenty-five years after the publication of The Tao of Physics, in the afterword to the fourth edition, Fritjof Capra takes up the theme of holism and its relationship to science:

> The new physics is an integral part of the new worldview that is now emerging in all the sciences and in society. The new worldview is an ecological worldview that is grounded, ultimately, in spiritual awareness. Therefore it is not surprising that the new paradigm, as it emerges in physics and in the other sciences, will be in harmony with many ideas in spiritual traditions.[46]

This expanded concept of an ecological consciousness that includes the spiritual dimension is precisely that which gives green medicine and healing its unique stamp and differentiates it from a mechanistic approach that addresses only the physical body.

In the days leading up to my father's passing I received numerous calls from family members regarding the urgency of his medical condition. While I had the clear sense that his time on this plane was coming to a close, others acted as if this was, hopefully, just another phase on the way to his eventual recovery. Like two people trying to communicate using different languages, I was presented with questions about what to do medically, but my answers were offered in the form of how we could look at the situation differently. During a phone call, in a moment of softening that I will never forget, my father let down his persona of bravery, and thanked me for not trying to impose my very different medical views upon him during this critical time. I believe this was a message of love, and an acknowledgment that although he understood rationally where I was coming from, he could nevertheless not fully incorporate the implications of my perspective into his own personal life. It is very hard to accept a new paradigm when one has staked one's life upon the old one. It does not necessarily invalidate the old; sometimes the old views need to find their proper place within the new framework.

Faced with the dilemma of when to visit my father, since I could not realistically jump in the car and make the four-hour trip every time I received a distressing phone call, I found myself trying to gauge when he was coming close to the end so that I could be there when it counted most. Believing that the end was near, confused, torn, and filled with grief I turned to the *I Ching* to inquire whether now was the time to be at my father's side. The response was powerful and personal, and I would like to share it with you, the reader, that you may witness an example of the oracle's wisdom. I received reading number fifty-three (See Figure 7.2) and, specifically, the sixth (top) line of the hexagram, which reads as follows:

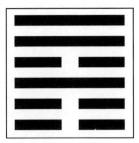

FIGURE 7.2: I Ching *Hexagram 53*

The wild goose gradually draws near the cloud heights.
Its feathers can be used for the sacred dance.
Good fortune.

And the explanatory commentary accompanying the lines read:

Here life comes to its end. A man's work stands completed. The path rises high toward heaven, like the flight of wild geese when they have left the earth far behind. There they fly, keeping to the order of their flight in strict formation. And if their feathers fall, they can serve as ornaments in the sacred dance pantomimes performed in the temples. Thus the life of a man who has perfected himself is a bright light for the people of the earth, who look up to him as an example.[47]

Please realize that, statistically speaking, the probability of receiving this one line all by itself can be calculated as one in 4,096. Clearly it was time to make my final visit, so the family packed and prepared to make the trip the next day. On waking the next morning, we found several messages on our answering machine that had come in through the night but that we had not heard while sleeping. My father had passed away around 2 a.m., with several of my siblings at his side. In the weeks following the funeral services, my wife purchased some goose feathers that she had found on an Internet Web site. We took the feathers to my father's favorite place on this earth, a lake in Upstate New York, where my wife and I and our children prayed and performed a ceremony in his memory and honor.

8

Advice and Dissent

Oz: Do not arouse the wrath of the Great and Powerful Oz!
Dorothy: If you were really great and powerful, you'd keep your
  promises!
Oz: Do you presume to criticize the Great Oz?
  Toto pulls the curtain aside . . .
Oz: You ungrateful creatures! Pay no attention to that
  man behind the curtain! The Great Oz has spoken!
  —*The Wizard of Oz*

At present, the medical profession itself has a monopoly on the
assessment of its standards and techniques. It is the judge of its
own productions—a situation which is fraught with the greatest
risk both for the physician himself and society.
  —Harris L. Coulter, *Divided Legacy*

PROPAGANDA AND POLITICS

It is perplexing to realize that in the United States criticism of most topics is tolerated and even encouraged, and yet it is rare to hear a genuine discussion that questions the basic assumptions of orthodox medical practice. We relentlessly question our political leaders, and there is a healthy degree of religious debate that takes place, but for some strange reason it is virtually unheard of to question scientific medical authorities. It is an indication, perhaps, of the degree to which we revere these authority figures. There is no real tradition of medical dissent other than what is depicted in the popular media's distorted overemphasis upon certain isolated examples, such as the Christian Scientist who refuses conventional treatment in the face of serious illness.

I am not talking about the debate over medical "reform" that restricts the conversation to the allocation of monetary resources and access to medical services. We continually move funding from here to there and back again, believing that this superficial shell game will somehow bring about progress. In the end, we remain stuck with the same old woefully inadequate medical body shop, which neglects our psychic and spiritual needs and increasingly serves and feeds off of only those who can afford this grand illusion of health care.

In early 2007, a controversy regarding a vaccine created to treat human papillomavirus (HPV) and promoted as a preventative against female cervical cancer raged in the media. As is typical of our collective cultural programming, the debate covered only certain aspects of this issue. We heard moral objections from the religious right regarding the promiscuity that would be encouraged among young women who would believe themselves prophylactically protected from this sexually transmitted disease (STD). We also heard from the voices of economic fairness, which decried the costs to those who can barely make ends meet. Those concerned with patient rights preferred the vaccine to be optional and understandably took issue with the prospect of yet another state-mandated medical intervention. And the defenders of the feminist perspective made the salient point that, once again, the medical patriarchy is trying to saddle women with the burden of dealing with an illness that is contracted primarily through sexual contact between a woman *and a man.*

Rarely did we hear anyone question the wisdom of such wholesale vaccination in terms of the health implications for an entire generation of American women. Not to say that there were not people out there voicing their concerns—they just did not register on the mainstream media's radar screen. It is not hard to imagine, ten, fifteen, twenty years from now, the standard "oops" emanating from the medical community after it has analyzed the latest data acknowledging the unanticipated consequences: "The Surgeon General has determined that women receiving the HPV vaccine are at significantly greater risk for developing kidney infections." I suppose that risk is not a bad trade-off compared to some of the more likely hypothetical long-term consequences of the vaccine, such as an increased incidence of infertility, or even an unexpected rise in uterine or ovarian cancer.

Who knows? Who has the medical wisdom to foresee the future? The only reference to health problems and adverse reactions that most people usually hear comes at the very end of a television report or newspaper article in a quick sentence or two, in effect, sending the subliminal message that it is just an afterthought and so you shouldn't worry your pretty little head because the scientists and doctors have taken care of all that hard thinking for you.

I do not want to get sidetracked by the general vaccine issue here as I will be taking it up later, but a few facts regarding this particular vaccine should illustrate the enormous blind spot that we seem to have when it comes to the latest medical innovations. First of all, and most controversially, there is no proof that HPV "causes" cervical cancer. There is only an "association." Because HPV is found in the majority of cervical cancer cells does not mean that the virus causes the cancer. This is merely a leap of logic taken by mechanistic medical science. It may be one factor among many but, as far as I am concerned, no one can determine its role as the main cause to be incontrovertible fact.

Suppose a data entry worker sits in front of his computer each day sipping coffee from a cup. I happen to pass by several times and notice that he is often complaining about pain in his wrist, a common ailment generated by the repetitive strain of excessive keyboarding. Is it reasonable for me to conclude that the coffee must be the cause of his pain? Or am I mistakenly confusing cause with association?

Listen here to the language used in a press release from the FDA's own Web site, dated June 8, 2006. Noting that the HPV vaccine, Gardasil, is "nearly" 100 percent effective in preventing precancerous cervical lesions, it goes on to say that:

> While the study period was not long enough for cervical cancer to develop, the prevention of these cervical precancerous lesions is believed highly likely to result in the prevention of those cancers.[48]

In my opinion, the term "precancerous" is one of those manufactured concepts that stretches the boundaries of known fact and serves the medical community more than it does the general population. So now we have a vaccine that was not tested long enough to determine whether or not it actually prevents cervical cancer, but which is claimed to treat a "precancerous" lesion that is "associated" with, and "is believed" to be "highly likely" to prevent cervical cancer. Are we to accept this as a conclusion drawn from rigorous scientific investigation? Or is it just a case of loose and wishful thinking? And perhaps if we told the data entry worker to drink tea instead of coffee, maybe his carpal tunnel syndrome would go away.

It is openly admitted that Gardasil will not prevent all cases of HPV-related cervical cancer, and thus there is no guarantee of success. Of course, there can be no guarantee with any medical therapy—without exception. Medical authorities also acknowledge that the vast majority of sexually transmitted cases of HPV infection will be successfully cleared by the individual's own immune system without ever causing warts or any other symptoms. Predictably, at the very end of the document, the FDA press release notes:

> *Most adverse experiences in study participants who received Gardasil included mild or moderate local reactions, such as pain or tenderness at the site of injection. The manufacturer has agreed to conduct several studies following licensure, including additional studies to further evaluate general safety and long-term effectiveness.*[49]

In other words, studies to determine long-term consequences, or in FDA language, long-term effectiveness, will be conducted after wholesale vaccination of the American female population has already begun. Well I am sorry, that is just a little too late for my taste. Furthermore, this rather bland assessment of risk by the FDA press release fails to mention some of the more serious events that have occurred upon and after vaccination. We are told that most reactions are mild or moderate, but this is essentially true of all drugs, and nothing is mentioned about more severe reactions. One of the more reputable organizations that offers consistently thorough reports on vaccines, their benefits, and their adverse effects, is the National Vaccine Information Center. Here, at their Web site, we find the full, unvarnished truth regarding the early track record of the HPV vaccine:

On June 8th 2006, the Food and Drug Administration (FDA) announced the approval of GARDASIL, and on June 29th the Advisory Committee on Immunizations Practices (ACIP) voted to recommend adding GARDASIL human papilloma virus vaccine to the Centers for Disease Control's national childhood recommended immunization schedule. On July 14 the first report of a serious reaction to the vaccine was filed with the federal Vaccine Adverse Event Reporting System (VAERS) ... Six months later, eighty-two reports of GARDASIL reactions have been submitted to VAERS on behalf of at least eighty-four young girls and two boys.[50]

The majority of reported reactions occurred on the same day as the administration of the vaccine, and all but three occurred within one week of the patient's receiving Gardasil. Some of the reported adverse reactions were neurological problems, including syncopal episodes (fainting spells), seizures, and a life-threatening form of paralysis called Guillain-Barre Syndrome. Additional reactions included arthralgic pain, joint pain, and other immunological symptoms.

Gardasil is a patented drug, and the only pharmaceutical company that can produce it is Merck, which is promoting it to the public as a cancer vaccine rather than an STD vaccine. Would you be more likely to consent to treatment if you felt it was preventing cancer or preventing an STD? At a cost of $360 for a course of three injections, Gardasil is also the most expensive vaccine ever marketed to the American public. Even though the original study was conducted on adult women, Gardasil has, nevertheless, been approved by the FDA for administration to girls as young as nine years old. Like dominos, a string of states have proposed or passed legislation *requiring* that young girls be vaccinated for HPV. On February 2, 2007, Texas Governor Rick Perry issued an executive order mandating the HPV vaccine be given to all schoolgirls entering sixth grade. After a group of Texas families filed a lawsuit, the Texas legislature overruled Governor Perry's order. It is important to note that the Governor's former chief of staff is a member of Merck's Texas lobbying team, and that Governor Perry has received campaign contributions from Merck in the past. Is it possible, at a cost of $360 for every young girl in the country, that Merck has something other than the public's health in mind?

A Reuters news agency article reported that data from the federal Vaccine Adverse Event Reporting System (VAERS) through November 30, 2008, revealed that Gardasil had been associated with 5,021 emergency room visits, 544 seizures, and 29 deaths.[51] As of June 1, 2009, the Center for Disease Control disclosed 14,072 VAERS reports of adverse events, 985 of which were considered "serious," including 43 deaths.[52] Regrettably, we are all too willing to line our young daughters up like lemmings and watch them plunge over the cliff into the unknown, which may bring the promise of freedom from cancer or, as is often the case with medical innovations, may lead to a variety of unexpected and irreversible consequences.

Yet few have questioned medical authorities or complained to our political leaders about why there has been so much urgency to get this vaccine pushed through the legislative process. Could it be that they do not want us to sit up and take notice and that there are significant financial and political perks coming to the various parties involved? No doubt, providing full and truthful disclosure to the public with adequate time for review would have generated significant resistance to mandatory administration of HPV vaccine. I suppose that a reasonable compromise would have been to make the vaccine available to those who choose to play Russian roulette with their health, but it is a travesty to require it across the board.

FEAR AND THE DENIAL OF DEATH

I believe that it is imperative to examine why the American public is so willing to relinquish its responsibility in the face of such critical medical decisions. Only when we come to understand our motivations can we begin to make real changes in our conditioned patterns of behavior. The answer, in this case, is complex and multifactorial, but the root cause of our abandoning our responsibility is fear. Another fundamental truth about contemporary allopathic medicine, in addition to its materialistic orientation and its mechanistic approach, is that it is based in fear. Fear pervades all aspects of conventional medical practice from top to bottom, from society to institution to doctor, all the way down to the patient. Fear is the force that drives the engine of mechanistic medicine, from its philosophical foundation to its practical application. While modern medicine has mastered the technical ability to control and suppress individual symptoms, healing is an altogether different thing, and genuine healing is rendered highly unlikely, if not impossible, within an atmosphere of pervasive fear.

As an example, consider what has become, to put it mildly, the ethically suspect marketing of medicine in modern America. Marketing prescription drugs directly to the public is a recent trend in our society. When I was a kid, a variety of over-the-counter products were advertised on television, and so the relatively benign Pepto-Bismol commercial urging me to drink pink stuff for an upset stomach was about as bad as it got. I still cannot get those old jingles out of my head. "Plop, plop, fizz, fizz, oh what a relief it is." I think that was Alka-Seltzer, and my memory for such minutiae is a testament to the power of advertising, not to mention to how much television I watched. But when the floodgates of direct-to-consumer advertising (DTCA) opened in the mid-1990s as a result of changes in FDA guidelines, I had a very bad feeling in my stomach that neither Pepto-Bismol nor Alka-Seltzer could soothe.

One estimate puts pharmaceutical industry expenditures for DTCA at $4.24 billion in the year 2005, approximately eleven times the amount spent in 1995.[53] Another estimate maintains that Americans spent $200.7 billion for prescription drugs in 2005, almost five times the amount spent in 1990.[54] In recent years, a class of drugs used in the treatment of arthritis called cox-2 inhibitors, which include Vioxx, Bextra, and Celebrex, had been some of the most heavily marketed drugs in U.S. history, until two of them were taken off the market because of increasing pressure over their association with an alarmingly increased risk of heart attacks and strokes. Amazingly, Celebrex remains on the market to this day.

The justification used at the time for DTCA was that it would allow for a better-informed public. We are now treated to a relentless barrage of prescription drug advertisements that has absolutely nothing to do with consumer education. I challenge you to find information of real value in pharmaceutical television advertisements—it is the exception to the rule.

We are instead treated to smiling people happily romping through fields of flowers as they testify to the efficacy of the latest anti-depressant, or suggestive images promising the rewards coming to me if I take their pill for erectile dysfunction. The problem though, just like those old jingles in my head, is that these ads have a powerful and often subliminal influence that seduces consumers into thinking that they need a product and that it will provide just what the advertisement promises.

Deceptive and flowery ads are not so bad as long as you are a discriminating person with the power to recognize when you are being fed pharmaceutical propaganda. What cannot be excused though, is the shameless and purposeful use of fear to scare people into believing that they must take a drug if they do not want something bad to happen to them. Nowhere is this more overtly the case than with the unabating parade of unscrupulous heart-disease-related pharmaceutical commercials. It is no coincidence, and it goes to the very heart of the matter (bad pun intended), that these ads target illnesses related to the organ most closely aligned with the human need for love, purpose, and meaning. They are used to wage a reprehensible campaign of terror that is ostensibly being conducted on our behalf, but in reality, serves primarily to benefit the pharmaceutical industry.

Thus, we in the United States endure a nightly prime-time deluge of images depicting what can happen if we do not control our blood pressure, or do not improve our cholesterol numbers. Overworked businessmen with distressed looks on their faces as they grab for the pain in their arms, and cartoonish portrayals of clots forming in arteries alternate with images of happy individuals who have remembered to take their daily dose of life-preserving company product. Words and images have power, and in this case, the power to induce fear, which becomes a significant factor, whether we want to believe it or not, in creating the very situation that the commercial claims to be protecting us from. The point here is to recognize the detestable form in which the message reaches us and the true ulterior motive of greed that underlies this message.

In addition, we are led to believe that the experts know best and that we should simply follow their advice, even when we have reservations. Our mechanistic worldview entails a universe of separate and unrelated parts, and encourages specialization and fragmentation of care. It follows that the uneducated layperson should defer to the doctor, who knows best. The doctor takes care of my body but I entrust my soul to the priest. The priest prays for me and the therapist tells me how to feel. The cardiologist lays territorial claim to my heart while the endocrinologist handles my thyroid. With each successive division of labor we gradually and progressively hand responsibility for our lives over to other people, organizations, and institutions.

These other professional groups and organizations are usually more than willing to participate in the delusion that they can accept responsibility for aspects of our lives that we do not want to own for ourselves. The modern trend toward professionalism and specialization virtually encodes these relationships and responsibilities into the very structure of society. Handing responsibility for our souls over to the priest and responsibility for our health over to the physician has come to seem downright normal. We actually begin to believe and actively participate in the collective lie that says we have no business caring for our own selves. Those who dare to act otherwise may come to be seen as odd, eccentric, or even subversive.

The more we nurture this type of societal arrangement, the more dependent and helpless we become. The more one defers or yields to the professionals, the more control and power they wield, and as power tends to corrupt, even the best intended of these individuals are inclined to resist when we begin to awaken and demand a role in the decision-making process. That health care personnel have unprecedented access to and control over our personal medical records compounds the problem. Even worse, medical information has become something that society expects the experts to safeguard and control on our behalf.

Acceptance of such a fragmented, specialized, and sub-specialized medical frame of reference in turn encourages us to avoid personal pain and suffering and, by extension, the larger issue of death. Mechanistic medicine would have us believe that pain and suffering are technical issues and that there is no need to think or worry about them because it is just a matter of time until science catches up, at which point we will be able to enjoy the fruits of our advanced technological civilization. The denial of death is pervasive in materialistic medicine and culture because, by definition, the most important aspect of life is our material existence, here and now.

If our dominant form of medicine treats only the physical body, what are we to do with spirit and soul? The overwhelming cultural response to this question is to not think about it, to delude and distract ourselves, to immerse ourselves in the physicality of now by greedily grabbing all that can be wrung out of life. When death finally knocks at our door, we desperately and angrily demand a cure, no matter how unrealistic, and then blame the system that failed us.

The killing of pain is a natural ally to the denial of death, whether the pain is physical, emotional, or spiritual. The pill-popping proclivity of modern America is a direct measure of the underlying fear of death that accompanies its materialistic orientation. The opportunities for growth that come from grappling with one's own personal pain are greatly diminished as a result. Consumer culture and its hollow promises have the net effect of lowering our tolerance for all forms of pain and suffering, which, in turn, increases our demand for medical services. Philosopher Ivan Illich explains:

> The reminder that suffering is a responsible activity is almost unbearable to consumers, for whom pleasure and dependence on industrial outputs coincide. By equating all personal participation in facing unavoidable pain with "masochism," they justify their passive life-style ... The new experience that has replaced dignified suffering is artificially prolonged, opaque, depersonalized maintenance. Increasingly, pain-killing turns people into unfeeling spectators of their own decaying selves.[55]

On the other hand, a genuine spiritual experience of ourselves and our place in the universe, and the acceptance of pain and suffering as natural and necessary components of growth and living, tend to temper the overwhelming fear of death that comes with a purely physical take on existence. A person who seeks firsthand spiritual experience has an opportunity to become acquainted with his or her own soul, thus allowing the development of a more realistic perspective regarding the fleeting nature of this physical life, and a sense of what comes next. Believers in reincarnation may see this life as just one phase in a long evolution of the soul, thus rendering death a natural and necessary step along the way.

The heroic and often grotesque battle against death at the end of life is responsible for by far, our greatest medical expenditures. Because it cannot satisfactorily contend with most forms of chronic illness, medicine is particularly proud of its ability to prolong life, even if that life is spent lying in bed or endlessly visiting doctors' offices. Prolonging life at all costs suggests that there is nothing worth valuing once life has expired. The very nature of modern medicine, along with its unconscious materialistic philosophy and core values, creates a milieu in which the physical body becomes the only reality, while the spirit and soul are an afterthought at best. And modern medicine becomes the perfect vehicle for taking advantage of the terror that such a perspective engenders in the face of death. The denial of death and loss of personal autonomy that result when we hand our lives over to the technocrats played out to a macabre extreme when in 2005 the federal government attempted to legislate the prolongation of Terry Schiavo's artificially maintained life, even though she had been in a persistent coma for over a decade.

We have forgotten that there is a vast difference between possession of volumes of facts regarding the physical body, and possession of wisdom. Wisdom is a quality of understanding, not a quantity of information. Green medical wisdom derives from a balanced overview of the various aspects of a given health situation rather than a specialized grasp upon a single part of the whole. In the final analysis, the relevant data combined with the requisite wisdom is much more likely to ensure satisfactory health outcomes.

While the surgeon possesses the superior technical knowledge and ability required to remove a gallbladder, the wisdom as to whether it should be removed at all is another issue, involving a complex multiplicity of factors. Recently a patient who had already been scheduled to have her gallbladder removed the following week came to see me in a last-ditch effort to avoid surgery. Conventional medicine, being what it is, offered no alternative, so surgery was the only logical solution. Instead, I employed an alternative combination of homeopathic and nutritional therapies, with much success. It is now one year later, and as she continues to improve, this patient has not required surgery. In fact, her attacks of pain are only a faint memory of what they once were.

When we learn to fear our own bodies, we are all the more willing to turn responsibility for its well-being over to outside authorities. Our cultural institutions encourage dependency, discourage personal responsibility, and tend to keep us from obtaining the necessary information required to help us develop our own judgment and wisdom. Fear arises particularly from not having enough information, when we do not understand, when we feel out of control, and when we are kept in the dark or we keep ourselves in the dark. The sterile, impersonal, specialized world of modern technological medicine becomes the perfect breeding ground for fear. Patients can be terrified by the forces set into motion when they are helpless and being wheeled down the hospital hallways toward their fate. Likewise, medical professionals, when challenged, can become fearful of losing their cultural status as authorities over their specified domains of technical expertise. In the 1970s, pediatrician Robert Mendelsohn wrote a simple, direct, and strong critique of medical practice, *Confessions of a Medical Heretic,* which everyone, especially physicians and residents in training, should read. In this passage he touches upon the topic of fear:

> *No wonder children are afraid of doctors. They know! Their instincts for real danger are uncorrupted. Fear seldom actually disappears. Adults are afraid, too. But they can't admit it, even to themselves. What happens is we become afraid of something else. We learn to fear not the doctor but what brings us to the doctor in the first place: our body and its natural processes.*[56]

LANGUAGE AND PROFESSIONAL CONTROL

The maintenance of the medical hierarchy of power tends to take precedence over the interests of the patient, which take a back seat. The power of language is one of the most powerful tools used to keep the patient in a submissive role, sometimes purposely, sometimes incidentally. Medical jargon may primarily be a language that medical personnel use to communicate with each other, but one of its most important functions is to keep patients in their place, at a distance, so that the authority of the physician is preserved. I came across two different definitions of "jargon," from the *Oxford American Dictionary* and *Merriam-Webster's Collegiate Dictionary*, respectively, that read as follows:

> *1. ... special words or expressions that are used by a particular profession or group and are difficult for others to understand.*
> *2. ... obscure and often pretentious language marked by circumlocutions and long words.*

Not once in medical school was I encouraged or instructed to communicate using terminology that the patient could understand. Quite to the contrary, a mastery of medical vocabulary was seen as a sign of learnedness that was to be displayed in order to impress the patient with the quality of the doctor. The clear but unspoken ulterior motive is that language can be employed as a tool to keep the patient ignorant and fearful and, ultimately, compliant and unlikely to challenge the physicians' authority. Back in the 1800s, the sharp-tongued Samuel Hahnemann was less diplomatic in his assessment of this predisposition of the medical profession, which has nowadays escalated to an extreme degree:

> *The physician's calling is not to make countless attempts at explanation regarding disease appearances and their proximate cause holding forth in unintelligible words or abstract and pompous expressions in order to appear very learned and astonish the ignorant, while a sick world sighs in vain for help. Of such learned fanaticism we have had quite enough. It is high time for all those who call themselves physicians, once and for all, to stop deceiving suffering humanity with idle talk, and begin now to act, that is to really help and to cure.*[57]

The sad reality is that medical jargon is frequently used to both intimidate and confuse. Even the well-educated patient can be easily cowed in the face of such technical mumbo-jumbo. It is a common experience to be made to feel embarrassed because we do not know what the doctor is saying. A patient's questions, aimed at clarification, are frequently rebuffed because the doctor's time, we are told, is more important than the patient's. The average patient is so well programmed by the medical-industrial complex that he or she often buys into this insidious myth. Add to this use of language as a weapon, the fact that the ailing patient is already in a highly vulnerable position, and you have a very potent combination. I remember the time a patient had visited her doctor with a complaint of tailbone pain. After becoming alarmed because the doctor told her that she had coccydynia, she made an appointment to consult me. It was a pleasure to see her look of distress turn to relief when I told her that coccydynia was medical lingo for tailbone pain! A green practitioner of medicine and healing must have the awareness, communication skills, and willingness to demystify medical jargon out of respect for the patient's need to be an equal partner in medical decision-making.

A few more examples may serve to illustrate the point. Receiving a diagnosis of "idiopathic hyperhidrosis" might cause you to break out in a sweat but, hopefully, the doctor will explain that this simply means excessive sweating of unknown origin. Perhaps you have been told that you have an "erythematous lesion." Translated into lay terms, that is a red skin thing. Let's hope you never come down with the dreaded "hypermetropia," meaning you are farsighted and might need corrective lenses. Do not panic if you develop "verruca vulgaris" because that just means that you have a wart. "Precancerous" is one of those terms that virtually guarantees the patient's absolute submission, even though it is a fabricated term for a nonexistent condition. Either you have cancer or you do not, and any doctor that claims to know with certainty that something *will become* cancer is not telling you the truth. But it sure makes the doctor's job a lot easier, and generates more business to boot, now that the patient is well on the way to developing an anxiety disorder.

It is in vogue among conventional physicians to warn that untreated heartburn can lead to esophageal cancer. Part of this successful campaign to achieve compliance comes straight out of the American political playbook. If you do not like something, make it sound bad or scary, as was done in renaming the estate tax the death tax. Thus, heartburn has now become gastro-esophageal reflux disease, undoubtedly a much more imposing and ominous title. In essence, the language of fear has changed what used to be an annoying symptom into a full-blown, scary disease with precancerous implications. Consequently, a sub-specialized medical niche is born, necessitating prescription drugs and regular medical evaluations, including invasive diagnostic measures such as upper gastrointestinal endoscopy. Even the frequently used term "compliance" implies a patient role of submission to the authority of the physician. Perhaps instead, the real goal of the enlightened green medical professional should be to seek patient "collaboration."

One telling phenomenon is the extent to which the general public has so thoroughly assimilated this medical lexicon and its accompanying mode of thinking. This becomes glaringly obvious when I conduct an interview in my office and find myself asking the patient to translate his medical jargon into actual symptomatology. Here, the roles are reversed. Some clients cannot do it, or cannot understand what I am asking them to do. People have become so programmed by the abstract thinking of medical science that their answers often reflect this. Correspondingly, they are sometimes so detached from the reality of their own experience of symptoms that they cannot describe them without a good bit of assistance.

We have come to accept the abstract diagnostic labels and mechanistic explanations as real, in lieu of our first-hand experiences. Add to this our propensity to pop a pill at the slightest inkling of a symptom and you have an entire society that has become disconnected from the distress signals being sent by our own bodies. This dissociation becomes even more evident when a practitioner tries to elicit information from a patient about psychological symptoms. A surprising percentage of people are incapable of identifying their own emotional states. Taking up the theme of medical control through abstraction, Ivan Illich, in his *Limits to Medicine*, eloquently implicates the role that language plays in the process of depersonalization. He describes how the patient's ...

> ... *sickness is taken from him and turned into the raw material for an institutional enterprise. His condition is interpreted according to a set of abstract rules in a language he cannot understand. He is taught about alien entities that the doctor combats, but only just as much as the doctor considers necessary to gain the patient's cooperation. Language is taken over by the doctors: the sick person is deprived of meaningful words for his anguish, which is thus further increased by linguistic mystification.*[58]

EDUCATION AND EMPOWERMENT

A common fear tactic wielded by physicians is the threat of discontinuation of services, although this is technically unethical because a doctor must have good reason to terminate a relationship. Nevertheless, the threat is commonly made. This is especially true for the type of patients that tend to utilize my unconventional medical services. They are often educated individuals with questioning minds who are unwilling to go blindly along with whatever their doctor says. This clash of paradigmatic codes can generate conflict between the authoritarian physician and patients who wish to actively participate in their own care. Many physicians do not like to be questioned about the wisdom of their choices and can become agitated when they feel their authority challenged. They may become angry, can threaten health consequences if their instructions are not followed, and some may even become abusive. Commonly, they tell the patient that it is time to seek help elsewhere.

Countless patients have told me stories of this nature over the years. I usually advise them not to burn their bridges and to try to maintain a relationship in spite of the unpleasantness. Sometimes the degree of antagonism coming from the doctor makes this impossible. It is strange to think that a patient's participation could be viewed as unwelcome, as the opposite is true when it comes to the form of medicine that I practice. I would likely become frustrated by a passive client who would prefer to defer to me on all matters. The emerging new age of green medical healing will seek to educate patients and enlist them as equal partners. Paradoxically, this will ultimately not undermine the role of the physician, who will still have valuable knowledge and experience to offer the patient—but the patient must be willing and motivated to participate if meaningful and effective healing is to take place.

Conventional medicine has expended its resources in seeking the holy grail of technological control over the symptoms and functions of our bodies. When we embrace this dangerous deception, we hand the responsibility for our own lives over to the so-called experts. The providers of mechanistic medicine are all too eager to accept this role, as it is a bottomless pit of financial reward because this arrangement rarely generates real health and healing. It can be shocking and overwhelming when a sick individual comes face to face with the false wizard hiding behind the curtain of technological omnipotence. When a patient confronts the reality that the medical world may not be able to deliver on the promises that it has advertised, the result can be disappointment and fear. A large percentage of medical malpractice lawsuits are initiated for this reason.

In my opinion, the true reason for the prevalence of medical torts is conventional medicine's egregiously overstated power to heal. The dangers of pharmaceutical and invasive procedure-oriented treatment, coupled with the consumer's naïve acceptance of medical propaganda, leads to highly unrealistic expectations, and ultimately tremendous disappointment. Having divested himself of personal responsibility, the "consumer" blames the "provider." Ultimately, the responsibility lies with both a public that is easily duped and a medical system with dollar signs as its bottom line.

Once placed in the defensive position of having to fend off lawsuits, the medical establishment that once employed language to intimidate and gain compliance now uses the same jargon to create a smokescreen of confusion. Research studies and statistics once used to convince, are now used to cast doubt and ambiguity. One study says this and another concludes that. Suddenly the certainty of medical fact transforms into a maze of medical confusion for which no one individual or institution is responsible. Our collective faith in scientific medical fact as truth is shaken when the flawed amalgam of mechanistic bias, tortured language, manipulation of data, and financially motivated marketing of medical product is revealed for what it is.

The proposed solution to the issue of negligence is almost always framed in terms of providing more and better medical resources, along with greater oversight and accountability, which translates into the bottom line of allocation of more funding. A true critique of the actual philosophy and practice of medicine is never forthcoming, at least in mainstream circles. The only time that meaningful debate about the substance of medicine occurs is after the fact, when the smokescreen of plausible deniability has been discredited, and when the casualties in terms of real lives have been counted. Only when a particular drug has failed and the adverse events are fully and openly admitted do we begin to question the wisdom that allowed it to be prescribed in the first place.

Unflinching honesty in education about the realities of health, illness, and the mechanistic paradigm to which our culture subscribes offers the only real way of changing the dead-end course that we are now pursuing. The word "doctor" derives from the Latin "docere," which means "to teach." Thus "doctor" means "teacher" in Latin. Doctor is the root of "doctorate," as in the degree one receives having reached the pinnacle of higher learning. The physician's primary role, therefore, should be as teacher. There can be no more effective health measure than proper patient education. Once patients are armed with the necessary information, they become empowered to make choices in their own best interests.

Unfortunately, the net effect of an encounter with the medical world resembles subjugation more than it does education. Popular culture tends to value and reward those with ego, those who control and possess, rather than those who benevolently and humbly serve. It is imperative for medical education to save its own soul by setting the example and returning to its roots to train physicians to be educators rather than obfuscators. Self-proclaimed medical heretic Robert Mendelsohn is not afraid to speak his mind:

> *Your hospital stay ... has a psychological effect on you similar to a voodoo curse. Whether you consciously acknowledge it or not, hospital procedures and environment encourage despair and debilitation rather than hope and support. ... The effect of all these psychological pins is that you relinquish any notion you may have had about having control over your health. Your captors isolate you, alienate you, scare you, depress you, and generally make you feel so anxious that you submit to their every wish. Your spirit broken, you are ready to be a Good Patient.*[59]

Remember our friend, the ibis-headed Egyptian god of writing, learning, and wisdom? In ancient times, magic and medicine were thought to be of equal importance in the hands of the healer. Thoth, the patron of scribes and physicians, wielded his medical knowledge and magical abilities through the power of language. (See Figure 8.1.) Today, we believe magic exists only in the minds of children or in Disney movies. Our jaded world scoffs at the notion of anything that it cannot grasp in its hands or measure with its devices. But thoughts have energy and thoughts have power. Words can enslave us and words can set us free. Words can kill and words can heal. I can tell a man who has recently developed asthma that he had better use an inhaler or risk suffocating to death from an asthmatic crisis, or I can note his obvious difficulty in breathing and offer reassurance that we will work together toward strength and better health. Carefully chosen words can infuse the mind with positive thoughts and energy, while poorly chosen words can fester and leave an energetic scar.

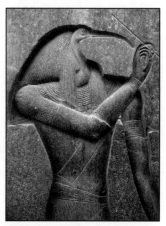

At first glance, it may seem that the magic has gone out of modern medicine, but the terrible truth is that the pervasive disdain for spirit, soul, and the mysterious, has allowed a form of black magic to worm its way into our medical institutions and our way of thinking about health and illness. We have become so crippled in spirit that we accept this black magic, even expect it, and, when our time has come, quietly submit to the medical-industrial complex and its greedy need for more

FIGURE 8.1: *Thoth, the Ibis-headed Egyptian God of Writing, Magic, and Medicine—Relief from the Throne of the Statue of Ramses II*

guinea pigs, money, and power. In *Limits to Medicine: Medical Nemesis, The Expropriation of Health,* Ivan Illich notes the influence of black magic that results from the split between doctor and priest:

> *Medical procedures turn into black magic when, instead of mobilizing his self-healing powers, they transform the sick man into a limp and mystified voyeur of his own treatment ... When doctors first set up shop outside the temples in Greece, India, and China, they ceased to be medicine men. When they claimed rational power over sickness, society lost the sense of the complex personage and his integrated healing which the sorcerer-shaman or curer*

*had provided. The great traditions of medical healing had left the
miracle cure to priests and kings.*[60]

Modern medicine relentlessly markets itself through fear, keeps uppity
patients in their places with fear, and defends and protects itself from critics with fear. This tenuous state of affairs has been allowed to proceed
unchecked for a very long time and those in places of authority have grown
accustomed to their status and their perks. They are not likely to relent
without having to face a good deal of conflict and resistance. It will take a
significant dose of courage for pioneering patients to demand a higher
standard of care and a greater degree of respect from those entrusted with
assisting them on their journey toward health and healing.

Fear is inimical to the healing process and should have no place in the
green practice of medicine. A green medical philosophy must include the
patient's fundamental right to dissent, to say "no." The use of language to
manipulate, intimidate, or obfuscate is reprehensible and must no longer
be tolerated. We must reject the traditional authoritarian medical model
and adopt an egalitarian approach that presupposes that patients must
always have a choice. All patients must be encouraged to play an active role
in the decision-making process. It is time to open up the debate, educate
our clients and ourselves, and pull back the veil that hides the human being
posing as the omnipotent wizard. We must take back our autonomous
power to heal ourselves.

9

The External Enemy

As Gregor Samsa awoke one morning from uneasy dreams he found himself transformed in his bed into a gigantic insect ... He feared, with a fair degree of certainty that at any moment the general tension would discharge itself in a combined attack upon him ... "We must try to get rid of it," his sister now said explicitly to her father ... "If this were Gregor, he would have realized long ago that human beings can't live with such a creature, and he'd have gone away on his own accord" ... Yet Gregor had not the slightest intention of frightening anyone, far less his sister.

—Franz Kafka, *The Metamorphosis*

THE OBJECTIFYING EGO

An enlightened green perspective assumes the interrelationship and unity of all things in the created universe. The dualistic mind, on the other hand, sees itself as the subject, and all things "out there" as objects. The ego perceives itself as alone and separate from all things other than itself. In psychological terms, we can say that the ego tends to project undesirable aspects of the self onto others out there. It is a peculiar weakness of human nature to blame others rather than owning up to our own responsibilities in life. Once convinced of our own rightness, the ego then defends itself when it feels threatened by anything that would remind it of the truth.

If I feel hurt by something someone says or does but I do not want to render myself vulnerable by admitting so, it is easier to simply project it outward by blaming or defaming the offending person. It requires a good bit more self-awareness, honesty, and humility to acknowledge that the other person hit a sore spot of mine and probably did not mean it. I need even more courage to take a risk by verbalizing this to the other person. Accepting the reality that the other person may respond in the positive or in the negative, I nevertheless admit having been hurt and ask the person to be more considerate and conscious of this the next time around. Even if the other person becomes defensive and responds poorly to my entreaty, I rest confident in the fact that I have chosen the high road, which resonates most closely with my own inner truth. Having overcome my pride, I have successfully withdrawn the projection of blame upon the other, and in the process have set a positive example that may be emulated by the other, which in time may strengthen and deepen the nature of our relationship.

The alternative is to deceive myself into believing that the other is responsible for my hurt feelings. It is not I that am sensitive, it is they who are insensitive, and it therefore cannot change until I receive a satisfactory apology, or worse yet, until I have exacted some form of retribution. In taking this tack, my ego has thus initiated an internal lawsuit. While I acknowledge that it is sometimes necessary to seek justice, I believe most psychological lawsuits are motivated by less admirable sentiments. My looking to even the score will adversely impact the relationship, and make the potential for healing ever the more distant. The *I Ching* refers frequently to "the inferiors," which can be roughly equated with the ego, and the "superior man," which can be interpreted as being the higher self. (See Figure 9.1.) In dealing with difficult situations of this nature, hexagram 56 of the *I Ching* advises us that the "superior man" ...

> *Is clear-minded and cautious*
> *In imposing penalties,*
> *And protracts no lawsuits.*

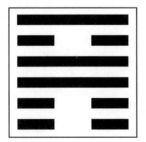

FIGURE 9.1: I Ching
Hexagram 56

This is what penalties and lawsuits should be like. They should be a quickly passing matter, and must not be dragged out indefinitely. Prisons ought to be places where people are lodged only temporarily, as guests are. They must not become dwelling places.[61]

In a holistic world, it is understood that thoughts have power, and so when I maintain an inner lawsuit against another I create the net effect of imprisoning that person. It is misinformation regarding a false conception of reality that allows the suit to continue. I maintain my projection and punish the other by refusing to yield my own delusion of innocence, keeping him or her imprisoned within my own mind. Over time, the object of my lawsuit ultimately becomes inflated into an enemy, something to be feared. My own internal division, resulting from my self-deception, is now reflected in an external division between me and the enemy against whom I am waging a war—and war, of course, entails a need to vanquish the enemy.

The dynamic of fear that keeps the engine of Western medicine running likewise needs an object to be feared. Once the object of our fear can be identified, then it becomes a simple matter of employing methods of waging war against it. Although this may not always be a consciously thought-out strategy, it is the operative and dominant belief at play in virtually all modern medical interventions.

SYMPTOMS AS IMAGINARY ENEMIES

On the most immediate level, this war is reflected in the prevailing tendency toward symptomatic treatment. All symptoms are predetermined, without forethought, to be undesirable, to be feared, and thus become fair game in the fight against disease. The ludicrous and dangerous extreme to which this policy has been taken is plainly evident in the long lists of prescribed medications taken by most senior citizens, who tend to follow their doctors' instructions with unquestioning obedience. The unwitting person with headaches, constipation, sore knee joints, itchy eyes, and spells of sad thoughts may emerge from the doctor's office armed with prescriptions for four, five, or more different, never-before-taken medications.

The medical world is full of doctors willing to treat toenail fungus by prescribing a particular class of medications that is known to be able to induce serious, life-threatening liver disease. Either their patients are being badly misinformed or they are ignoring the warnings, because a seemingly endless supply of potential victims are inclined to take that risk. I have certainly seen my share of patients who are disturbed enough by their toenail fungus that they are likely to do anything I tell them in order to treat it. Do you think the FDA's allegiance in this case lies more with the patient, whose health it is charged with safeguarding, or with the pharmaceutical manufacturer? Knowing the potential for harm, I will not prescribe these drugs, no matter how small I'm told that risk may be.

Consider this practice of symptom eradication in contrast to our previous discussion, which cast all symptoms as manifestations of the defense mechanism's attempt to heal itself. We will discuss the dire consequences of beating back our own symptoms at every turn in a future chapter, but for the time being, we must carefully contemplate whether viewing our symptoms as the enemy to be vanquished is really warranted. Is a symptom truly the unwanted outside invader that we think it is? And will ruthless subjugation of that symptom achieve what we are seeking?

The belief in an external enemy is so pervasive in modern society that we do not question its validity. And whether we like it or not, it encourages the false belief that our symptoms are not our own. They are something we contract, something we come down with, or succumb to, or are stricken by, as if they have wheedled their way into us from the outside and, consequently, it remains for the doctor to chase them away. They must originate from somewhere other than us, perhaps from a bug we caught, or bad food that we ate, or chemicals in the environment (not to minimize the reality of the unparalleled poisoning of the environment and food chain that is taking place). They are foreign intruders to be feared that can strike at any time without rhyme or reason.

This is the perspective that we are encouraged to embrace because it serves the agenda of mechanistic medicine. This view goes unchallenged when we accept that all things are random, unrelated, and without meaning, purpose, or connection. If we were to thoughtfully question this medical nihilism, the scientific establishment would be pressured to change its ways, to step out of its comfort zone and consider other possibilities. As it now stands, it will take significant effort to rouse the medical experts from their complacency.

DIAGNOSTIC DISTRACTION

Beyond the level of individual symptoms, the war is also waged against *groups* of symptoms. And this becomes the point at which the abstract mind takes us further and further from reality. Groups of symptoms can be arbitrarily and conveniently given names that carry various conscious and unconscious implications and agendas. The process of labeling creates the illusion that a given group of symptoms is an external entity that may one day try to invade us, giving us all the more reason to fear them. While diagnostic labels such as "pernicious anemia" or "pre-cancerous lesion," by the mere sound of their names, carry the implication of grave threat, most diagnoses induce fright simply because they are indecipherable to the layperson. A name can also be used to raise a symptom up to the level of a full-blown condition, as in the recently coined "restless leg syndrome." What was once a nervous habit now becomes an objectified enemy to be feared. In this case we have a "new" medical condition promoted specifically because a new drug can be marketed to treat it and, mind you, I did not say, "cure it."

A diagnostic name can also be used to deflect a patient's awareness from a doctor's inability to do anything about a condition. For example, while reassuring a patient that he or she does not have a more serious disease, the label "irritable bowel syndrome" satisfies the patient's need to know what the disease is, even though the available treatment options tend to be inadequate. It is as if receiving a diagnostic label is supposed to compensate for the lack of therapeutic satisfaction. Most important, a name can be used to convey the message that one should be concerned enough to seek the assistance and treatment that only a medical professional can provide. Whereas we all used to live, unknowingly, with some inevitable bone loss as we grew older, we are now subjected to a relentless campaign of fear urging us to seek medical help for the threat of "osteoporosis." And we all have that ubiquitous message indelibly stamped into our consciousness from having read countless medical labels over the years, "In the event that symptoms persist, consult your physician immediately."

If I have learned one thing from conducting detailed interviews of thousands of clients over the years, it is that the classical textbook description of a given diagnostic label rarely, if ever, presents itself in actual clinical practice. The proverbial round peg of the patient's actual illness seldom fits into the square hole of the diagnostic stereotype. Diagnostic labels are not real. They are approximations, abstractions, groups of symptoms lumped together for the sake of the diagnostician so that the illness can be classified and the illusion of control can be transmitted to the patient.

On the one hand, it is understandable why people fall for this sleight of hand. They naturally want to know the answer to the question, "What do I have?" At the completion of an intake, when a client finally asks me for a diagnosis, I often attempt to begin the process of reeducation by saying something like, "You just told me what you have. I think you may be asking me what label I would apply to it." Unfortunately, the relief that comes from having a name for what you have is short lived, as it rapidly gives way to, "Now what are we going to do about it?" The measurement and classification of diseases allows the illusion of them as external entities to seem all the more real. Ivan Illich explains:

> A taxonomy of diseases became possible. As minerals and plants could be classified, so diseases could be isolated and categorized by the doctor-taxonomist ... The use of physical measurements prepared for a belief in the real existence of diseases and their ontological autonomy from the perception of doctor and patient. The use of statistics underpinned this belief. It "showed" that diseases were present in the environment and could invade and infect people.[62]

It is tempting for the doctor to authoritatively announce the patient's diagnosis with absolute certainty. It makes the doctor sound smart and gives the patient a sense of control. Over the years countless people have reported to me the contradictory assessments made by the various doctors they have consulted. "Dr. A says I have asthma, Dr. B says it's reactive airway disease, Dr. C thinks it's hay fever, Dr. X believes it's laryngospasm, Dr. Y says it's chronic sinusitis, and Dr. Z thinks it's all in my head." While this may be a bit of an exaggeration, this sort of diagnostic discrepancy is much more common than you might think. This is particularly the case with chronic diseases that do not resolve of their own accord, because patients with chronic illness are the ones who tend to go from doctor to doctor in search of labels and the promises of solutions that come with them.

A diagnosis serves the need to objectify the enemy so that the delusion of "me versus my disease" can be maintained. But herein lies the dilemma—while the diagnosis of an external enemy helps ensure that the façade of dualistic medicine is maintained, the process often brings us no closer to a solution. Having arrived at a conclusive diagnosis often gives the false impression of medical success. Granted, an accurate diagnosis can often be of benefit, especially in acute and emergency situations, but just stop for a moment to consider how many people you know that have been given clear diagnoses and are still suffering from the consequences of their illnesses.

Technological medicine tends to tout its diagnostic successes precisely because its therapeutic options remain remarkably limited. Instead of hearing about the latest in medical *treatments,* we most often hear about the latest in *diagnostics*—like the shiny new open MRI machine. It can be disconcerting to consider the fact that the lion's share of our financial resources are channeled into advanced technology to diagnose illness rather than into actual treatments for those illnesses. Like the horse with the proverbial carrot held before its nose, we are led to believe that new therapeutic discoveries are just around the corner. But the new treatments that do make it into circulation tend largely to be marketing gimmicks. The lack of will to innovate results in the same old drugs being recycled with new names, shapes, and colors, with expanded indications to treat a wider range of illnesses.

The medical establishment is forever giving us the impression that it is on the verge of a breakthrough, but those breakthroughs are almost always new ways to figure out what it is that the patient has, not new treatments for what ails that patient. These diagnostic name games are the natural consequences of a form of medicine that has a very limited range of treatment options at its disposal. To give credit where it is due, I believe that the strength of conventional medicine is its diagnostic prowess in terms of the physical manifestations of illness but, unfortunately, its greatest weakness is in disease treatment. And while state-of-the-art physical diagnostic power is at our fingertips, modern medicine has little to offer the heart, mind, and soul.

The magical power of words—in this case, the power to label diseases—in and of itself carries no inherent ability to cure. Rather, it is the manner in which words are wielded and their context that gives them their potency. A colleague once told me of his horror after he witnessed a neurologist, who was obviously pleased with his diagnostic skill, announce to his patient, "Good news. We've figured out what it is. You have a brain tumor." Receiving a diagnosis of a chronic disease, rather than leading to the hoped-for cure, has the more likely effect of condemning the patient to accepting the irreversibility of the condition. Ironically, the notion of a disease as an independent invading enemy can be transmuted into its polar opposite when the patient begins to identify with the newly acquired diagnostic label. Thus the patient may accept the pronouncements of the experts and ultimately become the disease: "I am an asthmatic." "I am hyperactive." Along with such acceptance comes the finality of the physicality of particular diseases as viewed from the material paradigm.

GERM WARFARE

Nowhere is the objectification of an external enemy more clearly evident than in the basic tenets of germ theory. When Anton van Leeuwenhoek observed microorganisms through a microscope in the 1600s, the stage was set for more than one scientific pioneer to suggest that diseases could be transmitted or caused by these tiny entities. In 1854, British physician John Snow stemmed the tide of an outbreak of cholera by removing the handle of a pump in London when he realized that the source of contamination was in the water supply. In the 1860s, through a series of experiments involving fermentation, Louis Pasteur disproved the then prevailing belief in spontaneous generation, which contended that microorganisms could arise from inorganic or non-living organic matter. Because he found that the microbes that grew in broths during the process of fermentation in his experiments were not spontaneously generated from within the broth, he concluded that these microorganisms had to come from an outside source. This of course led to the practice of pasteurization, whereby liquids like milk are heated in order to kill the bacteria growing within.

These developments were the precursors for German physician Robert Koch's proofs that described modern germ theory, which today we take for granted. Koch is credited with isolating the organisms related to anthrax, tuberculosis, and cholera, and his students went on to discover those associated with diphtheria, typhoid, gonorrhea, tetanus, syphilis, and other diseases. Certain aspects of these rules of verification, which are referred to as Koch's Postulates, have since been refuted, but the fundamental concepts remain intact.

Renowned microbiologist, environmentalist, and Pulitzer Prize-winning author René Dubos, considered by some to be the father of medical ecology, is credited with coining the phrase, "Think globally, act locally," after his research led him to discern the parallels between the micro and macro environments and the importance of ecological balance. In his landmark book *Mirage of Health* Dubos makes an interesting observation regarding the historical concurrence of Pasteur's work with the development of Charles Darwin's theories:

> *Pasteur's first paper on the germ theory, the "Memoire sur la fermentation appelee lactique," appeared in 1857 just one month before Charles Darwin sent to Asa Gray the famous letter stating for the first time in a precise form the theory of evolution. Through this historical accident the germ theory of disease developed during the gory phase of Darwinism, when the interplay between living things was regarded as a struggle for survival, when one had to be friend or foe, with no quarter given. This attitude molded from the beginning the pattern of all the attempts at the control of microbial diseases. It led to a kind of aggressive warfare against the microbes, aimed at their elimination from the sick individual and from the community.*[63]

It is not that I dispute the obvious existence of microorganisms like bacteria and viruses, and I do not dispute that they play a role in disease development, but I do take issue with the overly simplistic notion that they are *the cause* of diseases. While it is true that a previously unexposed population can be profoundly affected by a new pathogen, this effect is largely a function of susceptibility. Once a population has been exposed, it tends to rapidly adapt, thus leaving most individuals resistant to the harmful effects of the very same bug. It is not that the virulence of the microbe decreases as much as that the resistance of the population increases. This is why devastating diseases of the past, like diphtheria and smallpox, no longer pose the same threat as they once did. Modern medicine would wish us to believe that vaccination programs deserve most of the credit for the eradication of many of these infectious diseases. I believe that vaccinations were a small factor, with the much larger factor being that as populations became exposed to these pathogens, they developed natural immunity.

If germs are not the causative factor in most cases of infectious disease, as is my contention, then the war against the microbial enemy is a misguided and losing battle. Simply because it can be technically accomplished, the medical establishment embraces a strategy of antimicrobial warfare at the slightest indication of infection. Bugs can be identified and antibiotics can be synthesized and employed, without forethought as to the repercussions of their usage. The usual modus operandi of conventional medicine entails a lopsided yang approach to health—and in the war against germs, we see the same basic strategy. Conventional medicine gives only one side of the picture serious consideration. As a result of this unholistic perspective, germs are identified, objectified, and labeled as enemy combatants. The very term "infection" has become one of those propagandistic scare words used to enlist participants in the war against microbes. They are undesirable entities separate from us, out there, and we do not want them in here. According to this medical viewpoint, if I have an infection, an antibiotic can be used to kill the bug and all should return to normal again. Unfortunately, the normalcy attained tends to be short-lived because the next infection, side effect, or complication is usually not far off.

The external enemy and the fear factor go hand in hand. As a culture we have become terrified at the mere thought of a variety of supposed threats, the gruesome details of which we are made never to forget by the media's relentless and repetitious sensationalism. Just turn to the television news on any given day to be reminded of the disease du jour that is supposedly on the verge of attacking and overwhelming the nation. Fear breeds more fear. It is no coincidence that this terror began to reach fever pitch around the time of the World Trade Center attack, when the designated enemy to be feared was anthrax. I have tried to recall the various epidemics of fear that have spread across the country in recent years. Undoubtedly you remember mad cow disease, Ebola virus, E. coli, SARS, West Nile virus, bird flu, and swine flu? I am sure there are others that I have overlooked.

Without fail, every winter we are ritually fed propaganda about the garden-variety flu, which strangely never meets up to its billing. Hyperbolic media reports about the shortage of flu vaccine feeds the hysteria, and yet, in contrast to this gross overkill, the actual prevalence and intensity of flu-like illnesses have been quite mild in recent years. While on the one hand, the pharmaceutical industry profits from the demand created by the hype, on the other, it is also very wary of being blamed by an American public that believes the hype and swallows the premise that if we accept the multitude of vaccinations offered we will all be safe. Both the media and medical authorities selectively downplay the prevailing scientific understanding that creating a vaccine that will correspond to a specific virus, which has yet to manifest itself, is a crapshoot. Viruses are unpredictable, can adapt, and can change and mutate. Odds are that a pre-made vaccine will not be effective because the specific virus cannot be anticipated. The media also looks the other way in not reporting adverse reactions to vaccines, which are rationalized away by medical authorities as the risks that must be taken in order to derive the benefits.

If we take a step back to look at the big picture, from a green perspective, microbes are not independent entities out there that have nothing to do with us except in the case of infectious illness. Most microbes are always present, in us and around us, and are part of the complex web of life. The interdependent relationship between human and microbe is a topic rarely discussed in popular culture. The threat that microorganisms pose, and the war against them, is a much more dramatic and sexy storyline than boring accounts of cooperation with our microscopic neighbors. Any truly successful campaign to eradicate microbes would surely result in the demise of many forms of life and perhaps even the human race.

The unchecked abuse of antibiotics, antifungals, and antivirals is not only polluting the environment and the food chain upon which we depend, but is insidiously destroying our collective immunological health. Since the medical patriarchy's predilection is for conflict over cooperation, the virtues of a more balanced approach seldom get an airing in the public forum. Mutually beneficial symbiotic relationships between human and microbe are not just common; they are essential. The mere presence of a microbe does not necessarily indicate that there is a problem or even the threat of a problem, for that matter. In 1959, microbiologist René Dubos wrote:

> ... the presence of pathogens in the body can bring about disease, but usually does not. The world is obsessed—naturally so—by the fact that poliomyelitis can kill and maim several thousand unfortunate victims every year. But more extraordinary, even though less dramatic, is the fact that millions upon millions of young people become infected with polio viruses all over the world, yet suffer no harm from the infection ... The dramatic episodes of conflict between men and microbes are what strikes the mind. What is less readily apprehended is the more common fact that infection can occur without producing disease.[64]

MAINTAINING THE TERRAIN

The high frequency of ear infections in young children is one of the more commonly encountered issues in family medicine. Over the years I have treated many ear infections without resorting to antibiotics, and not once do I recall a serious complication ever occurring. Recently, the pediatric protocol for treating ear infections has taken a 180-degree turn toward a "wait and see" attitude. It is understood that the majority of cases will resolve on their own without antibiotic therapy. Is it possible that the prior threat of meningitis was just a means to gain compliance?

In spite of this change in the standard of care, physicians continue to prescribe antibiotics unnecessarily. They also continue to prescribe antibiotics for of bronchitis and sinusitis, although research has shown that antibiotics are not necessary in most cases of either illness. The usual result of antibiotic misuse in pediatrics is diminished immunity, which predisposes these children to recurrent ear infections. In addition, kids with chronic ear infections and multiple antibiotic prescriptions usually show other signs of a weakened state of health, such as poor appetite, disturbed digestion, failure to gain weight and grow at a normal pace, chronic ear congestion, increased susceptibility to other types of infection, and even altered emotional states. Conversely, proper handling of an ear infection will usually prevent the vicious cycle of chronicity that is generated by antibiotic overuse.

The flip side of the issue concerns the terrain upon which microbes depend, where they are kept in check, or are allowed to proliferate. That terrain is nothing less than the microbe's entire environment and especially, for the purposes of our discussion, the human body with which the microbe interacts. The two bacteria most commonly associated with otitis media (middle ear infection) are *Streptococcus pneumonia* and *Haemophilus influenzae,* both of which are considered normal flora. In other words, these bacteria are commonly found in the upper respiratory tract, including the ears, of many healthy individuals. Together along with a variety of other microorganisms, they comprise the normal and necessary microenvironment of a healthy upper respiratory tract. This being the case, we are obligated to question the assertion that these are the bacteria that *cause* most ear infections and that killing them is the best therapeutic option.

If these bugs do not cause ear infections, then what does? This brings us back around to the neglected yin side of the health equation—the terrain in which the bugs live—our own human bodies. The health status of our own bodies may be the decisive factor that determines whether a bug is allowed to run amok or if maintains its normal function within the microenvironment. If a weakened immune system or stressor leads to an opportunity that a certain microbe takes advantage of, we can convincingly argue that the unchecked growth of the bacteria or virus is actually the *effect* that accompanies the condition rather than the cause. If this is true, a weakened immune system can be considered the cause, while microbial overgrowth would be the effect. Here again though, we must be careful not to fall into the simplistic either/or predicament of the reductionistic paradigm, which desperately seeks to definitively label the one and only causative factor. The successful prescription of an antibiotic in an instance of infection does not necessarily demonstrate the microbe involved to be the cause. Most disease states are the result of a complex constellation of factors and circumstances, some of which will never be known.

René Dubos used the example of insulin therapy in diabetes, perhaps the single greatest success attributable to modern medicine, to argue that the efficacy of the treatment does not bring us any closer to an explanation of the cause. Although insulin has kept countless thousands alive and well, it has not led to any greater understanding as to why or how the disease develops in the first place. Instead of medical science awkwardly imposing its explanations upon the mystery of human health, it must begin to open itself up to other possibilities by acknowledging what it does not know. Returning to our example of otitis media, we note that regular medicine makes a feeble attempt at holism by offering an additional causative factor other than the bacterium. The argument offered is that the Eustachian tube fails to function properly, allowing bacteria to build up and multiply, leading to an ear infection. However, this anatomical explanation is only one of many factors that can render a child susceptible to an ear infection.

If we consider the complex milieu within which bacteria are situated and we expand our consciousness to beyond the physical, we can easily enumerate a number of contributing factors that may play a role in the development of ear infections. For example, the nutritional status of the child, or even the nutritional status of the nursing mother can protect the child from, or render him or her susceptible to, infection. Perhaps the child is not being nursed and is instead being fed formula or cow's milk. Maybe the child was recently vaccinated and is now reacting by developing otitis as a response to this encroachment upon his or her immunological boundaries. It is not unusual for a parent to bundle a child up too warmly, or conversely, to expose a child to the winter cold for too long. An ear infection can even develop if a child is living in a stressful environment where the parents are arguing. Any or all of the above factors, and many others, can have an impact upon the constitution of the child, thus triggering a distress signal from the vital force in the form of otitis media.

Much of this is not new and may even seem obvious to some. Although understood by many in theory, it is not usually taken into practical account by practitioners of orthodox medicine who give lip service to holism and then proceed to employ the same old strategies. The inescapable fact remains that all things are connected, and attempts to reduce a situation to a few simple parameters can be a dysfunctional recipe for less-than-satisfactory results. Repeatedly treating a child's ear infections with antibiotics usually results in a variety of peripheral problems and susceptibility to further illness.

We have all heard that overuse of antibiotics can create resistant forms of microbes that have adapted and are therefore no longer susceptible to the standard antimicrobial drugs. Bigger guns are then needed to kill the bug, but these drugs can also do more harm to the patient, and ultimately, the evolving super-bug may then develop resistance to even the strongest of antimicrobials. It is also commonly understood that while an antimicrobial drug may subdue or kill the bacteria, fungus, or virus, it also tends to kill other beneficial microbes that constitute part of the normal microenvironment of our bodies. For example, when the normal gut flora is thrown out of balance, other microbes can move in to take advantage of the situation. When a child taking an antibiotic for an ear infection then develops diarrhea, the physician presumes that the drug has also killed some of the normal bacteria that inhabit the intestinal tract that are necessary for effective digestion. When an antibiotic prescription becomes necessary, many holistically educated patients will take the precaution of using probiotic supplements that contain beneficial lactic acid bacteria, like *Lactobacillus acidophilus*, in an attempt to pre-empt this disruption of the normal ecology of the gut.

It is incumbent upon patients to take such green measures because the majority of physicians are not inclined to prompt them to do so. Although these are well-known principles, even within conventional circles of thought, physicians usually ignore them, perhaps due to inertia, hubris, or lack of creative imagination. In spite of abundant evidence pointing to the dangers of antimicrobial overkill and to some simple remedies available to counteract this trend, the institutions charged with the responsibility for our health care nevertheless display a puzzling apathy. More thoughtful and effective long-term strategies of dealing with issues like this are neglected in favor of quick fixes. And pill popping suits the average American, who may grow impatient at the simple suggestion that staying home and resting for a few days might be the best medicine of all. (Heck, most people cannot sit still at home even when they have vacation time.)

The alternative to the yang approach of germ warfare involves the art of self-defense, which depends upon the host maintaining adequate resistance to the supposed invading enemy. The paradoxical result of maintaining good general health is that the former enemy ceases to be a threat and instead settles in to take its place in the balanced ecology of the human organism. While there is only one way to kill a bug, there are a multitude of factors to be considered and methods that can be employed to ensure peaceful coexistence with most microbial entities. The future of green medicine will be exemplified by an informed individual who is well acquainted with the workings of the vital force, its defense mechanism, and its inextricable interrelationship with the surrounding milieu. In this holistic scenario, antibiotics will be employed only as a last resort in situations that necessitate their use. Again, René Dubos, well before the new age of holism, argued in support of this philosophy:

> *A few microbes are considered 'good' because they do things which give satisfaction to men, and most others have a 'bad' reputation because their effects are considered detrimental in human affairs. This anthropocentric basis of judgment is of course philosophically questionable ... The view that some sort of ecological equilibrium can be achieved between microbes and their potential victims has not been popular among physicians and medical scientists ... It is rarely recognized, but nevertheless true, that animals or plants, as well as men, can live peacefully with their most notorious microbial enemies.[65]*

THE FUTILITY OF WAR

Diagnostic categorization and labeling, the abstractions of medical thought, and laboratory isolation of microbial entities together, conspire to lend validity to the illusion that a militaristic model of medicine that offers the promise of victory through force is achievable. The basic principles that apply to the microscopic world also apply to the macrocosmic world of people and their communities. The same dynamics also pertain to the psychological, spiritual, and cosmic realms. A fundamentally aggressive posture ensures that the avenue toward healing, balance, and reconciliation will remain closed.

The Hermetic tradition is considered by many to be the oldest spiritual tradition of the West, and the *Emerald Tablet* is perhaps the earliest and most important writing of Hermetic thought. In addition to being a spiritual body of work, the principles and practices of the Hermetic tradition are believed to be the historical and intellectual precursors to modern chemistry and physics. Although its age is unclear, varying sources place the tablet's origin with Thoth the Atlantean, thirty-six thousand years ago, while some consider it to be about ten thousand years old and of Egyptian origin. Hermes Trismegistus, who some believe was the reincarnation or spiritual descendent of Thoth, is believed to have authored the tablet, which was first mentioned in writing around 650 CE. Contained within the passages of the *Emerald Tablet* is a succinct expression of some of the most basic spiritual truths ever revealed to mankind. The tablet opens with the following words of wisdom:

> In truth, without deceit, certain, and most veritable.
> That which is Below corresponds to that which is Above,
> And that which is Above corresponds to that which is Below,
> To accomplish the miracles of the One Thing.
> And just as all things have come from this One Thing,
> Through the meditation of One Mind,
> So do all created things originate from this One Thing,
> Through Transformation.[66]

From this derives one of the most important and fundamental spiritual axioms of esoteric thought: "As above, so below." The macrocosm is contained within the microcosm. All that is out there in the universe is also reflected right here, within each individual. The waging of war may generate temporary gains, but it can never unify all parties into a peaceful whole. "Kill or be killed" is a limited and shortsighted philosophy of life and an equally ineffective medical philosophy. I can project my anger onto a convenient scapegoat but the dynamics of the human psyche and the cosmic laws of the universe guarantee that it will always come back to bite me in the end. Temporary antimicrobial success may win the battle at hand, but the health of the whole will suffer in the long run. The illusory external enemy is simply a reflection of our own internal state of affairs.

We often use words without understanding their derivations or original intent. One such word is "pharmacy," along with its variations: pharmacology, pharmacist, and pharmaceutical. In ancient Athens, the Greeks would conduct a ritual in times of trouble such as famine, illness, or plague. This usually involved a *pharmakos,* a person who served as a proxy for the particular scourge of the day. The pharmakos, which translates to "scapegoat," was often led out to the perimeter of the city where he was stoned, beaten and, some say, killed in a ritual act of purification. This expulsion of the symbolic source of evil and disharmony was believed to protect the city and its citizens from further harm. Here we find a direct parallel to the spirit in which modern drugs are employed in attempts to eradicate invading bugs. All undesirable symptoms, similarly, become scapegoats in the misguided war against disease. Jungian analyst and homeopathic physician Edward Whitmont draws a direct comparison between the masculine tendency to wage war against our enemies, and the pharmakos:

> *With the advent of the patriarchy, the propitiation and purification rites become guilt-riddance ceremonies. The prototype is now the scapegoat or pharmakos. Life becomes finite. The stress is no longer upon renewal, upon rejoining the light by passing through the darkness, but upon preserving light and life by ridding oneself of darkness, of what is held offensive to the gods and guardians of morality.*[67]

A one-sided, rational perspective falsely encourages us to believe that we can compartmentalize and choose to expel only those aspects that we do not wish to accept. In the short run this strategy creates the illusion of victory, but in the end it will always fall short. We are left with the fundamental fact that the only true, long-term answer lies in integrating all parts into their rightful places within the whole. Carol Anthony, author of an insightful exploration of the principles behind the *I Ching*, compares philosophies of East and West:

> *These two forces, Yang and Yin, are the primary opposites; their interaction is seen to give rise to all things. In Western thought, opposites are said to annihilate each other, but in Eastern thought they are said to arouse and complete each other, creating the eternal wheel of change.*[68]

Western medicine relies heavily upon the objectification of disease so that it can continue to prosecute its misguided war. Pharmaceuticals and surgical steel are the weapons used to wage the war against disease. If it's a symptom, stop it, if it's a germ, kill it—and if it's a dysfunctional body part, cut it out. It has become abundantly clear, particularly to many whose bodies have become the battlefield upon which the physician fights the enemy, that the war is an unmitigated failure. As with most forms of war, the repercussions are worse than the situation that led to the conflict in the first place. Rarely, a war is a justified affair, as when a Hitler must be prevented from marching across the globe. Similarly, a burst appendix requires the surgeon's intervention and antibiotic therapy before the entire organism is overwhelmed. But the vast majority of both acute and chronic illnesses never rise to the level of such do-or-die urgency. A multitude of more diplomatic measures can be taken, but the parochial closed-mindedness of conventional medicine usually prevents such measures from being brought to the disposal and benefit of suffering patients.

Neither of these conceptions, which equate the disease with the individual or regard the disease as external to the individual, has to be a true conception unless we allow it to be so. We do not have to subscribe to the existential quagmire that orthodox medicine would confine us to, like Gregor Samsa in Kafka's *Metamorphosis*, lying helplessly on his back ready to be squashed like the bug that he has become. There is another perspective, the outlines of which we have been tracing in this book, and it involves the notion of illness as an imbalance in the matrix of the body-heart-mind-soul. We can work with illness, rather than against it, if we perceive it as an energetic disturbance that requires recalibration in order to restore overall harmony. In this sense, illness becomes not our enemy but our guide pointing in the direction of healing and transformation.

The Annual Checkup

That phony saccharine Stepford wife voice on the drug commercial during the evening news reminds me that I need to make a doctor's appointment for my annual physical exam. I've been avoiding it but my employer requires that I get one. I think my last tetanus shot is still good, but I hope they don't make me get one of those colonoscopies. I dial the doctor's office and an automated voice answers. After following the steps as instructed, even though I know I hit the right buttons on my phone, I still wind up at a dead end. I hang up and try again but this time I don't follow the mechanical prompts. I just wait until the end of the message. Aha! I hear a ring, and a real person answers. I explain that I need a check-up but the earliest they can get me in is two and a half months away. I ask the person if she's sure she can't get me in sooner, but her voice grows irritated as she reminds me that the doctor has a busy practice. Having been put in my place, I agree to the time offered and thank her for her help.

Even though I responsibly marked it on my calendar a couple of months ago, the phone rings, and when I pick up, it's that mechanized voice again, this time reminding me of my appointment tomorrow. Figuring that if I arrive a little early they might take me in sooner, I plan to get there twenty minutes ahead of time. Much to my dismay, my strategy is for naught, as the waiting room is already filled by the time I arrive. I stand at the desk for a few minutes waiting to check in. The receptionist finally looks up after putting the phone down and tells me I have to fill out the new HIPAA (Health Insurance Portability and Accountability Act) form designed to protect my confidentiality. I've heard people talking about the new HIPAA law and how its real purpose is to make access to your personal records easier for medical professionals. I consider making a comment but it occurs to me that she may be the one that got impatient when I first scheduled the appointment. Instead I grab the only seat left in the room. The lady sitting next to me has a nasty cough—I sure hope I don't catch that. I try to read the privacy form but it seems to be written in legal jargon. I don't think I really understand it but what can you do? I sign it and get up to return it. The receptionist is on the phone again. I hope I don't lose my seat.

A half hour has passed and I can swear that only one person has been called in to see the doctor. Bored to tears I finally succumb to picking up a tattered six-month-old copy of *Time* magazine. A full-page ad of a guy on a bike with birds flying above and a dog following along encourages me to talk to my doctor about taking Celebrex for my arthritis. The small print on two more full pages acknowledges that it "may increase the chance of heart attack or stroke, which can lead to death." I wonder about the advertising costs to the makers of Celebrex for three pages in *Time.* I skim an article that tells me that the shape of my body should determine what I eat. Another two-page ad tells me to talk to my doctor about taking Vytorin to "treat the two sources of cholesterol." I shouldn't have eaten that meatball sub for lunch yesterday.

I told my boss I had a doctor's appointment but I hadn't anticipated that it might take all morning. I'll have to remember to ask the doctor for a note so I have a legitimate excuse. I hope I don't get in trouble. The nurse calls another patient in but I know that I got here before he did. A full hour has now passed beyond the time of my scheduled appointment, and finally the nurse announces my name loudly, in front of all waiting their turn. I wonder if that's included in the new privacy law, but grateful to have been called at all, I jump up from my seat. She leads me down the hallway to a small cubicle where I am told to take my shoes off. She measures my height and weight and takes my temperature, blood pressure, and pulse. She busily records numbers onto her clipboard and seems to have little time for chitchat. Before she leaves she hands me a paper gown and tells me to disrobe.

Having been momentarily lulled into thinking I was going to see the doctor I am quickly jarred back to the reality that this is now phase two of the waiting game—medical limbo or purgatory, if you will. Now alone, I try to decide how much of my clothes I'm actually going to take off. I'm definitely not taking my socks off—I don't care what she said. That shiny tile floor looks too cold. I fiddle around with the gown for a while before I figure out how it's supposed to go on. The examining table is covered with that white paper that reminds me of the stuff they wrap slices of ham in at the deli. I step up onto the stool and ease myself onto the examining table as the paper crinkles beneath me. I survey the white room looking for those ice cream sticks in a jar. There they are. There is a cartoonish poster of the human digestive tract hanging on the wall. Not much else. I know it's only been a few minutes but it seems like I've been sitting here for at least twenty. I hear voices and footsteps coming—maybe it's the doctor. No, the steps just pass on by. I feel like an idiot sitting here in my socks, underwear, and paper gown. They should make the doctor and nurse wear the same for just one day, so they know what it's like. I wish I'd brought that old copy of *Time* with me. I look up and begin to count the ceiling tiles to pass the time.

After an interminable amount of time the doctor finally comes in and apologizes for the delay, explaining that they had temporarily misplaced my chart. I guess I'm supposed to feel relieved. He calls me by my full name of Lawrence. The only other people that call me that are my parents—everyone else knows me as Larry. He asks me how I've been and I explain that I'm here for my annual. He pokes and prods me with his hands and various instruments while asking an array of questions, stopping at times to log the data into his new hand-held electronic gizmo toy. "Any pain when I press here?" "Having regular BM's?" "Have you been taking your cholesterol medicine?"

"No, yes, ummm sometimes," I respond.

"Your blood pressure is a little higher than last year's you know." He whips a pad out of the pocket of his white coat, scribbles something down, and tears off a sheet. "Well you're in pretty good shape but I want you to take this."

"What is it?"

"It's a beta blocker for your blood pressure."

"What's that?" I figure my blood pressure has gone up at least ten points just sitting here waiting for him.

"Trust me, it's very safe, and I want to see you back in a month to check that BP again. You can get dressed now." And just as quickly as he came, he is gone again, leaving me sitting there in my gown with a white piece of paper in my hand. Whew, at least I'll get out of here without needing a colonoscopy. I guess I'll go home after work and Google "beta blocker" to try and figure out what it is. Oh, crap! I forgot to ask for that excuse note.

Fin

10

Cultural Medicalization

I want a new drug
One that won't make me sick
One that won't make me crash my car
Or make me feel three feet thick
> —Chris Hayes & Huey Lewis, "I Want a New Drug (Called Love)"

I used to care but now I take a pill for that.
> —Bumper sticker message

All disease is a socially created reality. Its meaning and the response
it has evoked have a history. The study of this history will make
us understand the degree to which we are prisoners of the med-
ical ideology in which we were brought up.
> —Ivan Illich, *Limits to Medicine*

MEDICAL-INDUSTRIAL ORIGINS

When I began writing the preceding fictional interlude, I intended to depict the soul-robbing reality of what many experience when interfacing with the medical machine. To my surprise it started to take on a humorous tone, albeit a dark humor, of the absurdity of what we have come to accept as the price we pay for quality care. My special position as the "alternative" doctor has made me privy to countless stories of the medically absurd. It is only natural that patients dissatisfied with their conventional care tend to hold their tongues in the halls of science and then unburden themselves in my office. Since my practice is heavily dependent upon hearing patient's stories, their medical escapades tend to be part and parcel of the whole. The process is therapeutic in and of itself, as they are often surprised that I listen at all, and refreshed when they realize that I am in sympathy with and do not judge them. In all honesty, when I first started practicing twenty years ago I relished those stories as a critique of the mainstream and a vindication of the direction that I had chosen. I was immature and had set out on a lonely path, so every bit of affirmation helped, but now when I hear similar stories, I just cringe to myself, express my concern, and seek to teach patients to trust their own perceptions and intuitions.

The Industrial Revolution brought mechanized techniques designed to increase efficiency. Assembly lines and division of labor were great innovations; production soared and economic prosperity abounded. Specialized roles were assigned workers who became small cogs in the burgeoning new world of material production and consumption. The medical profession eventually came to emulate this highly successful model of production of material goods, and to this day, its influence pervades all aspects of health care, from top to bottom. But we have seen what happens when we try to apply this model to the field of human health—we wind up with a health care "industry." Ivan Illich and Robert Mendelsohn were two of the original maverick voices in the wilderness willing to acknowledge the obvious impact that this medical industry has upon society. Here, Dr. Mendelsohn makes the case in plain language:

> I believe that despite all the super technology and the elite bedside manner that's supposed to make you feel about as well cared for as an astronaut on the way to the moon, the greatest danger to your health is the doctor who practices Modern Medicine. I believe that Modern Medicine's treatments for disease are seldom effective, and that they're often more dangerous than the diseases they're designed to treat. I believe the dangers are compounded by the widespread use of dangerous procedures for non-diseases.[69]

Furthermore, he focuses on how the overutilization of pharmaceuticals and medical procedures is driven by a market mentality that treats patients as consumers:

> I believe that Modern Medicine has gone too far, by using in everyday situations extreme treatments designed for critical conditions.

Every minute of every day Modern Medicine goes too far, because Modern Medicine prides itself on going too far ... So when you go to the doctor, you're seen not as a person who needs help with his or her health, but as a potential market for the medical factory's products.[70]

Originally, hospitals were built as almshouses for the poor, but then doctors recognized their dual utility as centralized storage for their instruments of technology and convenient housing for the sick. We have now come full circle, as patients—often very sick patients—are discharged from the hospital as quickly as possible in the name of cost savings and efficiency. As with the military model employed in the war against disease, the industrial model is emulated to an extreme, and we are beginning to see the devastating results of this lopsided, left-brain approach to the practice of medicine. The modern human has become almost indistinguishable from the technologies that were supposedly created to serve humanity in order to make life easier. Lewis Mumford, the distinguished American historian of science and technology, referred to the integration of technological influence into the very fabric of culture as "technics." Here, Mumford points out the difference between using technology for our benefit and allowing it to penetrate all phases of life:

For note this: mechanization and regimentation are not new phenomena in history; what is new is the fact that these functions have been projected and embodied in organized forms which dominate every aspect of our existence. Other civilizations reached a high degree of technical proficiency without, apparently, being profoundly influenced by the methods and aims of technics.[71]

We now find ourselves contending with a medical technics that is evident in all phases of modern life, and that has come to exist, first and foremost, for its own economic benefit. Doctors, nurses, administrators, technicians, and all ancillary staff have, understandably, become dependent upon the institutions that generate their paychecks. When we are forced to subscribe to this monopolistic system for our own personal care, a problem arises. Our options are limited as the insurance industry, in cahoots with

,er medical institutions, dictates what medical practices are acceptable
d therefore what services are covered by our medical insurance dollars.

DISSENTER'S DILEMMA

If a patient is not fortunate enough to be of good health, then that person
must choose to either quietly submit to the indignities of a dysfunctional
and impersonal system or go kicking and screaming into the same. Those
who choose to opt out run the risk of being labeled as eccentric, or even
deviant, and may in some cases have to contend with legal authorities. The
heretic may even be judged by psychiatry to be unfit for society and thus
inadvertently thrown into the belly of the very beast that he or she was trying to avoid. Just a few years back, my local community was in an uproar
when a concerned father was reported by school authorities for taking his
child off medication for attention deficit disorder because of the side effects
that the child was experiencing. Child Protective Services threatened to
remove the child from the home if the parent did not comply. Basing their
action upon a physician's assessment of the situation, the school ruled that
in order to attend, the child had to take the prescription. This type of
Orwellian nightmare is just a stone's throw away from anyone who exer-
cises the inherent personal right to choose or not choose the form of health
care that best suits his or her needs.

We may become suspect if we choose to give birth to our children outside of normal medical channels. Never mind that for eons, childbirth took
place in the home, and that before the obstetrician, midwifery was the
norm. Now, if an at-home birth goes awry, charges can be brought against
midwives, who may not be able to legally practice in some states. (I highly
recommend the film *The Business of Being Born* to all those wishing to
educate themselves on the issues involved in home birthing.)

It is also customary and expected that a good parent will make regular "well-baby" visits to the pediatrician. The term itself exerts a not-so-
subtle influence upon any parent who might dare to think that there is no
need to visit the doctor since their child is doing just fine. Of course, the

ever-expanding list of immunizations that infants with immature immune systems are required to receive ensures an endless string of visits to the pediatrician anyway—both because of the vaccines themselves and the various illnesses triggered by taking those vaccines.

Once a child starts school, routine physical exams become mandatory for admittance and continued attendance. Woe to the parent whose child should then develop a case of pinkeye, because school administrators will panic and send the child home until "proper" medical care has been administered—as if a school should have any legal say in the type of medical care chosen by parents. I have always found the arbitrary designation of pinkeye as a scourge rather amusing, since croupy coughs, bronchitis, fevers, sneezing, and other ailments do not usually warrant the same degree of suspicion. The fear of pinkeye no doubt goes back to that cultural fear of infectious contamination, and we often see an added layer of hysteria if the condition in question carries the social implication of dirtiness or uncleanliness, as with lice or ringworm. Although several effective non-antibiotic methods of dealing with pinkeye exist, many parents will nevertheless succumb to the combined pressures of their workplace demanding their presence and schools acting as if educational administrators have the right to demand antibiotic treatment before the child is allowed to return to the classroom.

The revolving door at the pediatrician's office continues to turn when the child needs physical exams in order to attend high school. Likewise, school sporting activities require physical exams, and when you finally grow up and enter the real world, employers do too. Even if you are an independently employed adult, the system still has powerful methods for ensuring your dependence. Women are kept within medical grasp by virtue of the annual Pap smear, and men are supposed to get prostate exams. As we grow older, blood pressure checks and bone density tests keep us all coming back, as does the biggest cash cow of all, the cholesterol industry. Add to this, eye exams, mammograms, and colonoscopies, and you have a very effective means of keeping the masses in a state of medical dependency.

REDEFINING DISEASE

This deeply rooted reach of the tentacles of orthodox medicine into every aspect of our lives is a ubiquitous fact that most tend not to question. As medicine redefines previously normal aspects of life, such as childbirth, aging, and death, as being in need of medical intervention, its influence and control over our lives expands dramatically. This "medicalization" of our lives is often driven by the development of new pharmaceuticals that are in need of markets to exploit. Regular cholesterol checks and bone density scans would not be so heavily promoted if drugs did not exist to manipulate the quantitative outcomes of these tests. An exaggerated emphasis upon these lab values also serves medical professionals as a means of convincing themselves that they are actually doing something of benefit for the patient. As such, the numbers can become more important than the patient's actual state of health. By formerly non-medical issues being given diagnostic classification, these freshly manufactured medical problems become potential threats and begin to take on a newly found importance in the public eye. Thus, we become concerned about restless leg syndrome, jet lag, erectile dysfunction, seasonal affective disorder, gastroesophageal reflux disease, premenstrual dysphoric disorder, and many other diagnoses created by the medical industry. I am not denying the existence of these issues in some individuals, and the need for treatment in a few, but I am pointing out how diagnostic labeling serves the medical profession as a powerful marketing tool. Ivan Illich describes the extent to which medicalization reaches into our lives:

> Once a society is so organized that medicine can transform people into patients because they are unborn, newborn, menopausal, or at some other "age of risk," the population inevitably loses some of its autonomy to its healers. The ritualization of stages of life is nothing new; what is new is their intense medicalization ... This life-span is brought into existence with the prenatal check-up, when the doctor decides if and how the fetus shall be born, and it will end with a mark on a chart ordering resuscitation suspended.[72]

Many of these ostensibly necessary medical services are conveniently and euphemistically categorized under the heading of "preventive medicine." Thus, the conventional medical concept of prevention translates into making sure that we have not developed various diseases by using technologies to constantly check for them. This odd approach of waiting for medical conditions to blossom into full-blown diagnosable entities before taking genuinely effective preventive or therapeutic action suits the system well. It allows the physician to tell complaining patients not to worry because the blood work and diagnostic tests have revealed nothing of concern. Either a patient's symptoms fit neatly into a prefabricated diagnostic category or, for all practical purposes, they do not exist, and the patient is consequently out of luck. In the end, medicine justifies submission to this distorted concept of prevention by rationalizing that it will save health care dollars in the long run.

I sometimes wonder how often the average person would need to visit a doctor if the person went only when he or she had an actual complaint. It would also be very interesting to see how many health care providers would still be in business if excessive diagnostic measures were replaced by greener practices and true prevention. Just imagine if the American Medical Association threw its political clout behind programs that eliminated all junk food from schools and replaced them with organic foods, taught yoga and meditation techniques beginning in kindergarten, and taught methods of conflict resolution to all children. These simple measures alone would turn health care on its head. If we were really serious about comprehensive green prevention I can think of umpteen decent ideas just off the top of my head—like health care insurance for all, health care coverage of alternative forms of healing, paid leave for all new mothers, paid childcare for working mothers, serious regulation of the chemical and pharmaceutical industries (which poison our environment), mass transit development to reduce pollution and stress on commuters, promotion of organic food growers, and many others. To those who would claim that this is not feasible, I say let us not fool ourselves, as most of the money needed to fund the above could be easily obtained by funneling it away from our grotesquely bloated military defense budget. In the long run, true prevention would drastically reduce the cost of care for the chronically ill.

COMMODIFICATION OF MEDICINE

Let us also not deceive ourselves into believing that the medical-industrial complex exists for the benefit of the health of humankind. It is a profit-driven enterprise that serves pharmaceutical companies, the insurance industry, hospitals, and managed care companies first. Patient welfare is often the last consideration on the corporate medical boardroom agenda. I believe this to be the harsh and regrettable truth, regardless of how noble the intentions of the individuals working within the system may be. Doctors and nurses are actually very low in the medical pecking order, and higher powers often dictate to them what they can and cannot do. Decisions traditionally based upon the confidential relationship between doctor and patient are increasingly made by anonymous managed care bureaucrats whose bottom line is economic, not therapeutic. The autonomy of the health professions and their patients declines to the extent that medicalization prevails. Thus, the labeling and classification of newly manufactured so-called "diseases," coupled with new pharmaceutical products in search of markets, guarantees maximum exploitation by the various labs, hospitals, clinics, and administrative offices of the highly medicalized society.

Most patients who come to see me do so because they have tried the conventional route and are less than satisfied with the outcome. Nevertheless, they frequently describe the psychological pressure and stress they feel over disagreeing with, or going behind the back of, their regular physician, to whom they feel an understandable loyalty. Ironically, alternative forms of medical therapy are often accused by the conventional medical mainstream of being dangerous because, in seeking care from "unproven" sources, so the argument goes, the patient will waste valuable time and thus delay receiving the "real" conventional care that they need.

It is important that we question whether we would choose to give up our medical freedom to any medical system whatsoever even if it *could* guarantee the best outcome in all cases. While promoting regular medicine as the only existing form of effective therapy, its proponents must at the same time psychologically prepare its patients for frequent disappointments. Robert Mendelsohn emphasizes the need for regular medicine to downplay the expectations that patients should have regarding the outcomes of conventional therapy:

> *Of course, if the doctor were to admit that he had no power over the patient's affliction but that other powers—such as those of other healers or the patient's own—may, he would lose his control over the patient. Furthermore, since Modern Medicine's rites are not only growing less and less successful but also more and more deadly, it makes good business sense to prepare the patient for the inevitable results of the doctor's work.*[73]

As both autonomy and therapeutic success diminish, the masses become the perfect targets for even more commodified medical services. Because many consumers are unaware that they do have choices other than what the mainstream has to offer, a perfect storm of a medical marketplace is created. Diagnostic entities are created and defined by scientific authorities, medical language causes the layperson to feel inadequate and unable to ask questions, fear of the external enemy keeps the masses in submission, and medical products are marketed to consumers more than willing to purchase these promised "cures."

Practitioners of complementary and alternative medicine should not be immune from the same criticism. While herbal and nutritional supplements in most cases are safer than pharmaceuticals, they do not necessarily lead to any greater health simply because they are natural. Of course, the greatest hoax of all is the idea that health is a product, a commodity to be bought and sold, something out there that I can obtain to make me well again. Illich drives the point home:

> *The more time, toil, and sacrifice spent by a population in producing medicine as a commodity, the larger will be the by-product, namely, the fallacy that society has a supply of health locked away which can be mined and marketed ... The fallacy that society is caught forever in the drug age is one of the dogmas with which*

medical policy-making has been encumbered: it fits industrialized man. He has learned to try to purchase whatever he fancies.[74]

One way to measure the extent to which medical technics pervades American culture is to pay close attention to the topics of conversation when senior citizens gather. Next to the grandchildren, visits to the doctor and the results of diagnostic procedures come in a close second. The medicalization of the older generation is so thorough that they speak of their doctors, hospitals, lab tests, and medications with a devotion that only devotion to family can surpass. It is astonishing to see the ease with which these heavy consumers of medical services throw around medical jargon. On the one hand it is a good sign that they are educating themselves, but on the other, it is a sign of how well programmed they have become. While they do debate and question whether drug A or drug B is preferable and whether they should let Dr. X or Dr. Y perform the surgery, it is usually not congruent with their mindset to question if the drug or surgery is advisable at all.

Sadly, the most medicalized phase of life takes place during end-stage disease. At a time when the greatest concentration upon spiritual considerations is crucial for both patient and family, a macabre ritual of medical distraction takes place during which medical professionals convince themselves and the dying patient that there is still much that can be done. Often much energy is consumed discussing the latest blood tests, drugs and dosages, and what more can be done to stave off the inevitable, instead of on having quality time with family at the most important moments. As our willingness to spend health care dollars in this pursuit seems unlimited, our denial of death translates into the bread and butter of materialistic medicine.

Although many of us are intuitively reluctant to take pharmaceuticals, cultural brainwashing can often override our better instincts. We are programmed to trust the doctor and those brand-name medications that we have all grown up with. Tylenol is a name we have come to know and trust, but I wonder how many people realize that it and other acetaminophen-based drugs are the number one cause of acute liver failure in the United

States. Millions of advertising dollars are spent on reassuring doctor and patient alike that our drugs are safe and effective, even when they are not.

THE SICKNESS OF SOCIETY

Strangely, though, our society simultaneously wages a hypocritical war against drugs, as we are mandated to refrain from certain "recreational" drugs that are banned by the state under penalty of law. State sanctioned psychoactive drugs, some of which are well understood to be habit forming, may nevertheless be taken daily for years with a physician's approval, but we are just supposed to say "no" to those other drugs. You are encouraged, even expected, to take an antidepressant if you feel down, but if you are caught even once smoking marijuana as you try to unwind from the pressures of the day, it may spell the end of your entire career as teacher, lawyer, doctor, or bus driver. Prozac is good but marijuana is bad—so bad that it cannot even be used medicinally to help those that could benefit from it. The indoctrination is so complete that some parents will risk sending their own children to jail just to teach them the lessons of this schizophrenic cultural myth.

When the occasional person begins to get a glimpse of this deception, that is, begins to realize that it is the cultural milieu within which the medical-industrial complex thrives that is sick, that person may face a variety of strategies used to silence him. When, for example, the individual grows sick and tired of playing an uncreative role as cog in the great capitalist machine, he or she naturally is referred for care under the auspices of that very same medical-industrial complex. If the person dares to complain too much about the nature of a society that is creating the sickness, the tables will be turned and he or she will be called the sick one. This person must be made well again in order to return to being a productive member of society. An antidepressant may be prescribed to subdue the person's protesting mind. He or she had better not be too sick for too long or the risk of job loss will become real. One would assume the purpose of the medical system is to adapt and change as it seeks ever-improved ways of helping and healing, but it is usually the sick individual that must adapt and accept the onus created by a medicalized culture that demands passivity, punctuality, and productivity.

The naïve belief in science and technology as a panacea was on full display recently when I attended an academic awards ceremony at the local middle school for one of my children. Several on the bill, including the keynote speaker, glowingly described the opportunities on the technological horizon for those willing to pursue the dream. We were told that a world of scholarships and good-paying high-tech jobs was just waiting for those who studied their math and science— but nary a single opportunity for those whose areas of interest lay outside the realm of science was mentioned. My son's main interests are indeed in math and science and I suspect he may someday attend school to become an engineer of some sort, but I felt sorry for the poor parents and their children whose interests in art, music, languages, theater, history, and the humanities were swept aside as if they did not even exist. Half of humanity had been relegated to the dustbin before they even got out of the starting gate because their future fields of endeavor were not compatible with the collective objectives of the technocracy. Against all odds must that future music major pursue his or her dream, and when that student becomes discouraged and sick from swimming against the mainstream, he or she will likely be scolded for not having chosen a more practical profession.

By choosing cultural deception over personal integrity, a physician neglects his or her responsibility to fulfill the role of health advocate. It is a common sense, self-evident truth, requiring neither elaborate and expensive studies nor scientific proof, that our collective cultural health is on the decline. We are increasingly dependent upon pharmaceutical palliation in order to dull the cries of the body-heart-mind-soul as it protests against the dysfunction of a society that values aggression over cooperation, deception over truth-telling, and image over substance. There is something profoundly amiss when an estimated forty-five million Americans are without health insurance while some of our favorite sports heroes make $20 million or more per year. A society that preys upon its weakest and would strip away any semblance of a social safety net because that would be tantamount to the dreaded socialism, has lost its moral bearings to a dangerous degree.

While politicians bicker over perks and pay raises and pledge their allegiance to the highest corporate donor, the real reforms so desperately needed are eclipsed by societal priorities that worship superficiality and celebrity, violence and titillation, and egotism and vanity. The old and traditional are discarded for the new and novel, quantity trumps quality, and excess is pursued at the expense of balance. We are no longer human beings with foibles and frailties, but consumers in need of the necessary capital that we believe will allow us to purchase health and the American dream. Ivan Illich describes the futility of trying to purchase products for the killing of our pain, because pain is ...

> ... a side-effect of strategies for industrial expansion ... It is a curse, and to stop the "masses" from cursing society when they are pain-stricken, the industrial system delivers them medical pain-killers. Pain thus turns into a demand for more drugs, hospitals, medical services, and other outputs of corporate, impersonal care and into political support for further corporate growth no matter what its human, social, or economic cost. Pain has become a political issue which gives rise to a snowballing demand on the part of anesthesia consumers for artificially induced insensibility, unawareness, and even unconsciousness.[75]

Such an untenable state of affairs must, by definition, create increasing amounts of pain, suffering, alienation, fragmentation, and depersonalization. The solutions are not more drugs and medical services, but less. The answer will be found not by reinvesting in the medicalization of culture, but in reestablishing our autonomy as individuals who will decide what is best for our own mental, emotional, spiritual, and physical health. We must overcome the fear that paralyzes us and shake the delusion that we are not qualified to judge what is in our own best medical interests. Physicians must void their deal with the devil and return to their true calling, based in a genuine search for more holistic methods and a greener perspective that facilitates wholeness and healing. They must stop shilling for Big Pharma and return to advocating for their patients. They must relinquish the delusion that science and technocracy confers upon them that they are all-knowing and instead enter into a partnership with their patients, who are in need of the assistance that they are truly capable of offering. There, I've said it. Now I'll shut up and go take my medications before my head explodes.

The Illusion of Cure

*Suppression doesn't work in the long run. It is a form of resist-
ance, and resistance always fosters the persistence of what we resist.*

—Bob Frissell, *You Are a Spiritual Being Having a Human
Experience*

*The real origin of disease is uncertain; it is broadly societal, con-
stitutional, and cosmic. Real things are cured finally by a process,
not a particular medicine. Drugs, after all, are only a seeming
realization of the fantasy of solving all wrong things at once.*

—Richard Grossinger, *Planet Medicine*

SOME BRIEF CASE HISTORIES

I randomly thumbed through charts of patients that I have seen over the
years and selected the following partial case histories as examples.

Case One

A young girl noticed a puffy area of swelling on her forehead one day. It
spread to the bridge of her nose and then around one eye. A pediatrician
decided that it was an infection of the underlying tissues of the skin called
cellulitis and prescribed an antibiotic. Within a few days the girl began to
vomit and, as the vomiting subsided, she developed a very deep cough.
Soon the cough transitioned into wheezing that became worse during ath-
letic activities. Upon returning to the doctor, a prescription for an inhaler
was written for the girl's new diagnosis of asthma, which she had never
had before the onset of the swelling.

Case Two

A middle-aged man had been taking a commonly prescribed antihistamine during the previous year for his allergy symptoms of watery eyes and

runny nose. He awoke one morning with his upper and lower eyelids swollen. His doctor prescribed another antihistamine but the condition spread to his neck. Two rounds of a steroid called methylprednisolone (Medrol) were tried, each time giving only temporary relief, as the hive-like symptoms spread to his face, resulting in chronic swelling around the eyes. The doctor's new diagnosis was angioedema.

Case Three

In preparation for a trip overseas, an older man underwent a series of vaccinations. After one of them he suffered an immediate attack of dizziness, nausea, headache, sore throat, and malaise. Over the subsequent years he has had several episodes of severe vertigo (dizziness) lasting weeks at a time, requiring that he lie in bed until the attacks subside.

Case Four

A forty-year-old woman developed respiratory symptoms that were diagnosed as bronchitis. She was prescribed an asthma medication called theophylline. Her coughing and wheezing quickly improved but she immediately was stricken with a severe sharp pain running through her head from front to back. In the three years since the original diagnosis, she has had frequent headaches of a similar nature, which have been diagnosed as migraines. She takes two different medications for the migraines, which, nevertheless, continue to occur twice per week, and in recent months she has developed an arthritic condition that affects the joints in both arms and both legs.

Case Five

A young woman suffering from depression over a span of five years finally sought help and was started on antidepressant therapy. Within weeks she became overwhelmingly exhausted and could not get out of bed. In addition, she began to experience headaches, nausea, and chills. These symptoms have continued for years and have recently been diagnosed as chronic fatigue syndrome.

Case Six

A woman in her forties had been receiving allergy shots for over fifteen years. Her original symptoms were post-nasal drip, cough, sneezing, and eye swelling. Five years ago she began to have moderately severe coughing and wheezing attacks during the nights. Her original allergy symptoms are greatly diminished, her diagnosis has been changed to asthma, and she now needs three medications to manage her symptoms.

Case Seven

A pregnant woman agreed to a diagnostic procedure called amniocentesis, during which a needle was passed into the sac surrounding the developing fetus in order to obtain a sample of amniotic fluid. Sadly, this woman's womb became infected and she miscarried after four months of pregnancy. Another procedure called a dilatation and curettage (D&C) was performed to remove the remaining contents from the uterus, after which another infection developed that took four months to get under control, with the help of several courses of antibiotics. She has been unable to conceive another pregnancy in the four years since.

All of the preceding examples have one thing in common. Whether directly or indirectly, the health of each patient deteriorated over time subsequent to the medical treatment or procedure involved. Although some of these medical interventions provided temporary relief and some may have been necessary, ultimately the patient, in each case, was worse off in the long run. Rather than the rare exception, and contrary to what we would like to believe, this type of outcome is a common medical experience. We do not often hear about such outcomes, and this is due to the way that they are interpreted, spun, and whitewashed. The medical system's tendency to compartmentalize allows for the interrelationships between symptoms to be minimized and even dismissed without their potential connections being examined and reviewed adequately. A more well-rounded green perspective, while acknowledging the practical necessity in some instances for compartmentalization, nevertheless understands that it always entails a limited and distorted version of holistic reality.

In Case Four it is very easy to ignore the clear-cut link between the use of theophylline to treat bronchitis and its transmutation into migraine headaches. The conventional doctor has no philosophical frame of reference that would allow such a transmutation to make sense. Instead, it may be seen as an annoying anomaly and written off as mere coincidence. Or, as is commonly the case, the physician may trust the literature more than his or her own senses. The doctor simply believes that this symptom or that side effect cannot be caused by this or that drug because it is not listed in any medical reference books.

This type of denial is plainly evident in the event of vaccine injury when a perfectly healthy child becomes acutely febrile within hours after receiving a vaccine and shortly thereafter begins to exhibit previously unseen traits of autism. I do not know how many times this has to occur before conventional medicine will finally acknowledge the disgraceful truth about what is taking place. Rather than truth-seeking, the medical establishment is usually more concerned with face-saving. The political wheels of medicine are set into motion and we begin to hear dissembling phrases like, "There is no conclusive evidence," or, "Further studies are needed." Do I really need a study to prove that my big swollen black and blue thumb resulted from the hammer that I accidentally whomped it with a few minutes ago? The myopic nature of exclusively left-brained thinking gives rise to a tremendous capacity for denial. Medicine's lack of cohesive worldview, coupled with its tendency to rely heavily upon data and studies, provides it with convenient lines of defense that can range from conceit, to ignorance, to denial, to alibi.

The truth is that if orthodox medicine was forced to acknowledge the realities of its day-to-day interactions with its patients, it would be thrown into a serious existential crisis. Unfortunately, the matter cannot be forced— believe me, I have tried that strategy more than a few times. It cannot be expected that physicians, who have invested years of study and practice into their profession, can stop and turn on a dime to reconsider the very basis of all that they have worked toward. It will require a slow steady process of re-education and the receptive minds of younger physicians to bring about the necessary changes.

CONVENTIONAL IATROGENESIS

Broadly speaking, all of the cases above can be characterized as examples of *iatrogenesis*. The Greek *iatros* translates into *physician* so, technically, the term means anything caused by a physician, whether desirable or undesirable. In modern usage, the term refers to any adverse event or ill effect caused by the medical system. In short, iatrogenesis means physician-induced or medically induced disease. By extension, iatrogenesis can also be caused by any type of health care worker, medical intervention, or even non-physician healer or alternative practitioner. Iatrogenesis, therefore, is an immense source of morbidity and mortality. By some estimates, in the United States, medical care is the third leading cause of death,[76] following heart disease and cancer. Surgical mishaps, hospital infections, medication errors, and the adverse effects of drugs lead to hundreds of thousands of deaths per year.

The tremendous amount of iatrogenic pain and suffering induced by technological medicine is in direct contradiction to the medical prime directive of *primum non nocere*, the Latin phrase meaning, "first, do no harm." It is as if the priority of the patient's health now takes a back seat to the medical establishment's collective ego, which will acknowledge harm only as a last resort and only if it can be proven. For example, we often witness shockingly cold-blooded denials of harm when initial reports come out regarding the dangerous effects of some pharmaceuticals. Instead, we are told by media talking heads not to discontinue medications until we have consulted our physicians. Regardless of the seriousness of the threat uncovered, Big Pharma's spin machine will predictably tell us that the data is incomplete and more studies are needed before appropriate action can be taken. In essence, we are encouraged to continue treatment until harm is proven. By the time enough evidence is collected, thousands of lives have been damaged and millions more dollars have been harvested from the very victims of the defective product being foisted upon them.

Iatrogenesis is most often medically induced in the clinic and the hospital, but it can also be perpetuated and reinforced socially and culturally. The political trend in the United States that opposes providing a social safety net in the form of programs, such as school lunches for the poor, support for pregnant mothers, and day care for working parents, contributes significantly to iatrogenesis. Similarly, America's denial of death, avoidance of pain, glorification of violence, commodification of human sexuality, and commercialization of pharmaceuticals, can all be seen as trends conducive of iatrogenesis.

In Case Three it is clear that the initial attack of dizziness is an iatrogenic effect of the vaccine, although it may be easier for the medical mind to ignore common sense and deny the connection to the subsequent episodes of vertigo. Likewise, in Case Seven it is difficult to deny the iatrogenic infection caused by the amniocentesis needle, although it may be easier for the practitioner to convince himself that this had no relation to the woman's ensuing infertility.

Case One leaves itself open to claims of medical blamelessness because the two ailments seem so unrelated. After all, how can cellulitis lead to asthma? Mechanistic thinking commonly allows the medical profession to deny the reality of what has been observed firsthand. Although conventional medicine has no explanation for such a chain of events it is, nevertheless, what happened in this case. The empirical facts are that before the cellulitis there was no asthma, and after antibiotic treatment, the cough and subsequent asthma emerged from seemingly nowhere. As we shall see, there is a satisfactory explanation for this if we come to understand the true nature of the life force and how it responds when subjected to mechanistic medical treatment.

The certainty of an iatrogenic effect is a little less ironclad in Case Two. Although most observers would not make such a connection, I am of the mind that the chronic use of the antihistamine predisposed this person to the subsequent swelling of his face. Additionally, I believe that the antihistamine, in conjunction with the powerful steroid drug, encouraged the swelling to spread and turned it into a chronic condition, which now goes by the name of angioedema. The conventional medical argument would tend to be the reverse—that the condition spread and was destined to become chronic in spite of the physician's best efforts to control it. This is not unlike the case of the patient convinced to accept a cortisone shot for a chronically painful shoulder who then feels as good as new, until several months later, when the opposite shoulder begins to have the same kind of trouble, whereupon the patient is told that this is the natural progression of the disease. I would beg to differ.

Similarly, in Case Six one has to wonder at the wisdom of ten years of allergy shots if the end result is a newly developed case of asthma that requires three medications just to control it. Given this trade-off of asthma for allergy symptoms, continuing with another five years of the same allergy shots would seem to defy common sense. Here again, any reputable physician might feel perfectly comfortable in asserting that there is simply no connection between the two. While some would claim that the asthma represents a continuation of an allergic condition that has been resistant to treatment, I believe that the asthma, in this case, was caused by the prolonged course of allergy shots.

Along the same line of reasoning, was the depression in Case Five destined to become so overwhelming as to warrant the diagnosis of chronic fatigue syndrome, or was this woman's health pushed in that direction by the antidepressant? I am sure the doctor can point to lots of patients on the same antidepressant who did not fall victim to chronic fatigue, but this is no guarantee that it therefore cannot happen to anyone.

Is it all right in cases Two, Five, and Six to casually attribute the course of events to the progression of the disease as most conventional doctors would do, or can it be interpreted as resulting from the treatments employed in each case? This is far too important a consideration to simply leave to conjecture. It necessitates that we develop a framework of understanding that allows us to predict the likely outcome from such interventions and to also verify the validity of our predictions. Our understanding of the vital force and its patterns of response should provide just such a framework within which our observations and conclusions can be tested.

Contemporary medicine, to its credit, has come to acknowledge the role of some of the more obvious forms of iatrogenesis. Even so, its general reluctance to institute meaningful changes is likely to ensure that the incidence of iatrogenesis will not decline, at least in the foreseeable future. Most iatrogenesis is categorized as some form of medical error such as misread prescriptions, contaminated instruments, unanticipated drug interactions, or misdiagnosis. In other words, it can be argued that if these mistakes can be avoided then there is nothing wrong with the practice of medicine except when errors in its execution have been committed. This convenient but faulty line of thinking exonerates the practice of medicine from culpability and prevents a true self-examination of the substance of medicine and its real impact upon patients. Thus, to the medical mind, it becomes a simple matter of eliminating mistakes and errors, thereby evading claims as to the inappropriateness of its therapeutic philosophy and approach.

UNACKNOWLEDGED IATROGENESIS

If we accept orthodox medicine's definition of iatrogenesis, then the theoretical solution should amount to a simple matter of preventing medical error. However, there remains an unrecognized and unnamed category of medically induced illness that accounts for more harm than all other forms of iatrogenesis combined. As such, if the point that I am about to make is true, then education of the medical establishment and the general public regarding this basic truth would equate to a sea change that would profoundly alter the way medicine is viewed and practiced. This fundamental truth will be met with tremendous resistance in some quarters and, yet, may be deeply liberating to others. Given the practical implications that it holds for our collective health, I urge you to give serious consideration to the explanation that I am about to offer.

Allowing for the fact that iatrogenic disease, as it is understood by conventional medicine, is the result of appropriate medical treatment that has gone awry, it remains to explore the nature of what happens when a successful medical intervention has actually achieved its aim. We naturally assume that an effective medical treatment is a desirable treatment that results in a desirable outcome. After all, why should I complain if my headache goes away after taking Excedrin, or my arthritis clears up after a cortisone shot, or my sinus infection improves with an antibiotic, or my eczema disappears after using a topical steroid? These are typical examples of successfully executed medical therapies. In common parlance we would even venture to refer to them as medical "cures."

However, it is imperative that we be more mindful of the terminology that our impressionable, medicalized culture has uncritically come to accept. I recall seeing an old television commercial for an antifungal medication in which the young woman's reassuring voice proclaimed, "It cures my yeast infection every time." Skeptic that I am, I turned to my wife and asked, "How can it be a cure if it keeps coming back?" If my headache is cured soon after taking Excedrin, can it still be considered a cure when I get another headache the next day? If my arthritic knee feels like new after a cortisone shot, is it still appropriate to call it a cure if my other knee develops the same arthritic pain three months later? What if I continue to contract sinus infections after antibiotics clear them up each time? And what are we to think of the eczema that, after having magically vanished, returns upon discontinuation of the topical steroid? Far from nitpicking, the implications of these questions and their answers will have a far-reaching impact on the way we look at orthodox medicine and its effect upon human health and the life force.

Consider for a moment these potential cures for my ailing automobile. Driving down the road I suddenly notice that my tailpipe is emitting a large amount of thick, black smoke. I pull over, grab a rag from the back seat, stuff it into the tailpipe and continue on my way. Problem solved? Let's say I am driving along and I begin to hear an ominous knocking sound coming from the engine. I reach into the glove compartment for the earmuffs and place them over my head thus eliminating the disturbing sound. No worries? Assume that I know my car's alignment is off since a fender bender last week and it will likely cause uneven wear on my tires. No sweat, I'll just purchase new tires more frequently.

I think you get the point. These are obviously silly, superficial solutions that treat the symptom while ignoring the underlying issue. If this is so blatantly apparent when it comes to car care, why are we so willing to accept it as the standard of human health care? When a person's eczema recedes after a few applications of cortisone cream, is it a cure or just a temporary solution? Is it a cure if it stays away for a week, a month, a year? If the eczema was originally on the hands, is now gone, but then shows up on the knees, is it a cure? Did you ever know a person who had some warts burned or frozen off, only to have a bunch more crop up nearby? Is it fair to say that the old warts were cured but the new ones are just coincidental?

Furthermore, we know darn well that stuffing a rag in the car's tailpipe is not only not a cure, it is downright dangerous. Even medical authorities acknowledge that steroid drugs are immuno-suppressants—they work by suppressing the immune system. I know that cortisone is only a temporary measure because I have seen many people stop treatment only to have their symptoms return. Let us suppose that I have put up with eczema on my hands for several years and one day I decide to "stuff it" with topical cortisone. It works like a charm and the eczema vanishes but, to my dismay, my knees start to swell and become red and painful. My general practitioner runs a few tests and tells me I have the beginnings of rheumatoid arthritis. Did I unwittingly create a much more serious problem by suppressing the eczema? I ask my doctor about the connection but he quickly reassures me that cortisone cannot cause rheumatoid arthritis.

The regrettable truth is that we have been culturally conditioned to accept pill popping and symptom stopping as our primary forms of medical care. Our dumbed-down expectations and understanding of cure go no further than our increasingly shortened attention spans. If the eczema went away yesterday and my knees were swollen this morning, then we might be convinced to accept the linkage between the two. It would be much easier to dismiss if the knees were to swell six months or even a week later. The greater the distance that comes between two medical events the less likely we are to suspect that they have anything to do with each other—and the compartmentalization of mechanistic medicine does nothing to dispel our misunderstanding of such situations.

A change in medical terminology is in order. It does not serve us well to allow a term like *cure* to be so casually abused. The premise of the orthodox medical worldview and its consequent therapeutic game plan virtually guarantee that genuine cure will be a rare and otherwise accidental event. Remember, all symptoms are distress signals from the defense mechanism of a disordered and imbalanced bioenergetic life force. Treating the symptom amounts to shooting the messenger, and will, at best, allow the continuation of the underlying disorder and, at worst, intensify the imbalance.

Genuine cure implies not only full resolution of the condition in question but also that it will never come back, or at least not for a long time. A declaration of cure must also carry with it the obvious caveat that treatment should no longer be necessary. A daily dose of thyroid hormone for the rest of one's life does not constitute a cure for hypothyroidism, just as a daily dose of a beta-blocker will not cure high blood pressure. Additionally, cure implies that the subsequent health of the individual under treatment will be better than it was before treatment and, most importantly, it will continue to be better over time. Otherwise, why would we want to be cured? While this may seem a bold and daring demand to place upon a form of medical care from which we have come to expect so little, it is exactly what is needed, and it is imperative that we voice these opinions and concerns that they may some day be actualized.

From a fragmented unholistic perspective, we may believe my eczema to be cured if it does not return even after I stop applying cortisone cream. From a real-world perspective, in which I understand from the depths of my being that all things are connected, the subsequent development of rheumatoid arthritis is a clear-cut sign of deteriorating health and makes a powerful argument against the assignment of cure in this case. Even in the case of sinusitis, where an antibiotic is used to kill a bug that is presumed to be the cause of the problem, the true issue remains unresolved, as most individuals with sinusitis will tell you that it tends to recur at intervals. The killing of the bug cannot be considered a cure if it fails to address the underlying susceptibility of the life force, which allows the bug to recolonize to the point where it provokes successive episodes of sinusitis.

Thus, the vast majority of what contemporary standards consider cures are not cures at all. This conception of cure is an illusion, a shell game—trickery that not only fools the patient, but the doctor, too. Again, this is a very hard pill to swallow, and if accepted for what it is, would throw contemporary medicine into crisis. Therefore, realistically speaking, it is to be expected that this message can only be assimilated piecemeal, bit by bit, until the full impact will someday be appreciated.

CLARIFYING MEDICAL OUTCOMES

If we accept the premise that conventional medical cures are not what they seem to be, then we must employ more fitting terms that reflect the actual dynamics. Let us examine some of the terms that tend, in common usage, to be loosely applied to varying medical situations without regard for their specific meanings and implications.

Treatment is a relatively neutral word, which carries with it no suggestion of success or failure in terms of medical outcome. It simply indicates that something, rather than nothing, is being done for a given health condition. We can treat a cold that would mend on its own even if untreated, or we can treat heart disease that is chronic and possibly progressive. *Management,* on the other hand, implies that an ongoing situation is involved, a situation that must be managed. Although a short-term ailment can be managed, the term comes into play most often when speaking of chronic illness. Hence, the usual case of asthma is one that must be managed over time since it is not expected to be cured, and will therefore need to be dealt with periodically, if not daily. Since conventional medicine is unable to cure most chronic illnesses, it must manage them instead.

Palliation is an interesting term that is typically associated with end-stage disease when there is little or no hope of recovery and nothing else that can be done to ensure such an outcome. *Taber's Cyclopedic Medical Dictionary* tells us that to palliate is to "ease or reduce effect or intensity, esp. of a disease; to allay temporarily, as pain, without curing." The *Oxford American Dictionary* says that to palliate is to "make symptoms less severe or unpleasant without removing the cause" and to "disguise the seriousness or gravity of an offense." Terminal cancer patients are often given palliative care to relieve their suffering and make them as comfortable as is possible. By this standard, taking ibuprofen for a headache or acetaminophen for a fever should constitute palliative care, since both provide symptomatic relief, and neither, according to my line of reasoning, can be expected to cure the ailment being treated. We can reduce the fever or dull the pain of the headache, but this will not remove the cause.

Treatment of acute illnesses like a cold, bronchitis, or an ear infection may give the impression of effectiveness because, in addition to providing symptomatic relief, the person eventually recovers and appears well again. Thus, in acute illness, the illusion of cure occurs because the vast majority of cases are going to recover regardless of the treatment employed. Suppose I were to prescribe a seven-day course of an antibiotic for one person with bronchitis while I advised another to rest and drink plenty of fluids. Two weeks later, at their follow-up visits, the one that took the antibiotic reports feeling almost back to normal within one week. If the one that did not take an antibiotic tells me the same, is it reasonable to assume that the antibiotic helped the first person? Or would that person also have gotten better without treatment?

I believe this type of illusory cure to be the case in a significant number of antibiotic prescriptions. Even in cases where antibiotics are necessary and do work, a thorough assessment of the overall effect of treatment should take into account the subsequent health of these individuals as time passes. While it is true that an antibiotic can often extinguish an acute infection, the overall impact upon the vital force is usually to decrease immunity, which then encourages subsequent recurrence of illness. Antibiotics tend to cause the immune system to become lazy, sluggish, and dependent. In actuality, an individual who overuses antibiotics and symptomatic cold remedies often suffers diminished health and is render more susceptible to further infection and illness.

Since most conventional treatments provide only short-term relief and do not bring about long-term health improvements, the best that we can say is that the majority of these options are palliative. This is most obvious in relation to chronic illnesses like asthma and arthritis as evidenced by the fact that they must be managed over time, and are sometimes progressive in spite of treatment. Allopathic treatment of chronic disease usually provides only temporary relief, thereby necessitating daily doses of medication. I would argue that the conventional treatment of acute illness is usually unnecessary and likely to be palliative. In addition, subsequent overall health tends to diminish as a result of this approach.

In summary, most conventional medical treatment is palliative at best. Western medicine can offer only palliation in the vast majority of chronic diseases, and while acute treatments may help deal with short-term crises, they often negatively impact long-term health. This is actually a generous assessment of the net effect of the allopathic approach because, in reality, the situation can often turn out to be much worse. When a patient complains about an illness that recurs after conventional drug therapy, I am likely to remind that patient that he or she is lucky not to have developed a more problematic illness. It is preferable to have a recurrence of the same illness rather than come down with something completely new that is even worse than the original problem.

THE LESSONS OF SUPPRESSION

Let us return now to some of the cases from the beginning of this chapter. In Case One a young girl receiving antibiotic treatment for acute cellulitis wound up in the end with asthma. In Case Four a prescription of theophylline for bronchitis caused the immediate onset of migraine headaches. In both instances, treatment of an acute ailment led directly to the development of a chronic illness. Instead of temporary relief, we saw an actual worsening of health, so the term palliation is no longer applicable to these cases. If theophylline had improved the symptoms and the bronchitis had gone away only to return again three months later, the effect would have been predominantly palliative. The onset of migraines in displacement of the bronchitis, however, represents an undesirable turn for the worse. No matter how hard orthodox practitioners try to dismiss linkages like this as coincidental, they are emblematic of a very real, predictable, and commonplace problem with the everyday practice of Western medicine.

Because the effect we are now talking about is not merely temporary relief, or palliation, but a worsening of health, we need language that more appropriately reflects this iatrogenic influence. The term that best describes this dynamic is "suppression." Turning again to the *Oxford American Dictionary,* we find that to suppress is "to forcibly put an end to" and to "prevent the development, action, or expression of a feeling, impulse, idea, etc." Therefore, we are no longer just talking about the lessening of symptoms. We are preventing their expression and putting an end to them—and therein lies the rub. Remember, the same dynamic applies to all levels of mind, body, and soul. Psychological suppression is a commonly accepted phenomenon that entails the conscious inhibition of unacceptable memories. Many mental health issues can be traced to the suppression of undesirable thoughts or emotions. The suppressive parallel of using a drug to inhibit an undesirable physical symptom is clear, and although we are relentlessly urged to partake of this potentially harmful method of dealing with symptoms, modern medical standards tend not to recognize its dangers. We are seduced into believing that forcing symptoms into submission is the equivalent to cure, regardless of the final outcome.

As the popular cliché would have it, there is no free lunch, and so we cannot forcibly suppress symptoms without the possibility of creating an unwanted backlash. If the innate holistic wisdom of the life force chooses a particular symptom as a warning signal, then we must accept the reality that we proceed at our own risk when choosing to suppress that symptom. I am rarely surprised when I hear of larger health issues developing after the initiation of regular medical treatment. As a general guideline, any ailment that develops subsequent to a previous ailment that was treated by orthodox means and which has not come back is likely to be the result of suppression, especially if the new ailment is more troublesome or threatening than the original. There are no hard and fast rules, and there is no statute of limitations. Depression that emerges one year after steroid treatment for eczema can, in some cases, still be considered the end product of suppression. There can be a fine line between palliation and suppression; the difference is whether the condition under treatment returns or is displaced by a new condition.

When a suppressive medical therapy has successfully beaten back the defense mechanism, the vital force may appear to be quiescent for a period of time, until it regroups and gathers enough strength to generate the next best alternative to its original distress signal. Popular culture understands this phenomenon as it plays out in cancer therapy. *Metastasis* occurs when a particular cancer seems to go into remission only to recur in a new location at a later date. This concept can be more broadly applied to any symptom or condition that has been suppressed and that later manifests as a new symptom or illness. Metastasis therefore is the reincarnation, if you will, of a previously suppressed symptom or illness.

The medical establishment uses its usual mechanistic rationale to explain the reason for metastasis. According to this logic, metastasis occurs when all of the cancer cells are not killed by chemotherapy or radiation, and some have escaped and moved on to seed a new location where the cancer is now growing. To the contrary, I believe metastasis is often the logical result of suppression caused by the cancer therapy, and not a failure to kill all of the cancer cells. I am referring here to an energetic metastasis wherein the life force simply chooses another avenue to express its disturbance. Rather than an escaped cell finding a new place to grow a tumor, the vital energy is redirected to a new location where it again manifests as a tumor.

This dynamic applies not just to cancer but to all medical conditions that have been suppressed. The concept of energetic metastasis also elegantly explains how one symptom or condition can transmute into a new condition in a completely different anatomical location. Therefore, suppressive treatment in Case Four led to the displacement of bronchitis resulting in the metastatic eruption of chronic migraines. The increased rate of heart attacks associated with a class of non-steroidal anti-inflammatory drugs used to treat arthritis is a perfect example of metastasis. The most popular of these, Vioxx, was taken off the market. While the industry acknowledges the relationship, it does not understand the heart attacks to be a metastatic product of suppressing arthritis with these powerful drugs.

In some cases of cancer, suppressive therapy may be a reasonable choice of action that may buy a very sick person some valuable time. It is not at all unusual, though, that, while the cancer seems to go into remission, the person is subsequently stricken with another serious illness such as severe anemia, or a life-threatening blood disorder, and may even succumb to an acute infection like pneumonia. Regrettably, these are the metastatic outcomes of powerfully suppressive cancer therapies. While such powerful therapies may sometimes be justified as a last resort, they are a dead-end strategy for dealing with most acute and chronic ailments and virtually guarantee an endless maze of iatrogenic twists and turns. It may be necessary at times to forcibly intervene in the event of very threatening situations, as in appendicitis, severe pneumonia, acute asthmatic attack, and so on. But these interventions should be considered temporary, stopgap measures, to be employed only as necessary until safer and more effective non-suppressive solutions can be found. The conventional medical establishment must be willing to entertain greener alternative solutions that take into account long-term consequences.

In any event, palliative or suppressive measures are sometimes necessary, but the vast majority of medical conditions do not rise to this level of urgency, and so there is no need in these cases to resort to therapeutic methods that carry with them the risk of suppression and metastasis. Of course, palliation is almost always preferable to suppression but it cannot reliably be predicted whether an ailment under conventional treatment will metastasize or not. I am always uncomfortable and suspicious when I hear that an ailment treated by conventional means has not returned after time has elapsed. Conversely, when a client under my care reports the return of some old ailment that was previously treated by orthodox methods, then I am usually pleased by this development. I take it as a sign that the bioenergetic field was resilient enough to fight back by reinstating the original symptoms, which regular treatment tried to suppress. A weaker defense mechanism would have succumbed to suppression, thus requiring it to find a new avenue of symptomatic expression in order to register its distress.

Unfortunately, Western medicine has turned palliation and suppression into high art forms and it doesn't even know it. I propose to you that the Medical Emperor is wearing not a stitch of clothing beneath that white coat, and sadly, most of us are unable to see this because we are duped by propaganda and dazzled by the technological prowess of modern medicine. Although Western medicine may be largely unconscious of the effect the Emperor is having, it does not really want to know, because in the long run, it is good for business. If we accept the premise that orthodox treatment tends to encourage the development of deeper, more obstinate, and more chronic illness, then it follows that it also creates an endless source of renewed customers—customers who are deluded into thinking that they are receiving the best care the world has to offer. When we c
stand that the vast majority of medical interventions are at
and at worst suppressive, and that cure is a rare and uninte
then the ramifications become profound and disturbing.

Another interesting example of the inappropriate use of medical language is the term *side effect*. We are lulled into false complacency when we accept the subliminal message that a side effect is not a real effect or direct effect of a medication. Rather, we are encouraged to believe that it is just an annoying little symptom of peripheral concern that can occasionally occur in relation to a given medication. This convenient medical euphemism disguises the reality that a side effect is a direct and real effect caused by a drug. The propensity of the left-brain to compartmentalize allows regular medicine to convince us that the desirable effects are the direct, real, and intended result of a drug, while the undesirable effects are not the real effects but merely the minor, indirect, side effects of the product in question. We are programmed to believe that the desired effect of a drug is very common while side effects are atypical or even rare. This is far from the truth, and in fact, the reverse may actually be the case. It is not unusual for a patient to experience the side effects of a drug, such as the infamously toxic effect that some cholesterol drugs have upon the liver, while obtaining no benefit from that therapy, i.e., no improvement in the cholesterol profile. It is possible that an anti-hypertensive drug may cause the well-documented side effects of dry mouth and impotence while failing to lower the blood pressure. A lot of bad medicine gets a free pass when its actual effects are allowed to slide by under the innocuous rubric of "side effects."

Since the notion of a side effect is a fabrication of the medical mind designed to downplay dangers and increase compliance, we must begin the process of re-education by throwing this term out the window in the full knowledge that, with one major exception, all of the effects of any given drug are direct effects. That exception, of course, is the suppressive effect. The direct impact of an anti-hypertensive drug is to lower blood pressure, but if a patient subsequently falls into a depression we may accurately characterize this as the indirect, metastatic result of suppressed blood pressure. The depression is still linked to the drug but in an indirect way that medical science can easily dismiss as coincidental and unrelated. Similarly, while in Case One the direct effect of antibiotic treatment was the resolution of the cellulitis infection, the unfortunate suppressive effect resulted in metastasis, which manifested in the form of asthma.

Remembering that the life force of each individual is a unique energetic phenomenon, and that the dynamics that we have been discussing are general guidelines and not rules written in stone, it can sometimes be difficult to distinguish between a direct or suppressive effect. It is also entirely plausible that a healthy and resilient life force may rebound quite nicely and show no signs of being worse for the wear, even after the patient has taken an antibiotic or some other drug. Nevertheless, suppression is such a common and potentially devastating outcome from the use of pharmaceuticals that extreme caution must be employed so that most drugs are ultimately used only when absolutely necessary. When taking a medication leads to the worst case scenario, such as kidney or liver disease or a blood disorder, simply discontinuing use of the drug will usually not solve the problem since it is often too late to go back once the damage has been done. When future green practitioners look back upon our current era of suppressive medical therapies, they will marvel at allopathy's ability to ignore the obvious and the absurd lengths to which it pursued such a dead-end strategy.

SPIRITUAL ILLNESS

If these arguments regarding the vital energy and suppression are true, that is enough bad news to absorb in one sitting. But I am sorry to say that I have not yet even raised the most disturbing issue. If we return for a moment to the energetic gradient of the life force, which was discussed in an earlier chapter, you will recall that a hierarchical relationship exists among body, emotion, mind, and spirit. A healthy person will manifest symptoms and illness at the least threatening and most superficial level of the gradient, as exemplified by a rash, a cold, or a temporary mood. A compromised life force will manifest illness on a deeper level and often in chronic form, as typified by asthma, arthritis, or depression. The innate wisdom of the vital energy ensures the best possible outcome given what it has to work with and so it will, at all times, attempt to exteriorize the disturbance to the best of its ability. As the resistance of the energy field weakens, an illness may penetrate more deeply into the energetic interior of the individual.

With this natural hierarchical order in mind, it is very important to understand that suppressive treatments tend to push an illness, energetic disturbance, or imbalance further along that gradient, from exterior toward interior, and from body to emotion to mind and ultimately, to spirit and soul. While this may seem a controversial assertion, it must be named for what it is: The predominating use of suppressive therapies is the one most important factor accounting for the ever-increasing signs of emotional and spiritual illness that are so evident in contemporary society. This trend is further exacerbated by the imbalances of patriarchal and technological culture and its dissociative ability to ignore all but the most physical of realities.

This, to me, is the most important take-home point of this book and so I will state this as plainly as I can: Indiscriminate treatment of physical or minor emotional symptoms often leads to a greater likelihood of psychiatric and spiritual disease. A superficial preoccupation with treating surface symptoms, especially with potentially suppressive methods, as is the case with most modern pharmaceuticals and surgeries, encourages the development of mental, emotional, and spiritual illness. Even the seemingly benign treatment of a common cold with over-the-counter medicines can contribute to the possibility of illness on a deeper level. Although the cold symptoms targeted may appear to improve for a while, and all may seem to be well, this is only an illusion. Exerting pressure upon the outermost physical level of the gradient forces the energy of the system toward the interior, where it can regroup to generate new and more threatening health issues.

I make these claims with absolute sincerity and the utmost conviction, based upon years of observation and practical experience. I do not cite scientific proof or research to back up my claims because, as I have stated before, the parameters of conventional science are too narrow to grasp the nature of what I am trying to convey here. The reality of these energetic dynamics transcends left-brain concepts and methodologies. What is vitally important is that we begin to recognize the impact that mechanistic medicine is having upon our collective health. A simple understanding of these powerful truths can provide people with the confidence that they need, thus enabling them to say, "No thank you," when tempted by the many societal pressures to acquiesce to unnecessary health care interventions.

No doubt many will misunderstand this, and those who are motivated by fear to defend the dying paradigm of mechanistic medicine will twist it beyond recognition. So I must reiterate that I am not seeking to blame, disparage, or impugn the reputations of the many dedicated health care professionals who seek to ease the sufferings of humanity. Certainly, I am not suggesting that we dispense with all conventional drugs and surgeries. To the contrary, I am proposing a balance between right- and left-brain medical thought and methodology. I am pointing out the implications of a form of medicine that most of us have come to accept without understanding the nature of its long-term consequences. However, before balance can be achieved, the truth must be spoken regarding the pitfalls and dangers of this exclusively left-brained approach.

Every medical situation is unique, and the accumulated conventional, alternative, and esoteric medical knowledge and experience of humankind should be brought to bear in each case so that the most appropriate course of action may be taken, with the ultimate understanding and consent of the patient. Every individual has a different threshold for pain and suffering, and each illness carries with it its own unique degree of threat or harmlessness. Some individuals can easily forgo treatment where others may beg for relief. The physician's job is not to provide relief regardless of the consequences, but to ascertain the level of health threat that any given condition poses and to then educate patients regarding the short- and long-term consequences of the various available therapeutic modalities.

Instead, the prevailing health care mentality mirrors the superficiality and image consciousness of our culture, which has little tolerance for the slightest pimple, blemish, wart, sniffle, or runny nose. If we actually believe that an underarm sweat stain in the boardroom signals a lack of professionalism, then this fact alone indicates societal mental illness. The reality is that we all pee, poop, sneeze, and sweat, and no amount of medical technology will ever change that. A sober and clear-minded assessment of the suppressive nature of orthodox medicine will be a necessary prerequisite to meaningful changes that can lead to improvements in our collective cultural health. In the spirit of achieving that clarity let us continue with an example that illustrates the concepts that we have been exploring.

A COMPOSITE PEDIATRIC HISTORY

If I could paint a composite picture encapsulating the medical histories of some of the more common cases of childhood and adolescent illnesses that I have seen over the years, it might go something like this: A newborn boy came into the world by normal vaginal delivery, had good Apgar scores, and was sent home with a clean bill of health. After a few weeks, the child developed a mild diaper rash that was treated with talcum powder. The rash subsided for a while but eventually recurred, only this time with greater intensity. A pediatrician recommended that the mother apply zinc oxide ointment to the rash. To everyone's satisfaction, the rash promptly disappeared and all was well—until several days later, when the boy became mildly irritable and started waking more frequently at night. The pediatrician reassured the mother that nothing was wrong and suggested that the sleep trouble would probably settle down on its own. A few days later, after the sleep had improved, the child developed a sniffly, runny nose. Again the pediatrician opted to wait, advising that it was only a minor cold.

All was well for a while, until the child's first birthday when, after his first MMR (measles, mumps, rubella) shot, he immediately ran his first fever ever and became quite irritable. The pediatrician advised that this was a normal reaction to the vaccine and recommended Tylenol to reduce the fever. Within a few days the child seemed to be back to normal but, two weeks later, he ran another fever and this time was diagnosed with an ear infection. The doctor prescribed Amoxicillin, and within a few days the child recovered, although his appetite took two weeks to fully return to normal. Over the next eight months the child contracted four more ear infections, each requiring additional courses of antibiotics. By this time, even though the latest ear infection had resolved, the child had developed a chronically poor appetite, a stuffed-up nose, occasional loose stools, disturbed sleep patterns, and periods of irritable behavior.

As time passed, the ear infections faded and gradually morphed into what were now being diagnosed as sinus infections. These were characterized by a stuffed-up nose, thick yellow nasal discharge, a nasal-sounding voice, and occasional coughing. They occurred at least four to six times per year and were treated with decongestants and antibiotics. By the age of five this child continued to have a pretty picky appetite, periods of irritability, and was slowly becoming more prone to whiny, dissatisfied behavior.

During the summer of his eighth year, the child started to develop a runny nose, itchy eyes, and a bit of a cough. At the same time, he developed an itchy rash at the creases of both elbows. The pediatrician now determined that the child had both allergies and eczema. The doctor prescribed an antihistamine for the allergies and recommended a topical steroid for the eczema. Each application of steroid cream diminished the rash, but it would gradually return if left untreated. Likewise, the antihistamine partially alleviated the allergies, but they only cleared up fully at the end of the summer. The following summer, while rounding the bases during a Little League game, the child began to have difficulty breathing. Another visit to the pediatrician's office determined that the child was wheezing. The doctor made a new diagnosis of asthma and prescribed a daily steroid inhaler to be used along with another inhaler in the event of an acute attack of asthma.

The child's chronic whininess and irritability soon began to escalate. It now took him up to two hours beyond his usual bedtime to fall asleep. Sometimes he became downright defiant about going to bed. The parents tried a variety of strategies but were increasingly unable to manage his difficult behaviors. The child continued on daily asthma medication, and an antihistamine was added during the summers for the allergies. By the time the boy was eleven, reports began to come home from school regarding his behavior. One teacher observed him hitting a classmate, and another noted that he had failed to complete several assignments. The school psychologist was notified and, at a family meeting, the parents reassured school officials that there was nothing unusual going on at home and no marital disharmony that might be affecting the boy. They did acknowledge though, that their child's behavior was becoming increasingly difficult.

It was not long before a psychiatrist confirmed everyone's suspicions by concluding that the child's behavior was consistent with the diagnostic criteria for attention deficit hyperactivity disorder (ADHD). The doctor prescribed daily doses of Ritalin, and some of the difficulty in school settled down, but the child became rather subdued, almost lethargic, and at times appeared to be depressed. The child's already picky appetite took a nosedive, and the parents became concerned about the child's lack of growth and weight gain. The psychiatrist suggested the possibility of an antidepressant but the parents, whose frustration level had peaked by now, objected to any further medication.

Some variation of this scenario is unfolding right now in homes and doctors' offices across the nation, and while it used to be the exception, I believe that it is fast becoming the norm. Recent reports have associated ADHD drugs with an increased incidence of suicidal thoughts and hallucinations. This is not at all surprising and is the likely effect of these drugs' suppressive influence upon the symptoms of ADHD. Similarly, while antidepressants often reduce feelings and symptoms of depression, there are many who experience a decline in cognitive function while taking them. The suppressive impact of antidepressants can create a zombie-like effect, typified by a flat emotional affect, dullness of mind, and slowness of thinking. In essence, for some the trade-off becomes mental impairment in lieu of emotional impairment. While these are obvious examples of adverse drug effects, the suppressive nature of most drugs cause many other, more subtle and insidious effects that continue to go largely unrecognized.

Fortunately, somewhere along this dysfunctional chain of events, many people are beginning to question the wisdom of pursing an avenue of treatment that digs them deeper and deeper into a hole. Since the medical community usually does not offer alternatives, parents are placed in the position of having to look for answers on their own. They may begin to ask around among other parents of children that they know, and this is often how they wind up seeking help from alternative sources.

CREATING CHRONICITY

In the composite case above, even if you had no prior knowledge of the issues that we have been discussing, you can almost feel the suppressed and tangled mess of defense-mechanism distress as it gradually accumulates and snowballs out of control—like the ultimate game of symptomatic whack-a-mole—only here the mole with a diaper rash has mutated into a fire breathing dragon labeled ADHD. As orthodox medicine puzzles cluelessly over the reasons for rapidly rising rates of allergies, asthma, autism, and ADHD in our children, contemporary Greek homeopath, George Vithoulkas, summarizes the nature of the proverbial elephant sitting in the room:

> *It appears that almost no one within established medicine or society recognizes the fact that the development of chronic disease is neither accidental nor incidental, but is a strict, almost mathematical, sequence of events which many times originates from wrong treatment and the use of crude chemical drugs.*[77]

Since this dynamic applies not just to children with allergies and asthma but to all persons pursuing symptomatic drug therapy for their illnesses, the potential ramifications of this false form of healing are staggering. Keeping in mind that a healthy life force is more likely to produce an acute illness like a cold, fever, or flu, and that a weaker one is more susceptible to chronic disease, Vithoulkas reminds us of the general trajectory of societal illness over the past hundred years or so:

> *Statistics demonstrate quite clearly that the threat of acute diseases has diminished in this century, although not because of therapeutic effectiveness, and that there is a corresponding increase in crippling chronic diseases, cancer, heart disease, strokes, neurological disorders and epilepsy, violence, and insanity. Such is the inevitable result when the processes of Nature are ignored.*[78]

In terms of the prevalence and depth of mental and emotional illness, it is by no means a stretch to say that the United States, the country with the most advanced health care system, and the world's number one producer and purveyor of pharmaceuticals, may arguably be one of the sickest nations on earth. Although many other factors contribute to this trend, such as the stress created by the gutting of basic social services, the relentless emphasis upon competition, the go-it-alone pull-yourself-up-by-your-bootstraps mentality, and much more, drug therapies that produce symptomatic suppression may be the leading factor contributing to mental-emotional illness and spiritual emptiness in this country. What with antibiotics for every sniffle, steroid creams for every skin eruption, antihistamines for every itch, and a virtual avalanche of foreign substances injected into the body via vaccines, the vital energy of the average American kid does-n't stand a chance. In tiny increments, with each successive dose of over-the-counter or prescription medication taken, the center of gravity of the disturbance is slowly and progressively pushed away from the periphery toward the deepest levels of the organism.

The discerning eye can easily recognize the myriad manifestations of mental illness that permeate modern culture. The icy cold machismo exhib-ited by our Hollywood heroes and the shocking levels of violence displayed nightly on our television screens, the distorted and pervasive atmosphere of fear fomented by the sensationalist mass media, our frenzied and self-ish need to go faster, do more, own more, and consume more are all clear signs of a national psyche that has lost its sense of reality and perspective. Those who perceive the rudderlessness, narcissism, and lack of moral sen-sibility in society should be disconcerted. And it is truly scary to consider that all this is largely beyond our conscious control as long as we fail to perceive the role played by our prevailing mode of medical care.

The point of this discussion, therefore, is not to pass moral judgment upon the evils of technology and modern society, but to warn of the dan-gers inherent in embracing a mechanistic form of medicine that treats body, mind, and soul like a machine whose parts can be manipulated with-out concern for the impact upon the whole. Simply stated, from a holistic perspective, symptom suppression inevitably leads to deeper forms of ill-ness that are very difficult, if not impossible, to reverse with the conven-tional medical tools that we have at our disposal. It will take a significant shift of consciousness to allow us to collectively embrace the green med-ical paradigm before we can turn the tide in a positive direction. It will require that we step out of our comfort zone, shed our fears of the unknown, and come to see that all things are a manifestation of the One, and that running away from our problems, or suppressing them, are tem-porary band-aid approaches that will only lead to more complications and greater suffering.

Let us briefly review. Iatrogenesis can be defined as any treatment-induced illness and, although presumed to be the result of medical mis-takes, the far greater proportion of iatrogenesis is caused by what is believed to be appropriate medical treatment. The concept of cure in the practice of Western medicine is largely an illusion because most treatments do not lead to long-term health improvement. Treatment implies only that something is being done and carries with it no indication of success or failure. Management usually applies to chronic illness that cannot be cured and which therefore requires ongoing treatment. Palliation brings only temporarily relief and does not remove the cause of illness. Suppression occurs when a treatment forcibly prevents an illness from being expressed. In contradistinction to cure, suppression does not result in subsequent improvement of health. Metastasis is the backlash of suppression that occurs when an illness is displaced by a new manifestation of illness—one that is usually worse than the original. The vast majority of conventional medical treatments can be categorized as palliative or suppressive, since they rarely lead to genuine cure. Side effect is a euphemistic term used to downplay the unpleasant effects of a drug. There are no side effects, only direct effects, or indirect effects caused by suppression. Suppressive treatment forces the energetic expression of an illness toward the interior of the organism, resulting in a much greater likelihood of chronic disease and mental, emotional, and spiritual illness. This trend can be reversed if we think beyond the parameters of the material paradigm that ministers only to the physical body, and begin to perceive the realities of the unfulfilled needs of the body-heart-mind-soul.

Next, we will examine why it is so difficult for orthodox medicine to accept other modes of thought and perception. The answer has much to do with modern society's religious faith in technology and science, which, in turn, gives license to mainstream medicine to forgo the very scientific principles upon which it claims to be based.

12

The Sanctity of Science

MEDICINE AS RELIGION

The independent country doctor of the past has been replaced by large group practices, medical specialty clinics, medical laboratories, managed care bureaucracies, diagnostic imaging facilities, and those churches of medicine, our modern hospitals. In days long gone, churches were the largest and most centrally located buildings in many communities. The twentieth century saw the rise of the skyscraper, that monument to finance, industry, power, and wealth, which towered high above even the largest of churches. And we are now witnessing the runaway growth of the medical-industrial complex. While the buildings of this medical infrastructure may not stand as tall as some skyscrapers, the wealth and power that they represent are rivaled only by the military-industrial complex and the oil industry. Worship of the divine is eroding and is gradually being displaced by the glorification of capitalism, and the accumulation of corporate wealth has become heavily dependent upon the three pillars of weapons, oil, and pharmaceuticals. And modern medicine has increasingly come to resemble and fulfill the role of a form of religious practice, with its very large contingent of devout worshipers.

Most people view the barons of the oil industry with suspicion, and while many see the generals on the battlefield as heroes, they are heroes who are nevertheless answerable to the populace and government that they serve. The scientists and high priests of medicine, however, enjoy a unique status in modern culture, revered by the mainstream and mass media, and accountable to almost no one but themselves. As medicine expands seemingly without limitation, the patient and the patient's ills take a backseat to the needs and greed of the health care system. Worse yet, the patient who submits to the authority of the false gods of medicine often becomes less well off in the long run than when he or she first sought help from the system. Thus the benefits that accrue to the sick and suffering are a far cry from the status and wealth enjoyed by the system itself. I believe that in actuality they have an inverse relationship. The medical system maintains a parasitic relationship with its patients, upon whom it depends for *its* well-being. There is little interest, therefore, in seeing that the health of patients actually improves over time, since that would mean that they might become less dependent upon medical services.

The spiritual vacuum produced by our materialistic culture constitutes a vacancy that modern medicine has come to fill. Science, especially technological medicine, has usurped the role of spirituality, and in the process has *become* a religion to many. Not surprisingly, contemporary medicine exhibits all the earmarks of an organized form of religious practice. Medical buildings are our cathedrals, doctors our priests, and medical procedures our rituals. The doctor's white coat and stethoscope are symbols that carry greater significance for contemporary men and women than do the antiquated vestments and chalice of the priest. More important, the institution of medicine engenders a genuine faith and commands a subservience that many followers are no longer willing to pledge to organized religion. While organized religion has, to some extent, lost its power and authority over the general populace, medicine has not.

The patriarchal and authoritarian nature of Western medicine forms a direct parallel to the three monotheistic religious systems of Christianity, Judaism, and Islam. All are male-dominated faiths that claim the one true creator: God, Yahweh, and Allah, respectively. As to the identity of the god of medicine, I don't know—how about Big Pharma, or the Rational Mind? I will let you choose your own name. Just like the three big monotheistic faiths, medicine stubbornly insists upon its version of reality as the only true and viable perspective, while frequently seeking to discredit competing viewpoints. It routinely dismisses other methods of healing as naïve, unscientific, or irrational. Spokespersons for the mainstream periodically muster up the audacity to claim that alternative practitioners are just charlatans out to make a buck. Sadly, even sensible-minded people tend to swallow this propaganda without realizing the irony of such a claim.

When Western medicine is challenged with a particularly persuasive argument for the plausibility of another way, it may cite the sacred medical texts in order to invalidate the competing heresy. The "Scientific Study" represents the word of the god of science, and the final authority against which no person may argue. The familiar refrain, "Show me the studies," can silence even the most tenacious dissenter, who becomes intimidated and overwhelmed by the incontrovertible statistical truths of the "Sacred Studies." When the dissenter has the presence of mind to point out the ever-changing, ephemeral, and contradictory nature of the "Scientific Studies," the true believer in the infallibility of science is likely to respond by noting that this is the normal means by which scientific progress is made.

Similarly, when a patient insists upon the validity of personal symptomatic experience as evidence that may make a valuable contribution toward his or her own health care, medical church authorities are likely to dismiss this as mere "anecdote." The utterance of this single word puts the congregant back in a subservient place and transmits the unequivocal message that firsthand experience takes a backseat to the rational abstractions and statistical analyses of the Sacred Studies. The tenets of conventional medicine resemble a religious dogma that discredits opposing views and answers to no outside entity. Not unlike some authoritarian religious dogmas, orthodox medicine disempowers the individual and tries to convince us that true salvation can only be had under its auspices.

In a not so subtle way, the institutions of Western medicine can systematically strip the individual of all that is essential to the preservation of good health. Therefore, the average unsuspecting person, sometimes experiences a stay at the hospital for a simple procedure as a nightmare of humiliation designed to keep him or her in a submissive posture. Personal clothing is traded in for the generic white gown, a bland representation of the grade-school food pyramid replaces a healthy diet, sleep deprivation is induced by nurses following doctors' orders throughout the night, and the patient is there to listen and not to be heard. The priorities of the institution take precedence over the needs of the individual. In practical terms, these routine practices reminiscent of the industrial assembly line can make all the difference between a positive or negative outcome of a patient's struggle with illness. True empowerment of the patient remains an alien concept within the halls of medicine, where standard practices run contrary to the fundamentals of green medical philosophy.

MEDICAL FUNDAMENTALISM

The gods of modern medicine demand conformity and allegiance to an unnatural synthetic chemical armamentarium produced and supplied by a profit-driven corporate industry. Doctors surgically remove uncooperative body parts without a second thought. As medicine increasingly becomes a corporate endeavor, service with a personal touch becomes less likely, and patients are often faced with anonymous personnel who are less emotionally invested in the job at hand. All things natural and of the earth are viewed with suspicion. All causes are taken to be physical, leaving no room for the supernatural or spiritual. The one true material god of causality is worshiped to the exclusion of all other healing methods, persuasions, and belief systems. These are just a few of the sacred beliefs and practices of the "fundamentalist" doctrine of orthodox medicine. To think or act otherwise is to risk exposing oneself to ridicule and being branded an infidel.

As with all exclusionary dogmas, Western medicine needs an adversary to keep the forces of righteousness focused in the battle of good versus evil. As discussed earlier, symptoms are to be fought without quarter. All symptoms evoke a fear of the Evil One, Death, which serves to keep the faithful in line. The struggle against death is the unimpeachable banner under which the crusade against sickness is waged. Symptoms produced by the vital force and its natural wisdom are perverted into malevolent entities that might unleash their malignant influence unless they are stopped at all costs. Diplomacy, understanding, and cooperation with the vital energy are signs of weakness in this male-dominated arena where the false dragons are slain. Those who may begin to question the wisdom of church authorities are threatened with the withdrawal of the promise of protection from the scourge of disease.

When doubt begins to creep in, those "miracles of medicine" public relations stories are always there to shore up our wavering faith. One need only open the morning paper or turn on the evening news to find a glowing story about the grateful person whose life was saved by the latest development in surgical technique or medical technology. Not to take away from the value of some of these advancements, but the video clips and sound bites selectively produced for our consumption are rarely reflective of the whole story that plays out once the cameras are turned off and the reporters have gone home. We hear about the short-term miracle but not about the longer-term reality. Heart-warming stories paint rosy pictures and focus on the positive, while the everyday nitty-gritty details are rarely told. The front-page story trumpets the transplant as a resounding success but three months later a small notice on page ten tells us that the patient has died from complications. Our faith is undying and when the basket is passed at the medical church fundraiser, we give generously in support of physicians and institutions that continue to use the same old toxic chemical and surgical formulas to treat our physical ills. Ivan Illich weighs in on our belief in medical miracles and how they provide cover for the failures of the physician:

> *Public fascination with high-technology care and death can be understood as a deep-seated need for the engineering of miracles. Intensive care is but the culmination of a public worship organized around a medical priesthood struggling against death.*[79]
>
> *Medicine claims the patient even when the etiology is uncertain, the prognosis unfavorable, and the therapy of an experimental nature. Under these circumstances the attempt at a "medical miracle" can be a hedge against failure, since miracles may only be hoped for and cannot, by definition, be expected.*[80]

Microbiologist René Dubos views the belief in medical miracles with a similar critical eye:

> *Men want miracles as much today as in the past. If they do not join one of the new cults, they satisfy this need by worshiping at the altar of modern science.*
>
> *There are always men starved for hope or greedy for sensation who will testify to the healing power of a spectacular surgical feat or of a new miracle drug. They provide the testimonies of the new religions for which scientists with theories unproved or incomplete are always ready to provide the mystic language.*[81]

Our faith in the miracle of technology is understandable in the face of so much sickness and disease, as even those doing the "objective" reporting desire to believe in the inevitable triumph of the church of modern medicine over death and dying. Childhood indoctrination begins with early science education, as all good followers are taught that medical mistakes are to be pardoned because salvation ultimately lies with the progress of medicine through the trial and error of the scientific method. How many of us have witnessed the remaining days of a dying loved one spent as a guinea pig for the experimental treatment of the medical minister? Since it is heresy to admit defeat in the face of the Evil One, there is a small chance, we are told, that this latest concoction of toxic chemicals, which has never before been tried in this combination, may allow the patient to "survive" just a little while longer. In the end, when the patient succumbs, we are conditioned to understand that the good doctor did the best that could be done. And this is usually true—given the limitations that the medical priesthood places upon the doctor.

Ritual and ceremony, likewise, are performed to strengthen the faith of good churchgoers who, in turn, feel safe and protected by the gods of medicine from the threat of disease. As new rituals are instituted, devotees unquestioningly yield to the scientific authority of the medical clergy, and the list of tests and trials grows with each passing year. And so we submit to the annual physical exam, waiting patiently for hours in reception rooms, disrobing for strangers, having our blood pressure, temperature, and pulse checked, having blood drawn from our veins, urinating in cups, allowing our insides to be x-rayed, and our bone densities to be measured, sedating ourselves for colonoscopies, allowing breasts to be bruised for mammograms, and drinking radioactive sludge for expensive diagnostic imaging. In an act of supreme faith, many participate in perhaps the most important sacrament of all, as we open our mouths to receive "the body of Big Pharma." Whether helpful or harmful, these rituals inspire confidence in the true believer and provide an endless revenue stream for church coffers.

Paradoxically, even though orthodox medicine willingly assumes these religious functions for modern technological society, it refuses to accept the responsibility that comes with such a position of trust and leadership. When the going gets tough and its methods are questioned, and the promise of greater health remains unrealized by those with a growing sense of disbelief, the profession can always fall back upon the claim of scientific objectivity, which serves to shield the medical priesthood from all moral issues and their implications. After all, as you will recall, science is promoted as an "amoral" enterprise that is not subject to the considerations of good or bad, right or wrong. Rationalizations of this nature allow the health care community to have its cake and eat it, too. The physician is given the role and authority of priest but denies ethical and moral responsibility when the mad scientific experiment goes awry.

SACRAMENTAL ASSAULT ON THE IMMUNE SYSTEM

We cannot provide a thorough accounting of the pluses and minuses of conventional medicine without wading into the most sacred territory of all, the crowning achievement of medical science which, until recently, like the story of Christopher Columbus discovering America, no one dared to question. I am referring to that most revered medical sacrament, vaccination. Like many other medical rituals, the underlying assumptions that justify vaccination, its value, and importance are based mostly in faith, thus exempting it from genuine scientific examination and questioning. The greatest act of faith of all is demonstrated through the sacramental rite of vaccination, as great trust must be placed in any authority that would be allowed to routinely inject our children with an ever-expanding list of pathogens based upon the promise of protection from those very same agents of disease.

As it currently stands, forty-eight individual doses from a pool of fourteen different vaccines are administered to our children by the time they have reached the age of six, with more to come as they get older, and many more in the experimental pipeline that have yet to be produced and marketed. It is the truly fortunate individual that escapes unscathed from such a systematic and relentless assault upon the immune system. The strange silence in the face of the devastation that has been wrought is a testament to the unblinking belief of the general public. And when congregants complain, they must contend with the overwhelming moral force and legal authority of the medical church.

The administration of Hepatitis B vaccine at birth, before newborns even leave the hospital, has become the equivalent of modern medical baptism. This practice sets the stage for a lifetime of medical interventions, most of which are unwarranted, stand upon shaky scientific ground, and carry with them serious risks to life and limb. This first encounter with Big Pharma, together with the surgical practice of circumcision, constitute the initiatory rites of indoctrination that will be reinforced in a multitude of ways over the ensuing years. The laity is conditioned to conform to an arbitrarily arranged schedule of vaccinations set up primarily for the convenience of the pediatrician and the maximization of compliance and profit.

Thus, at two months of age, eight more vaccines are administered, seven more at four months, and eight more at six months of age. The infant, who surely would perish without constant attention to his or her every need by an adult, and who has barely begun to develop the most basic rudiments of a functioning immune system, is mandated to receive twenty-four vaccine doses by the time he or she has reached six months of age.

Let us consider for a moment this reality facing our children in its simplest terms. Virtually any substance whatsoever is capable of producing a mild to severe allergic reaction in certain individuals at any given time. There is no reliable way to predict who may react to what because, as we have already established, the status of the vital force and its susceptibilities is unique to each person. Most non-vaccine related allergic reactions are caused by contact of an allergen with the skin, mucus membranes, or digestive tract. Imagine now if those same allergens were injected directly into the blood stream or subcutaneous tissues. The potential for harm increases significantly when exposure to an allergen occurs in this manner, since it bypasses the skin and mucus membranes, which comprise the body's protective barrier and first line of defense against all foreign substances. It is not hard to imagine what devastation would occur if all those children that have been turning up allergic to peanuts were instead injected with peanut extract. Mandating injection with foreign disease agents guarantees a certain percentage of casualties.

The more familiar a substance is to our bodies and the more we come into contact with it, the more likely we are to adapt to it and not read it as a threat. The more foreign the substance we encounter, the greater the likelihood of an allergic reaction. Most children have never come into contact with these germs prior to being vaccinated. If every child is injected with close to fifty doses of foreign proteins, the expectation of allergic reaction should be very high indeed.

Truth and common sense are ignored in the name of medical progress and a religious fervor that views all bacteria and viruses as enemies to be eradicated in the misguided crusade against germs. Blind faith, in this case, trumps good judgment and rational thought. The war takes on a life of its own, with each aspect of the medical machine doing its part, yet none taking ultimate responsibility when tragedy strikes. Big Pharma manufactures the product, members of the medical profession send out the warning cry, and the mass media dutifully parrots this propaganda by broadcasting fear across the airwaves. Every autumn we are fed horror stories and dire warnings regarding the impending flu season, and told that we had better hurry on down to our doctor's office because precious vaccine is in short supply. Inexplicably, we never seem to hear about the wide range of adverse reactions, sad stories, and casualties that result from this poorly thought out medico-religious strategy.

To greater or lesser extent, all vaccines have been proven by conventional scientific studies and acknowledged by the orthodox medical establishment to be associated with a wide range of adverse reactions. There is no denying this fundamental truth. From the most immediate, obvious, and minor reactions that frequently occur, such as pain and swelling at the injection site, fever, rashes, hives, cough, runny nose, headache, sore throat, swollen glands, diarrhea, vomiting, irritability, sleep disturbance, and loss of appetite—all the way up to the more serious acute and long-term sequelae, such as prolonged crying, anaphylactic shock, jaundice, arthritis, blood disorders like thrombocytopenia, neurologic disorders like seizures, multiple sclerosis, encephalopathy, optic neuritis, Guillain-Barre syndrome, and even death—all of these are well documented phenomena that can take place anytime, from minutes to days to weeks after the administration of vaccines. These symptoms and sequelae, and many more, are clearly described in the *Physicians' Desk Reference* in the "Contraindications," "Warnings," "Precautions," and "Adverse Reactions" sections under the listing for each particular vaccine. But, as we shall see, this is only the tip of the iceberg when it comes to the threat that wholesale vaccination represents. Furthermore, the church of medicine loses much of its credibility when it periodically sends out its hollow and hysterical warnings regarding the dangers of "unproven" alternative therapies.

Evidence of the dangers of vaccination is so overwhelming that I am tempted to play the statistical game in order to prove my point, but I know that my battery of data is likely to be met with contradictory data and rationalizations intended to prove the opposite. In the end, I know that my standards of acceptable risk are significantly different from the usual left-brained "risks versus the benefits" arguments. For me, there is no amount of rationalization or statistical manipulation that can prove the safety or justify the necessity of any therapy that has been shown to regularly result in the deaths of patients who were healthy prior to that therapy. When adverse reactions do result in death, the authorities responsible need to acknowledge this reality rather than shifting into spin mode. If this were the case, parents could be on the receiving end of information that might actually help them decide whether they are willing to submit their children to such risk. As it stands, modern medicine directs significant medical resources toward downplaying the reality of those risks, thereby distorting the truth for the average person who does not have the time and energy to undertake a personal investigation. Being a parent is tough enough without having to stop and become an expert on immunization in anticipation of bringing children into the world.

My own experience tells me that not only are the mounting casualties from vaccine injuries very real and in many cases devastating, but the true extent of chronic and debilitating disease resulting from this public health crusade against germs has yet to be understood and acknowledged for the debacle that it is. The compartmentalized perspective of rational medicine easily considers a vaccine reaction, such as high fever, to be a one-time event that has come and gone and is therefore no longer relevant or of concern. Unfortunately, the vital force tends not to interpret these events in quite the same way. A vaccine reaction can leave an energetic scar that may have significant ramifications for the immune system and its future.

When the life force encounters an unnatural attack from a foreign antigen that has been injected, thus bypassing the body's normal protective barrier, its acute response to this grave threat can be intense, and the response pattern that sets in afterwards can, in some cases, cause a lifetime of chronic illness. In the short-term, patients can die, and in the long-term, their immune systems are dazed and confused. In the misguided attempt to create immunity to a particular germ, a single vaccine can cause the immune system to go haywire, resulting in immunologic chaos. I like to compare it to a car having electrical problems wherein the most unexpected and bizarre phenomena can occur. Similarly, there is no telling what type of immunologic dysfunction may arise, as it is completely dependent upon the interaction of the unique germ with the equally unique vital force. As such, a seemingly benign one-time event like a high fever after vaccination can be the precipitating factor that leads, even years later, to the development of chronic illnesses like rheumatoid arthritis, diabetes, or attention deficit disorder.

I firmly believe that this systematic assault upon the immune system is far and away the leading cause of autoimmune disease in our modern world. The unparalleled desecration of the Earth's ecosystems with an untold number of synthetic toxins and poisons produced by the chemical and pharmaceutical industries comes in a close second, but the destructive effects of vaccination are, in many cases, immediate and undeniable and, in some cases, long-term and potentially irreversible. Autoimmune attack of the body upon itself is the mechanism underlying nearly all of today's most problematic illnesses. There is little doubt in my mind that the frightening rise of childhood chronic diseases, like allergies, asthma, neurologic disorders, and behavior disorders, can be most directly attributed to this indiscriminate bombardment of the immune system. Amazingly, the church of medicine's public relations efforts have been more than adequate thus far at deflecting any and all blame. The public is shielded from the truth and the elephant in the room is ignored, while experts puzzle over our mysterious and unexplained epidemic of chronic disease.

A special note should be made regarding the startling rise of autism in our time. While the usual pattern of failure to develop socially and neurologically associated with autism remains somewhat of a mystery, a more specific type of "regressive" autism, in which a previously normally developing child suddenly or gradually decompensates, remains a mystery only to those who have their heads buried in the sand. Since many cases of this nature tend to occur between the ages of one and two, and also tend to occur in association with the development of fever and illness, the vaccines administered during this phase of life should be suspected as the most likely causative or triggering factors. I have personally consulted with more than a few parents who have related the stories of their normal children who, having been vaccinated, shortly thereafter became acutely ill, usually with high fever, and sometimes with vomiting and screaming, only to never regain health and never again behave in a normal manner. With a myriad of documented stories just like these, the medical establishment's political spin machine has the temerity to claim that there is "no conclusive evidence" or that "no link has been found" between vaccination and autism. These first-hand experiences of human devastation are often the ones dismissed by statisticians as "merely anecdotal" and therefore not relevant. One can either acknowledge the obvious or be deceived by the rationalizations, abstractions, and statistical manipulations of medical science.

To make matters worse, even if one were to find the time and energy to do the extensive research required to make an informed decision regarding the matter, one would find a number of obstacles in the way of obtaining clear unadulterated information. First and foremost, compulsory vaccination policies have made it very difficult to institute any meaningful changes in this most sacred ritual of the medical church. Although people do have some limited means to obtain an exemption from immunization, most are unaware of this possibility, and the church is not in any hurry to educate the congregation regarding their options.

CHURCH AND STATE ADJUDICATE

One might get the impression from the strength of my convictions that I would be a rabid anti-vaccination activist. Perhaps I leaned that way in the past but I have come to appreciate the complexity of the problem and the tremendous fear and pressure faced by parents wishing to do the right thing when it comes to the health of their children. So I make no effort to influence patients unless they specifically ask my opinion on the subject, at which point I will inform them of my bias while acknowledging that there are risks involved in either accepting or forgoing vaccination. If parents are not inclined to vaccinate I also inform them of their legal options, which vary from state to state. Some states offer "religious" exemptions, while other states have more enlightened policies, which allow for a more easily obtained "philosophical" exemption. A big part of the problem is that there is no in-between. You can either opt out of all vaccinations or must consent to the entire series of mandatory measures.

Although all states accept "medical" exemptions from vaccination, it is very rare that they grant this status. In actuality, in a most bizarre twist of logic, those persons that I would consider most vulnerable to vaccine injury are often the ones most strongly encouraged by public health authorities to be vaccinated. The young, the old, and the immuno-compromised are precisely the ones targeted by immunization proponents. For example, a child with asthma is, from my perspective, in an already weakened state and at heightened risk for serious complications from vaccination. Conventional wisdom turns this logic on its head and designates this child as the one most in need of protection from the infectious diseases that vaccines are designed to eradicate.

The U.S. government passed the National Childhood Vaccine Injury Act (NCVIA) in 1986 when vaccine manufacturers, because they were increasingly liable to lawsuits stemming from vaccine injuries, threatened to withdraw their products from the marketplace. This created a federal no-fault system in order to compensate victims of vaccine-related injuries and deaths. It should come as no surprise that the true motive behind this legislation was to protect the pharmaceutical industry, not the general public. Under the NCVIA, the Vaccine Adverse Event Reporting System (VAERS) was set up to track vaccine-related injuries, and the entire system was funded by a surcharge placed on each dose of vaccine sold. Those wishing to file a claim must apply for federal compensation under this system before pursuing a lawsuit against the drug company in question. The maximum payout for a vaccine-associated death is a meager $250,000. This represents a landmark coup for Big Pharma, which continues to reap the profits from the sale of vaccines while maintaining relative immunity from prosecution for the iatrogenic effects of its products.

As is often the case in legal arrangements of this nature, a number of conditions and obstacles are used to discourage the complainant from pursuing compensation. There are various statutes of limitation for the filing of claims and, most important, mechanisms of denial to reduce the number of "legitimate" claims. Our fractured left-brain cultural programming places doubt in the mind of the parent regarding the connection between vaccines and illnesses right from the start, and the chain of denial continues with the physician, who is mandated by law to report all vaccine-related injuries and events. In this way, the medical priesthood is placed in the role of making arbitrary and subjective judgment calls as to what symptoms and illnesses are considered to be vaccine related, and therefore reportable, and which are not.

Because it is understandable that no physician is eager to acknowledge that his or her actions may have led to a serious illness in a young child, it is estimated that a large number of these cases are dismissed by physicians in spite of parents' complaints. The physician who is pressed by a parent can refer to the *Vaccine Injury Table,* published under the NCVIA, which provides the criteria for the reporting of acceptable and admissible adverse events to VAERS. For instance, if a child experiences life-threatening ana-phylactic shock after receiving a DTP shot (diphtheria-tetanus-pertussis), the guidelines state that this must have taken place within the first four hours after administration of the vaccine, and if not, the burden of proof falls upon the patient to make the connection between the vaccine and the severe allergic reaction. In other words, if a severe reaction occurs *after* four hours, the medical system takes the convenient and unconscionable position that the reaction can not have been related to the vaccine. Fur-thermore, for patients to be eligible to file a claim, the effects of the vac-cine injury must have lasted for more than six months after the vaccine was given, or must have resulted in a hospital stay and surgery, or death. The injured party must jump over such a multitude of hurdles that it should come as no surprise that very few claims accepted for review under this system are ultimately compensated, and most are dismissed.

As if this is not enough, all guardians must sign an "informed consent" statement prior to allowing any child to be immunized. This charade is designed to create the illusion that the patient has rights in a process that is, in reality, mandated by law. There is no consent involved for the vast majority of people in most states, and the true purpose of these forms is to provide another layer of protection from liability. When parents con-cerned with the dangers of vaccination are faced with the threat of removal of their child from school for non-compliance, they find that they have no other option but to allow their child to be vaccinated. If a child were to become very ill shortly thereafter, thus compelling the parents to file a com-plaint, the medical system could then respond in its defense by noting that the parents gave "consent" for the child to be vaccinated. This consent process is a rather ingenious form of Machiavellian deception that is rationalized away by most within the medical field as a method of patient education.

Medical authorities tend to employ a number of predictable strategies when under pressure to deny or minimize the link between a vaccine and an injured child. They can argue that there are no studies to prove such a link or, as they are fond of saying, "there is no conclusive evidence." The pharmaceutical industry has authored plenty of research to prove the short-term safety of vaccines—although I take serious issue with that claim—in order to have them approved for the market. Once the vaccines are on the market, however, I suspect that the industry is not too keen to study the long-term effects of their products.

Another strategy is for the physician to lower the expectations of concerned parents by reassuring them that the high fever that their child develops after vaccination is a "normal" reaction, and should not be a cause for worry. The doctor may argue that the child's reaction was a fluke, or that it was just a "bad batch" of vaccine. The physician may also imply, for example, that it was the child's fault for being prone to allergic reactions and had the doctor known, he or she would not have administered the vaccine. The irony here is that, even when physicians are informed of a child's history of allergic tendencies, most will proceed to vaccinate notwithstanding. I have had more than a few parents tell me that they were encouraged by their doctor to have their child vaccinated in spite of a prior serious reaction, with the justification that the vaccine to be given was different from the one that the child had previously received. Sadly, some parents will acquiesce when offered this faulty logic and, tragically, I have seen the casualties that can result.

One of the biggest red herrings modern medicine has used in recent years to throw suspicious consumers off the trail has been to blame thimerosal, the mercury based preservative used in the manufacture of some vaccines. While it is true that vaccines containing this compound have a particularly reprehensible track record, the industry has seized upon it to convince the medical consumer that once this nasty little substance has been eliminated from vaccines, all will be right with the world of immunizations again. Thimerosal's toxicity is undeniable, but its removal does not in any way guarantee the elimination of vaccine injuries, which can be caused by a wide variety of other vaccine components.

NATURAL IMMUNITY

Conveniently, the same bad-batch argument is used when children who have been vaccinated against a given germ nevertheless come down with an illness related to the bug that they are supposedly now immune to. This is much more common than you would imagine and provides a segue to the next point in my critique of vaccination policy. In addition to the abundance of damning evidence pointing to the dangers of vaccination, I would contend that the supposition of the benefits attributed to wholesale immunization is built upon a house of cards. The notion that vaccination programs have been the leading factor in the eradication of infectious disease is a particularly egregious illusion promulgated by the church of medicine. While I would not deny that some degree of immunity can be conferred upon the vaccine recipient, belief in the claims of success in the elimination of certain diseases requires an irresponsible dismissal of much of the available evidence and our accumulated knowledge regarding the history and nature of epidemic disease.

I do not wish to get sidetracked into trying to prove this point, but I will provide some supportive evidence in favor of my argument. There is good reason to believe that the decline of certain infectious diseases has little to do with modern immunization practices and has everything to do with the natural life cycles of these pathogens combined with the improvements in living conditions and hygienic practices of contemporary cultures. The words of microbiologist René Dubos offer an apropos starting point:

> The spectacular decrease in mortality caused by infections during the past century bears testimony to the effectiveness of the measures aimed at the eradication of microbes. In
> role of these measures may not have been so
> believed. The toll of human lives exacted by
> to decrease several decades before control mea

260

germ theory were put into effect and almost a century before the introduction of antimicrobial drugs.[82]

Each epidemic disease has a natural rhythm, life cycle, and history that explain its rise, its decline, its virulence, and prevalence. Neither immunization campaigns nor the use of antimicrobials have significantly altered these diseases, mainly because their rise and decline took place well before the introduction of these medical interventions. By the time individual vaccines were developed, these illnesses had long ceased to be the threat that they once were. As a general rule, any population that has never before encountered a particular communicable microbe will, upon first contact, experience the greatest degree of virulence and highest rates of infection associated with that microbe. Thereafter, both virulence and rates of infection tend to decline as a function of a population's exposure to the microbe, which leads to natural adaptation and increased immunity. In spite of this reality, those who worship at the altar of technological medicine are reluctant to acknowledge that natural forces are usually more effective than medical interventions in encouraging the development of immunity.

Consider some of the following statistics in support of the inevitability of natural adaptation. In the period from 1911 to 1945, deaths related to the four leading causes of mortality among one- to fourteen-year-old children in the United States—measles, diphtheria, scarlet fever, and pertussis—declined by 95 percent. From 1911 to 1935, mortality rates from measles declined by 77 percent, deaths from scarlet fever went down 73 percent, pertussis deaths decreased by 73 percent, and diphtheria mortality rates dropped 88 percent.[83] Similarly, in England between 1860 and 1948, deaths from measles declined 94 percent, from scarlet fever by 99 percent, and from pertussis by 91 percent.[84] In addition, death rates attributed to polio from 1923 to 1953 declined by 47 percent in the United States. and 55 percent in England.[85] All of these trends took place well before the widespread use of vaccines and antibiotics, and in some cases, before the vaccines had ever been produced.

By the time a new vaccine has been developed and rolled out onto the assembly line, the real threats posed by most communicable microbes have come and gone. In fact, the immunity garnered by a population that has been exposed to a germ is far greater and more complete than the potential immunity gained through wholesale vaccination. Furthermore, because of the population's increased exposure in today's world of international travel and commerce, the dangers represented by new and never-before encountered microbes are greatly diminished. Ironically, the greater threat by far is the pernicious and malignant fear that drives medical and public health officials to institute compulsory administration of an increasing number of vaccines, the long-term effects of which are unstudied and unknown. The public is held hostage and forced to play a game of vaccination roulette, and the very same fear renders the majority into a mute mass of pliable subjects all too willing to be guinea pigs for this mad experiment.

While the intent of vaccine administration designed to boost immunity is conceptually admirable, it nevertheless is an abysmal practical failure. The notion that vaccination has led to the virtual eradication of certain communicable diseases is naïve and wishful thinking. Childhood immunization programs are the bread and butter that anchor pediatric practice, and they serve to indoctrinate all citizens into a lifelong dependency upon the medical-industrial complex. If the standards of evaluation used by conventional medical science are applied to current immunization practice then, when the truth is told, the risks and dangers far outweigh the potential benefits. The current state of affairs will someday be seen as one of the greatest medical scandals in human history. Entire books have been written about the wildly exaggerated benefits of vaccines, the downplaying of the serious dangers that they pose, and the medical hoax that they represent,[86] and so I do not wish to belabor the point. I will close the discussion with a quote from Barbara Loe Fisher, co-founder and president of the National Vaccine Information Center,[87] perhaps the most reliable source of truthful information regarding vaccines:

> We have become deathly afraid of viruses and bacteria which, in some cases, have been on this earth longer than humans. Instead of trying to find natural ways to enhance the functioning of our immune systems and come to an accommodation with microorganisms, we have blindly trusted public health offici
> like generals in a war, are determined to exterminate

evaluating the number of human casualties it will take. This cli-
mate of fear is the breeding ground for the draconian measures
being employed by, and powers given to public health officials. It's
very dangerous.[88]

When one forsakes critical judgment and bases the rightness of his or her position on faith, the questioning of this faith can often generate an angry and defensive response. The flaws inherent in this most revered of medical sacraments are often defended with an irrational and dogmatic ferocity. As such, the intensity of the denial can be understood to be in direct proportion to the reality of the unacknowledged dangers. When legal authority conferred by the state backs the power of the medical church, the potential for abuse is significantly magnified. As with this and other issues of importance to the health and well-being of our planet, the medical priesthood must begin to accept that it does not have a monopoly on perspectives and potential solutions to these problems.

The materialistic orientation of the church of medicine dismisses the role of spirit in healing and concerns itself primarily with the technical repair of the physical body. The needs of the soul are seen as superstition and the search for the purpose and meaning of illness are deemed to be unscientific considerations. Contemporary medical fundamentalism assumes the form and function of a religion but believes in nothing but the physical here and now. If orthodox medicine remains closed to change it will, sooner or later, become obsolete. It must learn to shed its dogmatic authoritarian tendencies and embrace a genuine spirituality that respects all beliefs and their role in health and healing. The new medical paradigm will turn orthodox Western materialistic medical philosophy on its head and bring together the best of spirit and science. The green medical revolution will be characterized by an ecumenical spirit of inclusiveness that recognizes the unique diversity of humankind's struggles and illnesses, and the amazing variety of healing modalities at its disposal. The way forward will require a medical philosophy of unity through diversity.

Healing the Rift

Know the male,
yet keep to the female:
receive the world in your arms.
If you receive the world,
the Tao will never leave you
and you will be like a little child.

    —Lao-tzu, *Tao Te Ching*

Isis, Creator of the universe,
Sovereign of the sky and stars,
Mistress of life,
Regent of the Gods,
Magician with divine wisdom,
Female sun,
Who stamps everything with her royal seal!
Man lives on your order,
Nothing happens without your agreement.

    —Inscription in the Temple of Isis at Philae

Jesus said to them, "When you make the two into one, and when
you make the inner like the outer and the outer like the inner, and
the upper like the lower, and when you make male and female
into a single one, so that the male will not be male nor the female
be female ... then you will enter the kingdom."

    —Marvin Meyer, *The Gnostic Gospels of Jesus*

TWO PEAS IN A POD

It should come as no surprise that I have my share of differences with the scientific establishment and the medical status quo, but now that my critique has reached its peak, I would like to change the tone in the name of finding common ground for the benefit of the sick and the suffering. I have felt it necessary to be honest in my criticisms because I believe they represent a perspective that rarely gets an airing in the arena of public discourse. An honest assessment of the current state of affairs is a necessary prerequisite to genuine reforms that will someday encompass the best of conventional medical and alternative healing perspectives. The two need to learn to come together in an attitude of mutual respect and understanding so that the resulting whole will be superior to the sum of its parts.

My buddy Rob and I were best friends growing up as kids on Long Island. We were like two peas in a pod. In retrospect, it seems that our common bond was our authoritarian fathers. We did everything together, until high school, when something funny began to happen. We continued to be good friends but we gradually began to part ways. He took the conventional path, conforming to expectations. He played football, graduated from a good Catholic university, married his high school cheerleader sweetheart, went to medical school, and eventually followed in his father's footsteps by becoming an orthopedic surgeon. Rob remains to this day a highly esteemed physician residing with his family in the same community in which we grew up together.

I, on the other hand, took the unconventional route. I rebelled strenuously against my authoritarian upbringing, left town to go to college, hadn't the foggiest notion of what I really wanted to do in life, traveled around Europe after college, subsisted in a number of dead-end jobs, visited monasteries looking for answers, and eventually enrolled in osteopathic medical school. Once there, I remained unsettled, considered psychiatry, explored a variety of alternative medical fields and, by the grace of God, found homeopathy and settled into private practice.

I have sporadically kept in touch over the years. We had a great ple of high school reunions, and in recent years, I saw him r's death and he visited me at my father's wake. Both times we reminisced over our trying times with those two stubborn old coots. Having come full circle, we still have that same instant rapport. He, the exemplar of mainstream medicine, and I, the healer who has taken the road less traveled. The fascinating thing is that whenever we come together, those professional personas quickly fall away, and we are just two old friends that have taken different paths, which have ultimately led us back to similar places in life. We are both engaged in trying to help our patients as best as we can in our own unique ways.

Over the years, from time to time Rob has appeared in my dreams, especially in times of crisis or transition. He is usually there lending a helping hand, sometimes literally reaching a hand out for me to grab, as if the cosmic forces are telling me that I am getting too far out on a limb and I need to come back over to the conventional side for awhile. In one dream I was riding a unicycle and the road crumbled in front of me. I wound up hanging to the side of a cliff, when Rob came along, stuck out his hand, and pulled me to safety. The concepts presented in this book are the byproduct of a lifelong struggle to come to a greater understanding of health and illness, and the message conveyed by this dream is the perfect metaphor for a significant piece of the solution.

I know that I am not alone in my struggle. Many patients have come to me disgusted over their encounter with the conventional medical world. At those moments I find myself in the unique position of mediator, trying to gently explain why they should not burn any bridges with allopathic medicine, and how regular medicine can be helpful if they use its services judiciously. My role becomes counselor, as patients visit their regular doctors, undergo exams and tests, return to me, and with the information obtained, ask me what I think they should do. Should they consent to this procedure? Should they take that drug? Should they find another doctor?

Many who genuinely need mainstream services resist because of some prior negative experience. It is common for people to come away feeling they have been dehumanized, frightened, spoken down to, misunderstood, treated like a lab value, or not given adequate time to explain. If physicians only knew how many patients sat quietly and respectfully through their medical visits, only to leave afterward in disgust, tempted to throw the scription they have received into the trash can. Many of these comp are completely legitimate, and if truth is spoken to power, mainstream medicine must come to realize that its cultural and financial status does not give it the authority to treat those whom it is intended to serve in such a manner.

As something has obviously gone wrong, serious consideration must be given to the issue of how to right the situation, and I believe that the theme we have been exploring in this book goes directly to the heart of the matter. The masculine, analytical, dualistic left-brain cannot operate as a functioning healthy whole without a partnership with the feminine, intuitive, holistic right-brain. In a given situation, one function may come into play more than the other, but both are indispensable and deserving of equal respect. A successful solution to a patient's dilemma may be discovered by virtue of a bit of data, an exercise of logic, through a strong feeling, an intuitive hunch—or all of the above. The problem begins when the rational mind declares that feelings should not enter into the scientific equation of health care. In response, the intuitive function senses the dissociative nature of this clinical approach and recoils from its lack of respect for the other half of human experience.

I firmly believe that the future of medicine hinges upon our recognition of this unnatural divide and our genuine intention to heal the rift. A problem cannot be solved until it is identified, acknowledged, and understood for what it is. The sweeping critique laid out before you is not intended to bad-mouth Western medicine, but it is deliberately calculated to raise consciousness about the faults in its design and delivery. Only when the problem is understood in all of its ramifications can meaningful changes be implemented. So where do we begin to bridge the gap? How do we attempt to heal the divide? How can we encourage conventional medical personnel to meet alternative practitioners halfway, and vice versa, in order to create a healthier, greener, holistic medical profession?

THE EVOLUTION OF CONSCIOUSNESS

A discussion of the process of the development, maturation, and evolution of the human psyche may be an instructive starting point. In the beginning of human life there is no "I." The consciousness of a child in the womb is that of oneness with the universe. The child does not and cannot differentiate itself from its mother, or its mother from the rest of creation. The child is unaware of itself. All is one. It experiences what its mother experiences. The next phase, from birth onward, involves the gradual process of individual ego development. The child gradually grows up to realize that it and the mother are not one and the same. The ego develops self-awareness, and this becomes the foundation of the inevitable and necessary phenomenon of dualistic thinking. The ego comes to identify itself as apart from all others. The adolescent begins to develop a unique identity, and in the process, comes to experience him- or herself as alone, separate, an independent entity. The once-concrete mind develops the capacity for abstraction and comes to see itself not only as separate from others but also identifies the mind as different and separate from the body.

The development, maturation, and evolution of humankind parallels this process of individual development, thereby demonstrating one of the fundamental precepts of all creation: "As above, so below." What we find true in the microcosm is also true in the macrocosm, and vice versa. The cultures we often refer to as "primitive" tend to be ancient or native cultures that have retained the awareness of oneness, of unity with the universe, and their customs and practices reflect this belief or mode of consciousness. Just as mother and child are one, so too, God is everywhere—in the skies, the winds, the birds, and the stones. All thoughts that are thought and actions that are taken have an impact upon all the rest of the universe because, by definition, all is one. But as time marched on, through eons and generations, the human mind developed the ability to abstract, analyze, and differentiate all of those individual persons and parts from one another. The modern scientific mind has broken the universe down into an unending array of parts, particles, and components, thus creating the illusion that all of these bits and pieces are isolated and separate entities, just as we see ourselves as isolated and separate beings.

Thus, the world begins in the maternal feminine womb where all is one, after which the patriarchal masculine process of growth and maturation into a differentiated individual takes place. Both on an individual and collective basis the matriarchal precedes and then transitions into the patriarchal phase of life. The catch, the snag, here and now in our modern world, is that the patriarchal phase has been taken to its extreme and the result is an unfounded presumption of superiority to the matriarchal influence. Overemphasis upon the rational, scientific, dualistic, materialistic, reductionistic, cause-and-effect left-brain of the masculine threatens to bring civilization to its knees by refusing to acknowledge the other half of human existence and cosmic law. The trick, the key to the solution, is to realize that the processes of human and cosmic growth and transformation are incomplete. There is much left to be accomplished. When we come to understand this, the meaningless dissection of the universe into an infinite array of bits and pieces regains its power and purpose as we realize that we are now called upon to put it all back together again.

We are now witnessing the early stages in the next step of the evolutionary maturation of humankind. As we begin to come full circle, we are aware of the many fragments but we are also recognizing the unbreakable interconnections that bind them all together. We can celebrate the uniqueness of each human soul while at the same time acknowledging that as human beings we cannot act or think as if we are not connected to the whole of creation and beyond. We are coming to see the world holistically just as the child sees all things as one, but we can also choose to exercise our rational and analytical faculties as differentiated beings to assist us in discernment.

Gareth Knight, an authority on the subject of magic, in his book *Magic and the Western Mind* compares the transformational process involved in alchemy with the evolution of consciousness. He writes that the alchemists:

> ... *saw all forms of existence, even the inanimate, as rooted in one basic ground of beingness and capable of growth, evolution and transformation. This is exactly the same pattern that we observe in our theory of the evolution of human consciousness. Consciousness starts as an apparently confused elemental mass of group consciousness, it distills into individualized and eventually spiritualized separate parts, which then attain to a higher synthesis of unity-in-diversity instead of unity-in-mass. The spiritualized units can then act as a focus of transformation for less developed units about them.*[89]

The matriarchal leads to the patriarchal which leads back to the matriarchal, in a giant loop of cosmic evolution toward a more holistic comprehension of life, its trajectory, and its purpose. It is not that one way is any more valid than the other. They are both relevant and true. They are simply different modes of perception—different but complementary modes of perception which, when combined, create a synergistic effect superior to the individual capacities of their parts. Left-brain and right-brain working together as the unified whole that it is. A well-developed and secure ego can work in concert with feeling and intuition. When our powers of perception and understanding are highly developed, we come to know and experience things of a higher order, on other cosmic planes. The higher self, which is capable of seeing the bigger picture, can enrich our lives in ways that the ego cannot comprehend. From the vantage point of the higher self we find the lessons learned from fields of endeavor such as parapsychology, spirituality, and mysticism to be edifying, humbling, and transformational.

Without the ability to abstract and break the universe into its component parts the medical scientist would be unable, for example, to identify and isolate penicillin for use to treat infections. Without the complementary and the equally important understanding of the unity of all things, the single-minded production and overuse of a long line of antibiotics can lead to an environmental crisis in the world of germs, as is the case with dangerous forms of mutant microbes such as methicillin-resistant staphylococcus aureus (MRSA). Even with this crisis at hand the medical world is still unable to conceive of new solutions, as it continues to pursue the same strategies that led to the problem in the first place.

It is not sufficient to assume that the medical scientist's job is done once it has been determined that penicillin can kill germs. Before we can consider penicillin a safe, reliable, and desirable method of dealing with infectious disease, we must explore and understand the practical, short-term, long-term, immunological, ecological, energetic, ethical, philosophical, and spiritual implications to the best of our abilities. Just imagine the potential results if we were to develop and use all of our faculties to solve these problems in our quest to heal the sick.

As a practical matter, we understand that there are left-brain and right-brain dominant individuals. This is normal and natural. It is the difference between the scientists and mathematicians of the world on the one hand, and the artists, musicians, and linguists on the other. The problem lies with a culture that overvalues the one and marginalizes the other. In the best of circumstances, our educational system conspires to accentuate the differences by funneling the two factions into separate curricula. In the worst case, left-brain activities are considered superior, and the arts languish because they are perceived to be of no practical purpose. As we increasingly come to embrace the green value of well-roundedness, we will seek to teach balance by encouraging left-brain dominant individuals to develop right-brain functions, and vice versa.

This is of particular relevance to medical training because left-brain dominant students are usually the ones selected to become our future doctors. So there is an understandable explanation when a patient complains that a particular doctor has all the warmth and communication skills of a stone. Likewise, when the technicians of medical science dismiss practitioners of alternative healing arts as irrational and unscientific, they reveal their bias. The notion of trying to "prove" the value of holistic healing methods in scientific terms is oftentimes an absurdity, because many of these modalities operate from within a different conceptual paradigm, stand on their own merit, and are not amenable to being studied in the proverbial petri dish. Those who can memorize, analyze, and manipulate mathematical problems in their minds may be well suited to be technicians, but they are unlikely to be effective healers unless they first learn to embrace the feminine, synchronistic, vitalistic, qualitative, intuitive, spiritual half of the equation.

STRENGTHS AND WEAKNESSES OF MEDICINE

Before a genuine reconciliation of opposites can be fulfilled, a frank discussion of the strengths and weaknesses of each must take place. Since it is not the purpose of this work to inventory all aspects of every medical and healing modality, I will venture to make some general statements and assessments, but it is important to understand that there are always exceptions to the rule. With this in mind, I will begin with what I believe to be the most valuable and least harmful practices of Western medicine.

Undeniably, conventional medicine has expended a good deal of its energy in, and achieved a high degree of success with the development of diagnostic technology. From my vantage point, this is the health care system's most valuable feature. There is no doubt that blood tests, the culturing of germs, X-rays, MRIs, CAT scans, ultrasonography, mammography, pyelography, endoscopy, and the like are of great value in determining the physical nature of the problems facing our patients. However, the information gathered through the old-fashioned medical interview and physical exam is increasingly undervalued and neglected. The problem occurs when technologies are over utilized and the physician becomes dependent upon them. It is not unusual for my patients to undergo diagnostic procedures at the urging of their regular physicians, only to have the resulting information confirm what the patients and I had already concluded by virtue of the information obtained from the interview and physical exam. The clear value of these diagnostic measures notwithstanding, the modern physician has come to trust in technology more than in his or her own perceptions, intuitions, and judgment.

Another clear strength of conventional medicine is its handling of acute, urgent, and emergent physical health problems. Broken bones, ruptured appendixes, hemorrhaging arteries, serious burns, cranial bleeds, amputated appendages, bullet wounds, lacerations, fibrillating hearts, and advanced infections are a few such conditions best left to urgent-care medicine. Broadly speaking, conventional medicine is the most appropriate option in the event of physical trauma and advanced life-threatening illness. Allopathic medicine is great in emergencies, and it can keep you alive. It has mastered the art of temporarily keeping the physical body from falling apart.

There is a wide variety of surgical procedures and some are indispensable. Others are fundamentally cosmetic, and many are dangerous, unwarranted, and opportunistic. No surgery should ever be considered routine or foolproof. Surgery should always be a last resort once all
have been exhausted.

From a pharmaceutical perspective, the most valuable contributions made by conventional medicine are insulin for diabetes and thyroid hormone for hypothyroidism. Both preserve life in chronic illness and come with a minimum of side effects. Drugs used to treat anaphylaxis are lifesavers in the event of serious allergic reactions. Antibiotics are very useful in some cases, although flagrantly over utilized in most cases. Asthma medications can keep patients safe and breathing, but are of no use in curing the condition. Arthritis drugs may ease pain and discomfort, but will not cure the condition, and its risks are not worth the benefits in many cases. Antidepressants should be prescribed only in the worst of cases, as there are many other options of equal or greater value. These are some of the most useful medications. Many other commonly prescribed drugs are of questionable merit, are essentially suppressive in their actions, cause serious side effects, and can be replaced by other, safer treatments of similar or superior benefit.

While diagnostics, acute care medicine, emergency medicine, and trauma medicine are allopathic strengths, the treatment of run-of-the-mill common illnesses and chronic illness remain its weaknesses. As previously discussed, the mending of most minor colds, coughs, headaches, runny noses, fevers, rashes, aches, and pains are best left to time and nature. Pharmaceutical intervention may provide relief by suppressing symptoms but will increase the possibility of turning a simple acute ailment into a more serious condition. Holistic methods tend to be safer for minor illnesses, are less likely to suppress, can assist the vital force in its goals, but are also usually not necessary.

As a general rule, most drugs designed to manage chronic illness are more problematic than the conditions they are intended to treat, and the bulk of human suffering falls into this category. All that modern medicine has to offer are suppressive medications, which force the energetic disturbance of the vital force toward deeper levels, thus contributing to more serious illness. The most lucrative aspect of the medical-industrial complex is the treatment of chronic disease because it creates a vicious cycle that almost guarantees an endless supply of human misery in need of relief. Once patients start down this road they commonly wind up needing drugs for the effects of the drugs for the effects of the drugs, if you know what I mean. I am not being cynical or disingenuous when I argue that most people, with some exceptions, would be better off in the long run without the drugs prescribed for their chronic illnesses. Again, to summarize this very important point, the vast majority of human suffering falls into the category of chronic disease, and the greatest weakness of conventional medicine correspondingly lies in the treatment of chronic disease. Allopathic treatment of chronic illness almost guarantees the continuation and complication of human suffering, thereby ensuring that it remains medicine's greatest source of revenue.

By contrast, it is precisely in the sphere of chronic illness that most forms of green medicine and healing are of greatest value and present much less of a risk than conventional measures. While drugs and surgeries cannot cure the majority of chronic diseases, there is reasonable likelihood of achieving this aim through holistic approaches. Chronic back pain is far better served by chiropractic, osteopathic, acupuncture, massage, or yoga, than with muscle relaxants, painkillers, or surgery. Most cases of asthma can be cured through homeopathy, meditation, and relaxation, while conventional medications can only be used as a temporary means of keeping patients safe. Nutritional therapy, exercise, homeopathy, and yoga are far safer and more effective in helping many cases of arthritis than commonly prescribed anti-inflammatory drugs. While antidepressants may suppress depression or numb the emotions of patients so that they can function in their daily lives, other methods such as energy healing, spiritual guidance, light therapy, and exercise can frequently achieve better results.

A CASE OF LYME DISEASE

The experience of a young woman that I once saw serves to illustrate the point. Joan explained to me that four months earlier she had become severely ill after finding a tick attached to her foot. She developed the worst headache she had ever felt, "bone crushing" fatigue, achy joints, chills and sweats, heaviness of the limbs, and pains shooting up the ankle from a swollen red toe at the spot where the tick had been found. After consulting an allopathic doctor, she tested positive for Lyme disease, and Doxycycline, the standard treatment for Lyme, was prescribed. Although she completed a twenty-five day course of the antibiotic, she had felt better within twenty-four hours after the first dose. My experience has taught me that Lyme patients who receive treatment before or soon after the onset of symptoms do the best in the long run. However, once the condition becomes chronic, in other words, once the symptoms have had a little time to take hold, they tend not to respond to antibiotics anymore. Sometimes, established cases of Lyme disease may respond briefly, only to quickly relapse after longer courses of stronger antibiotics, thus illustrating the phenomenon of temporary suppression followed by the resurgence of an illness.

In this particular case, Joan had experienced complete relief by the next day—until two months later, when the fatigue, joint pains, and heaviness began to return. This time she noted that the heaviness was localized to the right arm and leg, as if "the muscles don't want to obey." Based upon the pattern of her symptoms I prescribed two doses of a homeopathic medicine called Gelsemium, which is strongly indicated for illnesses that involve great fatigue and heaviness of the limbs. When I saw her five weeks later she reported that she had felt "very, very crabby" that evening after taking the medicine. Interestingly, Joan's husband noticed that she felt very hot the whole night during her sleep, and was concerned that she might have a fever, although she was unaware of this. Upon waking the next morning, all of her symptoms had vanished and she said that she had "felt excellent ever since then."

She also reported that her old tendency toward sinus congestion had acted up since the Lyme symptoms had subsided. This is an example of how a curative response encourages the vital force to redirect the energy of an illness by trading off the deeper, more threatening manifestation for more superficial, less serious symptoms. By her own admission, she much preferred the sinus congestion over the fatigue and paralytic limb sensations. Here we have a straightforward example of a chronic condition that orthodox medicine has little to offer except more of the same antibiotics. If the medical establishment were to acknowledge its limitations and concede to its poor track record with chronic illness, then a safer and more effective synthesis of conventional and green healing modalities could become possible. The perfect blend, in this case, was an immediate course of antibiotics and follow-up homeopathic care.

RECOVERING THE FEMININE

A thoughtfully balanced health care system should emphasize preventative measures and patient education first and foremost, in spite of the fact that this may not be very glamorous or financially rewarding in the near term. Right from the start, all children should be taught some form of mental/spiritual discipline like meditation, yoga, or Tai Chi. Proper nutrition is crucial to the prevention of chronic illness, and physicians should assert their moral authority as front-line advocates in this area. There is simply no excuse for the processed and genetically modified foods, chemicals, and preservatives that constitute the American diet. When some food additive is linked to a health problem, we are likely to hear the familiar refrain that more studies are needed. When the medical establishment fails to take a stand on issues like this and instead offers weak rationalizations, it loses its credibility in the eyes of the general public.

Western culture is the product of the past several thousand years of patriarchy. There is no denying that we live in male-dominated times that emphasize the values of competition, possession, expansion, war, and a linear way of seeing the world. These values permeate all aspects of education, work, religion, and recreation. The feminine values of cooperation, communication, nurturing, sharing, and healing may be given lip service but are, in reality, ruthlessly trampled in the collective rat race to become one of the boys with the most toys. To this point, the emancipation of women has been framed largely in terms of obtaining the same rights and privileges that men enjoy. And many women have become very successful at competing in a man's world, but the problem is that they are still playing by men's rules.

True respect and appreciation for the feminine, and the fact that it can be expressed and embodied by both men and women, have yet to seep into mainstream consciousness. I am not talking about superficial window dressing like hospital rooms with pretty pictures and flowery wallpaper. I am referring to a significant change in values and perspective. But it is on its way, and Edward C. Whitmont, physician, homeopath, and Jungian analyst, has written one of the most important works on the subject, *The Return of the Goddess*. It opens with this inspiring passage:

> *At the low point of a cultural development that has led us into the deadlock of scientific materialism, technological destructiveness, religious nihilism and spiritual impoverishment, a most astounding phenomenon has occurred. A new mythologem is arising in our midst and asks to be integrated into our modern frame of reference. It is the myth of the ancient Goddess who once ruled the earth and heaven before the advent of the patriarchy and of the patriarchal religions.[90]*

If we are to begin to heal the rift, we must first look to our spiritual roots. While we in the West have been taught that "civilization" essentially began in ancient Greece and Rome, the history of human life extends far beyond this into the distant past. Although the historical record correspondingly becomes thinner, there is abundant evidence pointing to the universal existence of female-oriented and female-dominated cultures, religious practices, and civilizations. Academic science, indoctrinated in patriarchal ways, is reluctant to acknowledge the overwhelming evidence of matriarchal history represented by thousands of artifacts and archeological finds. It tends to diminish this information by referring to it as evidence of ancient "fertility cults." Some have interpreted the word "cult" as carrying the negative connotation of something sinister that is shared by only a small group of people. Erich Neumann, analytical psychologist and contemporary of Carl Jung, is author of *The Great Mother*, a monumental work on the archetype of the feminine. Here he reminds us of the true origins of human civilization and the modern patriarchal psyche:

> *Moreover, because the patriarchal world strives to deny its dark and "lowly" lineage, its origin in this primordial world, it does everything in its power to conceal its own descent from the Dark Mother and—both rightly and wrongly at once—considers it necessary to forge a "higher genealogy," tracing its descent from*

heaven, the god of heaven, and the luminous aspect. But nearly
all the early and primitive documents trace the origin of the world
and of man to the darkness, the Great Round, the goddess.[91]

The Goddess's influence was considerable in ancient times. There are literally hundreds of different female goddesses and deities that are now known by virtue of oral history, religious texts, and artifacts and statues of great antiquity. The Egyptian goddesses Isis and Hathor; the Roman Venus and Minerva; Greek goddesses Artemis, Aphrodite, and Persephone; the Celtic Danu, Airmid, and Morrigan; Hawaiian goddesses Pele, Papa, and Lie; the Chinese Kwan Yin; the Aztec Chicomecoatl; the Mayan IxChel; the Lakota White Buffalo Calf Woman; and the Christian Mary are just a sampling of the abundance of feminine deities, many of whom are still worshipped around the globe to this day.

In some cases, gods and goddesses were of equal importance, and in others, goddesses were the primary deities of matriarchal societies. Perhaps the most continuous and complete goddess tradition originated with the Hindu customs of India. Some believe India is the most ancient seat of all civilization, and that it has influenced all subsequent cultures. It appears that prior to the advent of patriarchy the female goddess—Mother of the Universe—was revered in almost all parts of the world. Over the centuries, her influence in the West has been eclipsed by the masculine gods of Christianity, Judaism, and Islam.

Let us return again to the woman with Lyme disease, because there is more to her story. Almost as an aside, and with a bit of reluctance, Joan told me that after she began to feel better she had a very strong psychic/spiritual experience. It happens that she had seen a friend at church and during their conversation she put her hand on his shoulder, whereupon she felt something strange. She wondered what was wrong and he told her that his brother-in-law had recently been diagnosed with cancer. Naturally, she was surprised and she expressed her sympathies.

Joan then described to me what had happened when she awoke the next morning, after hearing this news. "My head was awake, but my body was not. I saw the Virgin Mary, who I recognize as the Egyptian Queen, Isis, in a shrine backlit by candles, carrying a child. She filled my whole self." Mary assured her that the brother-in-law was in her care. Joan explained to me that she believed all goddesses are the one goddess, who travels by different names throughout history and culture.

Joan told her husband that morning that she needed to go to the church to light a candle, but as is often the case, life can become busy and she did not get around to it. A few days later she bumped into the wife whose brother was sick. Again, she related her condolences and debated whether she should tell her about her "vision." Overcoming her fear of seeming a little foolish, Joan felt it important to say something. Upon hearing about the vision, the wife acted unfazed, because she assumed that her husband had told her of his brother-in-law's experiences. She went on to explain that since his illness, her brother had been having frequent nightly visitations from the Virgin Mary! Needless to say, my client hurried down to the church where she lit a candle at a shrine of Mother Mary.

No doubt some receptive doctors out there might respond the way one would hope. But imagine for a moment if Joan had relayed her story to the average conventional physician. Would he ask if she has been having a lot of these "visions," refer her to a psychiatrist, prescribe a sleep aid or antidepressant, or make a note on the chart regarding her odd behavior?

I was deeply affected by Joan's vision of Mary/Isis and engaged her in a fruitful discussion of intuitive, psychic, and spiritual experiences and beliefs, and encouraged her not to neglect this opportunity for personal growth and change. The healing of her Lyme disease had been accompanied by the opening of a cosmic doorway. She had to decide whether she would step across the threshold. I referred her to my shaman friend from Vermont, whom I had consulted years earlier, because I felt inadequate to guide her and to do justice to the potential rewards and blessings that she could receive and abilities that she could develop from such a powerful apparition.

It is interesting to note that after Christianity became the official religion of the Roman Empire, the Egyptian Temple of Isis remained open until the sixth century, in spite of the fact that Constantine closed all pagan temples by decree in 331 CE. (See Figure 13.1.) Isis came to be associated with the Virgin Mary, and some believe that early Christian iconography

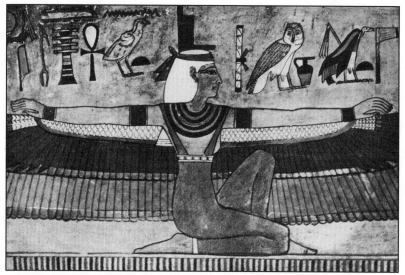

FIGURE 13.1: *Egyptian Queen Isis, from the Tomb of Seti I, Valley of the Kings*

of the seated mother and child is influenced by images of Isis holding the child Horus.

A sourcebook on Egyptian gods and goddesses describes some of the attributes of Isis:

> *Courageous, loving, loyal, resourceful, clever, pitiful as a victim, stubbornly refusing to accept defeat, Isis is portrayed in the myths as the most psychologically complex of all the Egyptian deities, seemingly as humanly vulnerable as she is supernaturally powerful and indestructible ... The popularity of Isis was, and still is for her thousands of modern devotees, largely due to her personal qualities, her ability to empathize with human suffering on account of her own tribulations on Earth, and her willingness and power to help those in distress by means of her magic.*[92]

This bout of Lyme disease may have contained a deeper meaning, one hidden from the patient and me. The energetic backlog represented by Joan's Lyme disease had transmuted into a new awareness of a neglected part of her psyche that was demanding recognition. This could not have happened if she had continued with more antibiotics in a futile attempt to suppress the disease out of existence. Whether we believe that she had cosmic contact with Mary/Isis or we say that she was experiencing the Mary/Isis goddess energy within herself does not really matter. The implications remained the same. Her task now was to tune into her feminine side, which was calling her to a spiritual dimension of herself that resonated with a friend of hers who was also suffering in a time of illness. Thus her own illness had been transformed into a capacity to help another in need. This again touches upon the theme of the wounded healer, which we will be taking up in more depth in a short while.

MYTHIC SUBSTANTIATION

I have always puzzled over the conspicuous absence of the feminine in the Christian idea of the Trinity. Strangely, a cross with four arms is used to symbolize its three aspects. Father, Son, and Holy Spirit form the three arms of the sign of the cross, and yet there is fourth arm that goes unnamed. This fourth and longest arm points downward, toward the earth. Father and Son are obviously masculine, but Spirit, too, is of masculine nature, and looks upward toward the sky, toward the light, toward Father Sky or Father Sun. Despite Mary's prominence in the story of Christ, she is afforded no place on the cross. I believe this is more than a mere metaphor, rather it is clear evidence of the patriarchy's denial and dismissal of the feminine. A great deal of suffering has been perpetrated upon humanity as a result of this inability to integrate the feminine into the whole. My personal remedy for this imbalance has been to turn the trinity into a quaternity, and so, long ago I decided to sign myself in the name of the Father, Mother, Son, and Spirit. The feminine is still outnumbered, three to one, but at least my method represents a partial solution to an issue that holds great significance for me. Perhaps Father, Mother, Spirit, and Soul would constitute a more accurate rendering of holistic reality.

Furthermore, if we compare the role of the Church of the one true male God with that of the Church of Medicine, we become aware of two irreconcilable positions that place Westerners in a peculiar double bind. While medicine, on the one hand, acknowledges the reality of the physical body and disavows the place of spirit and soul in healing, the religious patriarchy, on the other, minimizes the importance of the physical body and, in some cases, views it with shame and revulsion. This schizophrenic disconnect places many in an untenable situation. What are we to believe? Which church shall we choose? Is the human body with its physical brain as command center our only reality, as contemporary materialism would have us believe? Or is the physical body an essentially irrelevant and temporary vehicle to be tolerated on the way to a more desirable afterlife as spirit?

Such is the conundrum of a dualistic perspective that insists upon an either/or answer. Our cultural conditioning prevents the realization of the more feminine conclusion that all is one. In reality, there is no conflict because the notion of body as separate from soul is an illusion. It is the product of a fractured mind out of touch with its spiritual essence. The way to heal this split between doctor of the body and patriarchal keeper of the soul is to invite the Goddess back into our lives. Her gentle loving touch of kindness and inclusiveness is the perfect counterbalance to the hard, cold factual worldview of the rational medical mind.

Upon closer scrutiny, we find there is another level of dissociation that begs for reconciliation. Let us return to the caduceus, the medical symbol of two snakes wound around the staff. Much of the available historical, mythological, and archeological evidence points to an intimate relationship between the Goddess and the serpent. The Minoan Snake Goddess of ancient Greece is one well-known example. Archeologists on the island of Crete have found a number of figurines dating back to 1600 BCE of a woman holding two snakes. Many believe that Minoan civilization was matriarchal, and that snakes were treated as virtual household pets and revered as sacred symbols of the Goddess. Many Goddess images from around the world are depicted with snakes as their allies and, in fact, some scholars believe that the serpent is one of the most ancient symbols of female divinity.

The fact that Western religious traditions hold the snake to be a symbol of evil, and that conventional medicine fails to comprehend the significance of the serpents associated with its own emblem, form a metaphor for modern humanity's divorce from its own feminine right-brain attributes and potentialities. This artificial and unnecessary divide stands in the way of the newly emerging green medical paradigm, which is beginning to recognize that unification of the opposites is the only means of achieving genuine and lasting healing of the sick individual and of the sick system itself.

The biblical account of Adam and Eve is another example of how the mythic stories of human history can have such a powerful impact upon contemporary life. The allegory is particularly relevant to our discussion, as it illustrates how different versions and interpretations can result in very different worldviews. The popular version of the story paints Eve as the weak female tempted by the evil serpent to taste of the forbidden apple from the Tree of Knowledge. She in turn tempts Adam, and once the evil deed is done, they feel shame and cover their genitalia with fig leaves. Both are then cast out of the paradisiacal Garden of Eden by a displeased God.

In 1945, a large number of previously unknown Gnostic Christian scriptures were found buried in a sealed jar in the city of Nag Hammadi, on the west bank of the Nile River in Upper Egypt. When Elaine Pagels's introduction to the Nag Hammadi texts, *The Gnostic Gospels,* was published in 1979, a glimpse into the historical censorship and selective construction of the composition of the Bible by Christian orthodoxy became accessible to the general public. Here we find a startlingly different version of the Adam and Eve tale—one that goes to the heart of a spiritual understanding that facilitates the leap of faith required when transitioning from the old medical construct to the new green paradigm.

In one of the Nag Hammadi texts, the Goddess assumes the form of the Tree of Knowledge in the Garden, and she sends the serpent as a messenger to rescue Adam and Eve from bondage and ignorance. Once they have partaken of the apple, they receive the knowledge of good and evil. They also become aware that God, out of jealousy, did not want them to discover their own divinity, because this would have the effect of elevating them to the status of His equals.

Thus, the patriarchal version would have us believe that the female temptress and evil snake colluded to bring man down, into his fallen state. Once Adam and Eve have come into possession of this forbidden knowledge, the angry male God ensures that humankind is banished from the

Garden and burdened with shame. The other, matriarchal version tells us that the Goddess Herself, in the form of the World Tree and in collaboration with the wise serpent, dispenses the fruit of wisdom that enables the achievement of enlightenment. Author Linda Johnsen, in her book *The Living Goddess,* comments on this remarkable 180-degree turn in perspective:

> *The Gnostics turn the Bible inside out, praising the intelligence, courage and ultimate divinity of Eve, the most reviled woman in the Western religious tradition!*
>
> *For the Westerner, eating that apple is the worst possible sin; questioning why God would deny us a share in his divine nature is the worst possible blasphemy. For the Easterner, not reaching for that apple is the greatest spiritual failure.*[93]

We may come to understand some of our attitudes toward the orthodox medical priesthood more clearly with the help of this primordial myth regarding the relationships of man and woman to God and to each other. The physician represents a privileged caste, and is keeper of the secret knowledge. Modern medicine expends much effort to ensure this status, and keeps the layperson in the dark and feeling ashamed about wishing to know more. Having a primary role in one's own destiny, through self-knowledge and self-healing, becomes the forbidden fruit. The serpent is the evil influence of illness and disease to be crushed and is intimately associated with Eve, the symbol of all things feminine. The most dysfunctional potentialities of a dualistic worldview inevitably become realized when the scientific patriarchy does not honor the feminine qualities of intuition, receptivity, inclusion, emotion, patience, love, and holism.

This reinterpretation of the Adam and Eve myth provides a signpost pointing in the direction of the new medical horizon. The feminine and the serpent become allies in the healing process that ultimately involves growth, change, self-knowledge, and the awareness of one's own divinity. This is not mere role reversal, because the masculine does not become subjugated but is reduced to a role that is equal and complementary to the feminine. God and Goddess together, like left-brain and right-brain, form a balanced whole, representing and respecting all energies of the universe, positive and negative.

Seen from this perspective, the exclusion of any one element becomes the seed from which disharmony and disease can germinate.

For this balancing to take place, the medical mind must begin to loosen its grip on its position as king of the hill. The feminine cannot be incorporated into the whole without an equivalent diminution of the ego of medical science and its rational perspective. The road map toward genuine health rarely forms a straight line, seldom conforms to conventional logic, and often involves a bit of the mysterious and magical. Letting go of the ego's need for control can be frightening, but as Dr. Edward Whitmont would advise us, the rewards are available to those with the requisite receptivity:

> *In the drinking of the Goddess's waters the ego's personal claim to power is renounced. Indeed, the ego acknowledges itself as but a recipient and channel of a destiny flowing from a deep, mysterious ground of being which is the source both of terror and revulsion as well as of the beautiful play of life. This power flowing from the sovereignty of life is to be handled in a reverential fashion if the protection of the Goddess is to be gained.*[94]

In the end, the experience of our own separateness is just an illusion promulgated by the tunnel vision of the rational mind. The right way, the wrong way, the true god, and the false god—are all products of dualism. This limited conception of reality is the cause of untold human strife, misery, and suffering. To attempt to isolate the "secret ingredient" is to miss the point. There is no one-size miracle drug that fits all and there never will be. Factionalism takes us further away from respect, truth, love, beauty, health, and healing.

All of the bits and pieces of the universe—those electrons, protons, and neutrons, waters, stones, plants, and animals, planets, stars, and comets—are bound together by one invisible energetic matrix. So too, the bones, muscles, organs, blood cells, and neurons of the human body are animated by a unifying vital force. Taken as a whole, they make possible the myriad shapes, sizes, colors, and races of human life, birth, death, and rebirth. Similarly, all of those gods, goddesses, angels, and spirits are but aspects of the

Whole, the One, the God/dess of all creation, and together, they represent an expression of the incredible diversity of human culture and spirituality.

These ideas regarding separateness, wholeness, dualism, and holism constitute more than just philosophical speculation. Although they may operate on an unconscious level, they lie at the conceptual foundation of the entire medical-industrial complex and permeate the everyday practice of conventional medicine. One's spirituality, philosophy, and psychology ultimately inform the practical nature of medical strategies and healing methods that he or she chooses. Dysfunctional practices originate from spiritual, philosophical, and psychological misunderstandings. True, meaningful, and lasting change will require practitioners and healers to be increasingly aware of the origins of orthodox medicine's motivations, rituals, and practices. Individuals must also become aware of their personal relationship to this system in order to make wise and informed decisions regarding their own health and care.

Up to this point we have examined how the energy of the vital force can manifest symptomatically as illness and poor health. Let us now turn to a discussion of the process of healing. We will explore what this process looks like in real terms when someone has been blessed by the return of health after its absence.

The Direction of Cure

Ultimately, healing the physical form does nothing unless there is a complementary change of consciousness. All healers know this. If this does not take place, the physical form will return rather rapidly to the state it was in.

—David Spangler, *Explorations: Emerging Aspects of the New Culture*

The Greeks did not even think about enjoying happiness without taking pain in their stride. Pain was the soul's experience of evolution.

—Ivan Illich, *Limits to Medicine*

Jesus said, "If you bring forth what is within you, what you bring forth will save you. If you do not bring forth what is within you, what you do not bring forth will destroy you."

—Stevan Davies, *The Gospel of Thomas*

REDUCTIONISM AND EMPIRICISM

Perhaps the nearest conventional medicine comes to an appreciation of the defense mechanism and its resistance or susceptibility to illness is when it considers the topic of immunity. The entire field of immunology has developed from our understanding of the aspects of the human body that are summoned up in its resistance to disease, and so we hear much about white blood cells, T cells, antigens, antibodies, and other micro-components of the immune system. Medical terms like "immuno-suppression," "autoimmune," and "immuno-compromised" demonstrate an awareness of this protective function of the immune system and how it can be undermined and weakened by a variety of factors. This is all well and good, we've gained much valuable information from the study of the immune system, but it nevertheless represents a gross underestimation of the nature of the defense mechanism of the bioenergetic life force. It is, in essence, a reductionistic depiction of the defense mechanism in its physical manifestation in a very specific and limited way. To reduce resistance to illness to the biological components of the immune system is to severely underestimate the innate healing capacity of the human organism.

Remember that biology is driven by chemistry and that chemistry is driven by physics. In the end, all things in the physical universe can be defined by their energetic properties and are driven by the laws, as far as we understand them, of physics. Taken a step further, this use of the term "energy" is also a convenient and palatable way to describe an even more profound concept, which most scientists are just too uncomfortable to accept and assimilate. Because beyond the scientifically explainable world of physics lies the intangible human soul and its spiritual essence.

As we have previously seen, indigenous cultures have viewed illness as a sickness of the soul. Many formal religious traditions would concur that spiritual illness is a fundamental reality that requires a non-physical approach to be adequately addressed. Ritual, meditation, prayer, self-discipline, and divine intervention are just a few such ways for healing the spirit and soul. According to the mechanistic line of thinking, an exorcism would be the spiritual equivalent of an allopathic approach that attempts to banish, eradicate, or kill the supposedly external invading enemy. In any event, if we acknowledge our present appreciation of the dynamics of health and healing truthfully, we must admit that we have but an inkling of insight into the mysterious nature of the body-heart-mind-soul unity and its resistance and susceptibility to disease.

Despite the limitations of our knowledge, I will press on and attempt to express a view of healing as I have come to understand it from my studies, personal struggles, and clinical experiences. First and foremost, I feel we must come to trust what we see with our own eyes and experience with our own senses. Our perceptions, intuitions, and judgments are critically important. When a person with disease A is treated with drug B, and disease A completely disappears but the overall health of the person declines with the passage of time, it is unacceptable and cannot be considered a viable method of treatment, let alone a form of healing. The compartmentalized approach of the rational mind would have us believe that drug B is successful, simply by virtue of the fact that it seems to eliminate disease A. When we consider the bigger picture, we come to know better, and yet we continue to patronize, support, and invest in a medical system that tends to follow this basic shortsighted formula of symptom eradication without forethought as to its consequences. The vast majority of regular medical interventions lead to palliation, suppression, or metastasis, and contribute to a net decrease in overall health, well-being, and immunity.

A medical therapy makes little sense if it does not lead to greater health, vitality, and personal and spiritual power. And so there must be a better way. The good news is that there is and, in fact, there are a variety of better ways. As we shall see, these better ways all have several things in common—they follow the holistic principles of a green medical perspective. The first of these is the manner in which the life force is approached. Ignoring the energetic defense mechanism by remaining unconscious of its patterns and propensities is the incorrect approach. We can continue to wage war against it out of this fundamental ignorance or we can work with it, respect its needs, and learn from it.

If we choose to work with the vital force and seek to trust our own perceptions, then we must take one important first step upon encountering any individual suffering from poor health or illness. We simply ask that person about his or her condition. We do not, on the other hand, give someone one minute to answer, run a bunch of tests, and then presume to tell the patient what is wrong. Again, we ask *the individual* about his or her condition. Perhaps one of the most critical and powerful moments during an interview occurs after the client has had a chance to describe the main ailment or complaint. This is when I look the person in the eye and ask why he or she thinks this illness has developed. If the client begins to answer in the materialistic medical terms that have been unconsciously assimilated over a lifetime, I immediately stop him or her and say, "No, I'm asking *you* why *you* think you have become ill."

Having been conditioned by the pervasive influence of the old medical paradigm, it is not surprising that many people do not trust their own instincts. However, with a little encouragement, they will often go right to the heart of the matter. Although this technique of eliciting the client's opinion about the reason for his or her illness may not always work, sometimes the answers can be quite illuminating. Statements such as, "I know it began after I caught my husband cheating on me," "My dog died a month before I got sick," "When I saw the pictures of the bombing on TV I felt sick," "I swear it was that medication I took for my heartburn," "It's the building resentment that I feel toward my mother-in-law," and "I've never felt the same since I had my gallbladder removed two years ago," are just a sampling of the potential responses that can point directly to the source of a problem. These are the very same answers that a regular physician is likely to dismiss out of hand because they are of little relevance to the conventional materialistic framework from which he or she operates.

Practicing this primary principle of trusting the expressions of the individual and the individual's life force, rather than an abstracted cookie-cutter version of this information in the form of a conventional diagnosis, is the most immediate and direct way of respecting the uniqueness of each person's body-heart-mind-soul. This empirical, experiential, individualizing approach of accepting that "what you see is what you get" is the polar opposite to the need of the rational mind to interpret, quantify, and filter the information it receives. An empirical approach can quickly lead to the core of an issue that can be generating a variety of peripheral symptoms and difficulties. This is not to say that conventional diagnosis is of no value. It is important to factor in the information received from such a diagnosis and, depending upon each situation, it may be of great value—or it can be relatively inconsequential.

PROCESS AND CURE

If a core issue can be identified, a healer can use it as a yardstick against which to gauge all subsequent progress. As an example, consider the young woman with arthritis who also admits to feeling that she has failed in her desire to become an accomplished artist. We can judge any therapy that diminishes the arthritic tendency to be ineffective unless it is accompanied by some form of headway in how she feels about her artistic ambitions. If she returned to the doctor to report less joint pain and a renewed motivation to pursue her interests, then I would be more inclined to judge the therapy as a positive one. If she reported that she had much less pain and had come to a new perspective regarding her art and now felt that she had given it her best try and genuinely did not consider herself to be a failure anymore, then I would be very pleased. Indeed, I would even venture to call it a curative response.

This brings us to the next important green principle. All signs and symptoms are, by definition, connected and must therefore be treated as the whole that they represent. Any therapy that isolates a symptom or part of the body and attempts to treat it without consideration for the larger whole will most likely fall short and turn out to be palliative or potentially suppressive. We cannot, out of convenience, ignore the woman's increasing sense of failure and consequent depression because we wish to focus on the arthritis. They are one and the same and cannot be separated. If the arthritis is improving while the depression is worsening then it is reasonable to investigate whether this is being caused by the chosen therapy. Likewise, treating the arthritis with an anti-inflammatory drug and the depression with an antidepressant would not constitute treatment of the whole. It would simply be a form of double suppression. An effective therapy must honor and reflect our conception of the seemingly separate bits and pieces of the universe as an actual integrated whole. Anything that has an impact upon one part can potentially have an effect upon all other parts. An ecological outlook of this nature is much more likely to result in a positive outcome and fewer unforeseen complications.

Technically speaking, if we want to nitpick, there is no such thing as a cure. How do we know that the "cured" individual will not develop an even worse condition a week, a month, or a year after treatment? If this turns out to be the case, can we fairly say that the patient had been cured? The truth is that we will never know for sure, as we cannot predict the future. What we can be reasonably assured of is the direction that someone's health is taking over time. The process of healing can be judged to be moving in the right direction or the wrong direction. The goal of cure is a theoretical endpoint in the process of healing, and this endpoint is an idealized construct that is rarely ever reached. We cannot judge the process to be completed even at the time of death since the soul continues after the physical body has expired. Some believe the soul subsequently reincarnates at a later time to continue growing, changing, healing, and learning its evolutionary lessons through the vehicle of another physical body.

There is no magic pill that will someday cure us of our ills once and for all. The achievement of health is always a work in progress. Otherwise, if there were a concrete endpoint, life would come to a standstill and would lose all sense of purpose and meaning. Since growth, development, and change are requisite characteristics of human evolution, we can only judge an individual to be stuck, declining in health, or moving in a positive direction toward greater health. In reality, the trajectory of the average person's health history tends to look like a roller coaster ride with its ups, downs, and straightaways. The most that we can hope to achieve is to make sure that the coaster does not get hung up and is moving smoothly forward in the proper direction.

Let us consider another example to help illustrate this concept of directionality. Suppose a woman traces the onset of her eczema to the breakup of her marriage after she found out that her husband had been cheating on her. She has eruptions on her arms and legs that can itch, especially if she becomes agitated and emotional. She notes that her previous allergic tendency toward itchy eyes and runny nose seemed to recede right around the same time that the eczema started. Careful interviewing reveals that she feels quite bitter over the fate of her marriage, and she admits that she has had a hard time trusting the men that she has met since then.

Now, we can surmise that the shock of her husband's infidelity induced enough distress to her vital force as to cause it to get stuck at the point of anger and mistrust, such that she continues to react to current relationships as if she were still back in the original situation. It is reasonable to believe that the vital energy has chosen to manifest this distress on the surface as an itchy and annoying skin eruption as a reminder of the issue that keeps getting "under her skin." Given this interpretation, would it make sense to address our treatment to the itchy skin condition? Or does it make most sense to help her at the point of stuckness?

Let us assume that a doctor prescribes a topical cortisone cream and, as expected, her eczema virtually disappears. On the other hand, she reports that she is also feeling noticeably more irritated and impatient toward the people around her. Should we be surprised when the perceived "cure" of her eczema results in an overall decrease in her general happiness? After all, we know that cortisone will not serve in any way to address her anger and mistrust. From our previous discussions, we know that suppressing the itch is likely to force the energetic disturbance of the life force toward the deeper interior, thereby intensifying this person's irritability.

What if we instead choose a therapeutic intervention designed to address the underlying source of her unhappiness? Now she reports that her emotions came to a cathartic climax one day as she became quite angry and then melted down into a torrent of tears as she grieved the betrayal of her husband and the loss of her marriage. Almost simultaneously, her itch intensified until it was almost intolerable. But just as the anger let up and she broke into tears, so too, the itch diminished and no longer seemed to bother her. In the following days, she felt a letting go of the anger and a renewed ability to forgive her ex-husband in spite of his clear-cut trans-gressions. Not surprisingly, she also reports that her allergic itchy eyes and runny nose returned just as she was beginning to feel better emotionally.

Shouldn't we be pleased with this latter scenario, and doesn't it seem to indicate that she has been released from the grips of the stuckness of her vital energy? That her allergic tendency has reemerged serves as an additional indicator of a return to the less threatening state of health, which had existed prior to the emotional trauma that threw her life force out of balance. The bioenergetic life force has moved away from stuckness and in a positive direction toward greater flexibility and renewed emotional freedom, thus allowing her to take risks again. Now she can be receptive to a new partner that she can relate to with an open and genuine feeling of trust. Relying on a principle that we have already discussed, one sure-fire way to determine whether this return to allergies is desirable or not is to ask the patient how she feels about it. If she indicates that she prefers her current allergies to the anger and itchiness, then we can believe that the changes manifesting are in the correct direction, the direction of cure.

All green therapeutic modalities that honor and work with the life force have in common the fact that they trust the uniqueness of the individual and the individual's own perceptions about his or her health. Green med-icine assumes the truth of the interconnectedness of all things and there-fore all symptoms on all levels, and its modalities strive to assist the energy of the life force to move in a direction toward greater health and vitality, the direction of cure. This direction is opposite to the direction of suppression. Remember our previous conceptualization of the life force and its movement along the physical, emotional, mental, and spiritual levels of the bioenergetic gradient? The center of gravity of the expression of an illness can move in a negative direction, toward the deepest spiritual level, or in a positive direction, toward the outer physical level. Any symptom or health condition can be made to move in either of these directions, depending upon the nature of the particular therapeutic method employed.

When a health condition is encouraged to move in the proper direction we can be assured that this is also the direction of strengthened immunity, increased vitality, and a more stable state of balance. The right direction also implies the unsticking of the life force from its prior state of stubborn inflexibility, which is what all ongoing chronic health problems are about. The vital force has, in essence, become stuck in a negative feedback loop, thereby causing the same symptoms to persist and repeat themselves over and over. The annoying itch hanging onto Joan, the woman in our example, will persist until it is improperly suppressed or until something helps release her from her unforgiving anger and mistrust.

It is important to understand that these states, as a general rule, are not voluntary—they are usually not consciously chosen. If they were it would be as simple as saying, "I forgive you," and being done with it. Forgiveness should be the norm in any mature relationship. One person transgresses, the other person is hurt, the offending party apologizes, and ultimately the other can find forgiveness. This behavior is the sign of a healthy vital force. But when a particularly shocking transgression inflicts a significant blow to the life force, a person can become stuck, and in spite of all genuine attempts to forgive, can still feel anger and hurt every time something reminds that person of the original shocking event. Those around the individual who grow impatient with the sufferer's inability to let go may not understand and demand that the person "just get over it." This attitude is a reflection of our left-brain cultural bias that insists that one can simply will oneself into wellness again. Sometimes this is possible, and many times it is not. In fact, this masculine "tough it out" mentality can lead to significant health complications when it convinces the mind to temporarily override or mask the distress signals of the life force, potentially making matters worse in the long run.

It is of great import for any healer to ascertain where the suffering individual has become stuck. It is advantageous to locate this core from which most symptoms are being generated. Identifying the core allows for the possibility of outside intervention to help reset the bioenergetic field of the ailing person back to a flexible state of balance. Achieving this balance lets the vital energy flow freely again to respond to whatever comes its way next.

The innate wisdom of the life force leads it to manifest its signs and symptoms of distress in the least threatening way possible. Suppression of these indicators encourages the development of deeper illness. The process of cure involves assisting the defense mechanism to bring the energy of the disturbance to the surface in order to resolve it so that balance can be restored. Spiritual, mental, and emotional health are more important than the elimination of superficial physical symptomatology. Paying respect to the direction of cure, from inside to out, from interior to exterior, will ensure an overall increase of health, vitality, and freedom to embrace change.

A CASE OF ASTHMA AND INFIDELITY

I have been working with a client recently whose course of treatment vividly reflects this concept of direction of cure. Bill is a tennis pro in his mid-forties who came to me for treatment of his asthma, which had begun three years earlier after a bout with pneumonia. He is very health conscious, eats a clean vegetarian diet, and regularly runs. In spite of these commendable health measures, he is unable to resume his regular physical activity unless he takes an asthma medication called Advair. Even with this medication, he can tell when he runs that his breathing is not quite normal, and he must sometimes resort to a second drug, called albuterol.

When I asked him why he thought he had contracted asthma, Bill responded with these exact words: "Unscientifically speaking, I was under a lot of emotional stress." Right away, the unconscious psychological pressure that patients face when dealing with the medical establishment was evidenced by his feeling compelled to justify himself because he had no scientific evidence to back up his claim. And this was with me, the so-called alternative doctor, with whom, I would like to think, he should have found it unnecessary to defend his own assessment of himself. But our social programming is very strong and we absorb many unconscious messages during our lifetime, including, "Don't trust your own perceptions," "The professionals know better," and "I can't compete with science."

When I inquired about the nature of his stress, he told me, "I have two girlfriends stressing me out. Women and me are not a good combination. I have no boundaries to protect myself." When I asked what he needed to protect himself from, he offered, "I protect myself from shame, guilt, abandonment, and emotional pain." Our ensuing discussion made it apparent that Bill had no qualms about having two girlfriends. He saw no inconsistency in this, even though he acknowledged that he had to keep one from finding out about the other. I thought to myself that it was no wonder he was having trouble breathing.

He had previously spent a good number of years in psychotherapy working on issues from childhood, including the shame that he had felt because his mother had suffered from mental illness. In addition, Bill had a tendency toward sinus infections, a feeling of chronic tightness in the right sacro-iliac region, and an extensive rash that was originally located on his chest. After his rash was treated with an antifungal medication, it relocated and now covered most of his back. After proper deliberation, I asked him to quit drinking coffee, prescribed a homeopathic medication, and advised that he continue with his usual routine of health-promoting behaviors.

To my delight, at his return visit one month later, Bill announced that he had stopped taking his Advair one week prior. Since then, he had twice run two and one-half miles without any trouble breathing. "I used to wheeze on exhaling. Now it's almost normal. I can't believe it. I'm ecstatic!" He noted that he'd had more trouble breathing than usual during the first two days after seeing me, but then this difficulty had subsided. This was similar to the "healing crisis" experienced by the mistrustful woman with the itch that had reached its crescendo just before her health took a sudden turn for the better. Most practitioners of the alternative healing arts and sciences are well aware of this phenomenon. An exacerbation of symptoms is often a prelude to their subsequent improvement and resolution. A comparable parallel occurs when someone experiences a significant loss like the death of a loved one. It is often not possible to simply get past it and move on. One must first experience the grief of the loss in its full force before it can ultimately be released.

My client Bill also reported a little improvement in his sacro-iliac tension but the rash was unchanged. And I was encouraged when he told me that he was feeling more energetic on the tennis court. Most important, he indicated that a change was occurring at the deepest level of his dilemma. In referring to one of his girlfriends he said, "I've pulled back and now she's coming forward. I have more objectivity and safety in myself." Although he was still not questioning that he had more than one ongoing relationship he nevertheless seemed to be reconsidering the nature of those relationships.

After two months, he noted that there had been a "drastic improvement," and he had increased his running routine to two and one-half miles every three days without need for any medication. The rash, however, remained unchanged. In between visits to my office he had an episode of mildly increased breathing difficulty, which, after subsiding, was immediately followed by a headache with a lot of sinus pressure. Concerned that this was a sinus infection, he consulted his regular physician. Bill's words were as follows, verbatim: "The doctor scared me. He said it could be fatal." Hence, without my knowledge he had taken a ten-day course of an antibiotic.

In the weeks following the antibiotic treatment his breathing began to decline again. He resumed taking Advair and stopped running. He was still struggling with girlfriend issues but there was a slight twist in the plot: he became upset that one girlfriend was not willing to be exclusive with him. I reflected back to him that this seemed rather unfair, given his own non-exclusivity. I made an adjustment in the homeopathic prescription and advised him to continue his regular medication unless he felt noticeably improved again.

One month later, Bill reported his breathing had improved again. He had discontinued his medications, had started jumping rope, and was working out with a punching bag. Interestingly, his rash had gotten worse, spreading back toward the chest, where it had originally begun. He said he felt generally better emotionally and that relations had improved with the one girlfriend he seemed to be focusing more of his attention on. I felt that we were able to have a more candid discussion about the problematic nature of having more than one committed romantic relationship.

The following month, Bill had resumed running and described "a feeling of well-being" in his lungs. Unable to resist, he had dabbed just a little bit of an antifungal cream on the rash that had spread to his chest and, mysteriously, the entire rash subsequently disappeared, even from his back, where he had not applied any of the cream. "I'm definitely better emotionally," he reported. And then he said something remarkable. "I have infidelity problems. I can't be fully honest. I'm moving away from that. I can breathe easier."

Admittedly, this is a case in progress, and we may have some ups and downs to navigate just yet, but overall I feel very confident in stating that Bill's health is heading in the direction of cure. Considering his lifelong psychological issues, he has made some surprising changes in attitude and these have been accompanied by a distinct ability to breathe easier. The overall trend of his physical progress has gone from asthma to sinusitis to skin rash. In fact, at one point his rash intensified as his asthma subsided. It is notable that in the course of these physical changes he has gradually altered his perspective regarding the deeper emotional issues that had been preventing him from breathing freely.

By keeping in mind the interconnectedness of all of Bill's symptoms and problems, and taking care to encourage his vital energy to move in the proper direction, we have been able to achieve positive results thus far. On the other hand, it is instructive to note that his life force had begun to push the energetic disturbance from one physical manifestation, the asthma, to another less threatening one, sinus congestion. This was a favorable development and, had I known about it, I would have advised him to be patient with the changes taking place. But the antibiotic directed at the sinuses deprived the vital energy of its escape route, so to speak, thus pushing the energetic disturbance back inward toward asthma again. This example of suppression was no coincidence. It is the dynamic that lies at the root of why most allopathic medicines should be reserved only for situations that demand them as an absolute necessity.

THE NATURE OF HEALING

The example of Bill's case provides an appropriate jumping-off point for drawing distinctions between conventional medicine and other forms of healing. We tend to casually interchange the terms *treatment, cure,* and *healing* with little appreciation for their differences. Now we may begin to compare and contrast them with greater precision. Treatment, as we have previously indicated, carries with it no connotation of positive or negative outcome. Cure is a hypothetical ideal, an endpoint to a process that is always ongoing. In a more limited sense, cure can be provisionally attributed to a given condition if it has gone away for a long time and is accompanied by a general improvement in the health of the individual. Healing is the actual process that takes place as the person changes and transforms on the road to recovery, better health, and well-being. Healing takes place in the direction of cure, and while there may be setbacks and breakthroughs, we can view the total process as the winding path of the healing journey. In this sense, healing is never complete, as there is always some physical, emotional, or spiritual issue that can be worked on or improved. In this sense, healing becomes nearly synonymous with growth and change.

The unfortunate reality is that conventional medical treatment is almost always just that, treatment. Conventional treatment is not conscious of the differences and does not emphasize healing. It concerns itself with the repair of the physical body, and in doing so may provide time for actual healing to occur. One may pursue healing in addition to conventional therapy but orthodox treatment alone is usually not sufficient to create healing. Healing may occasionally be the inadvertent result of orthodox medical or surgical intervention but this is not its intent. Most conventional doctors do not concern themselves with the whole; they tend to consider the job done when the specific part in question is no longer generating symptoms. Repairing the physical body is a method designed to maintain the status quo. As for psyche and spirit, this territory is left up to the therapist, psychologist, psychiatrist, priest, minister, rabbi, or imam.

Herein lies the crucial distinction, as illustrated in the preceding case. Authentic healing is almost always accompanied by change and growth of consciousness. Let me repeat this key point, which is the decisive difference between mere treatment and genuine healing. *Authentic healing is almost always accompanied by change and growth of consciousness.* And genuine healing is the hallmark of green medicine. Not only is growth part and parcel of healing, it is the actual purpose and goal of the process. Illness, therefore, becomes the spur that should lead one to seek growth and change. Most people become conscious of this role of illness only when they are properly educated about its function and purposes. What would be the purpose of "treating" my client's asthma if it simply allowed him to continue to behave in ways detrimental to himself and others? It would be like performing a liver transplant so that someone could continue to drink alcohol. Of course, we may not always reach the intended goal for all of our patients. Some are contented with a diminishment of symptoms, are no worse for the wear, and continue essentially unchanged. Nevertheless, it is my hope to help all those who seek genuine healing to learn and to raise their awareness about the process.

Illness is an opportunity that can be embraced or resisted. Allopathic medicine always stands ready to assist those who would prefer to resist. Conventional medicine is pain avoidant, averse to suffering, and generally in denial regarding the nature of life, death, illness, and disease. While it prefers to pursue the illusion of clinical perfection, some uncooperative bug or unforeseen issue always manages to bypass its sterile fortress to gum up the works. And its misguided solution is usually more of the same—it invents more powerful drugs, increases the dosage, and intensifies the war in the false belief that the enemy will someday be vanquished.

Please do not misconstrue my intent here. I am not suggesting that we should seek out suffering and revel in pain. Martyrdom and masochism are neither the purpose nor the goal. The philosophical perspective and practical approach in dealing with pain, illness, and disease can make all the difference in the world, though. We must acknowledge that the pain is there to tell us that change is required. We can float along in blissful ignorance, popping a pill every time something threatens to burst our bubble, or we can embrace the unfolding journey of life, death, and rebirth. We can dabble with surface symptomatology or we can plumb the depths to the core of our illness. We can benefit if we pursue the path and go with the flow of the vital force as it reveals its hidden mysteries, which can potentially free us from unnecessary suffering. True healing takes place from the source, and its rewards are often life changing, enlightening, and deeply gratifying.

Bill's asthma provided him with the opportunity to learn how to nurture a deeper and more satisfying relationship. In similar fashion, Joan's annoying itch gave her a chance to reconsider her angry and mistrustful view of relationships. All illness, especially chronic illness, carries the seed of potential transformation that can bring about physical, emotional, mental, or spiritual growth. It is sufficient that we understand the call and embrace the challenge. Whether we succeed or fail is beside the point. We cannot control our own destiny. We can only pursue the path in hope of finding our place and our purpose.

Pain or illness often accompany even normal physical growth, as when a child has teething pains or an adolescent has growing pains. These milestones are usually concomitant with emotional and developmental changes. It is no coincidence that the overwhelming changes that the average teenager faces in high school or upon heading off to college, can become bogged down into a prolonged illness like mononucleosis. It is as if the life force needs adequate time to process the profundity of the transformations taking place. Lying in bed for days or weeks can serve a person as an incubation phase for adequately absorbing the full impact and meaning of the time. Our fast-paced and demanding cultural attitudes can be counterproductive at these sensitive times. If such an adolescent does become stuck, we can call on a variety of healing modalities to assist in making the transition a successful one.

There are no medical coincidences. Illness is a synchronistic clue pregnant with potential meaning if we can appreciate its significance and are willing to receive the gift it has to offer. It is not there to be feared. Illness may be mysterious and perplexing, but it holds within it the key to unlock the door, the understanding that can dislodge the vital energy from its fixed state of rigidity, the change of consciousness that can restore balance to unbalanced circumstances. Visionary priest and scientist Teilhard de Chardin states the case with poetic elegance:

> *Human suffering, the sum total of suffering poured out at each moment over the whole earth, is like an immeasurable ocean. But what makes up this immensity? Is it blackness, emptiness, barren wastes? No, indeed: it is potential energy. Suffering holds hidden within it, in extreme intensity, the ascensional force of the world. The whole point is to set this force free by making it conscious of what it signifies and of what it is capable.*[95]

THE SACRED DIMENSION OF HEALING

The direction of cure entails a green philosophy that values the individual uniqueness of each situation, recognizes the reality of all that lies beyond the physical, assumes the connection between all things, and honors the potential, if not discernible, meaning behind each human being's illness and struggles. All therapies that follow these principles can be of use in the pursuit of healing. The acceptance of the challenges posed by illness can result in men, women, and children who are more kind, loving, healthy, mature, balanced, and enlightened.

The uniqueness of our time is that we are approaching the endpoint of patriarchal dominance. The limited perspective of the left-brain has created more problems than it has solved. The prevailing disbelief in cosmic and spiritual realities and the consequent atrophy of knowledge and understanding of the principles that govern these realms have created a desperate need for wise men and women to lead us out of these dark times of dense materialism. Disrespect for history, tradition, our elders, and the departed have left us seeking superficial material answers, which are not to be had. This lack of mature spiritual guidance often leads the individual down dead-end paths, and sometimes the only way back is through significant pain and suffering. Bill Plotkin explains how the rigidity of the rational mindset can precipitate crises in need of solutions:

> *All too often, the soul finds one day that the ego has become too hardened, too entrenched in its routines, so that almost nothing can budge it. In contemporary Western culture, our egos often develop in such a way that we are both underdeveloped and overly*

hardened. If, in our youth, there had been elders about, they would have provided initiatory experiences to soften us up or crack us open. Without elders, the soul waits for—or creates—a trauma, something extreme that will loosen the ego's grip on its old way of belonging to the world.[96]

The wisdom of our elders has become unavailable to us because we are no longer willing to listen. When we do not listen, we delay the maturation process and cannot make the necessary adjustments and changes needed to maintain balance. Technological culture encourages and enables the ego to persist in its delusion of control. When the ego is unwilling to concede, the wisdom of the life force may forcibly bring about change through illness. We often perceive such illness as the enemy rather than the redeemer that it is.

The interplay of opposites serves the same fundamental purpose. The creative dance of the masculine and feminine keeps the energetic flow going and promotes balance. The empirical complements the rational. Heart and mind, the cosmic and the microscopic, and synchronicity and causality all work together as one. If one begins to dominate the other, the restricted component may begin to make itself known through symptomatology as a reminder that balance must be restored if peace is to be achieved.

Real physical healing, as opposed to mere suppression, is accompanied by growth of consciousness. Purpose and meaning are absolute essentials in the ongoing healing process, and the avoidance of pain, whether physical, emotional, or spiritual, is counterproductive to this process. Incarnation of the soul into a physical body allows it to heal, grow in consciousness, and evolve. Self-healing facilitated by an understanding of these green principles will promote healing of our communities and our Mother Earth.

Native American tradition was such that the family would thank the buffalo spirit for the food and clothing that they had received from the hunt. Likewise, the native healer invokes the spirits of plants used in ceremonies, and thanks the spirits of herbs administered in healing rituals. The administration of Western medicine, by contrast, is a strictly secular enterprise. It defines itself in material terms, is devoid of meaning, and has been stripped of its sacredness. Authentic healing is a meaning-filled process that involves the raising of consciousness, and this cannot take place if we take into account only the material body.

Now let us summarize some of the main points regarding the direction of cure. The first prerequisite to healing is that we trust our empirical perceptions and the unique expression of the vital energy rather than a preconceived notion of disease categories. All signs and symptoms are by definition one, and together they form a more complete picture of the distressed vital energy. Treatment of the whole will yield better results than treatment of a symptom, and it can be of great benefit to identify the core issue from which most of a person's distress arises. The elimination of symptoms cannot be considered productive unless it is also followed by improved vitality and well-being.

Cure is a hypothetical ideal. There is no endpoint. The achievement and maintenance of health are always works in progress. The direction of cure is opposite to the direction of suppression. It involves extricating the life force from its negative feedback loop, thus allowing the expression of symptoms to move from interior to exterior. *Healing* is a *process* that leads in the direction of cure, toward greater health, vitality, and balance. Authentic healing is almost always accompanied by change and growth of consciousness. Illness, therefore, is a synchronistic opportunity to embrace change that can lead to greater health and well-being.

All healing is, in essence, a sacred endeavor. I often pray quietly for divine guidance and assistance when trying to help my patients. I fear if I did this out loud in front of them that half of them might never return. Perhaps I underestimate them. I envision a day when we may once again openly invoke the spirits of our medicines and pray with conviction for divine intercession for health and healing. Genuine green healing, in the end, is a sacred privilege that involves body, heart, mind, and soul.

We turn now to one of the greatest mysteries of healing. The alchemists of yore were onto something very important when they sought to uncover the secrets of the transformative process of turning crude metals into gold. As we shall see, modern-day alchemists carry on the tradition, and their best work is reflected in the principle of the "wounded healer."

15

The Alchemical Key

Alchemy, the secret art of the land of Khem, is one of the two old-est sciences known to the world. The other is astrology. The begin-nings of both extend back into the obscurity of prehistoric times. According to the earliest records extant, alchemy and astrology were considered as divinely revealed to man so that by their aid he might regain his lost estate.

—Manly P. Hall, *The Secret Teachings of All Ages*

What happens in the spirit world is a reflection of what happens in the physical world. In healing, it is easier to make the changes in the energetic or spirit world. According to the "as above, so below" tenet, those changes are reflected back into the physical body, and healing happens according to natural law.

—Nicki Scully, *Alchemical Healing*

ACHILLES HEAL

So the legend goes that when the Greeks, under the command of King Agamemnon, set off to find Troy to partake in the Trojan War, they unwittingly landed in Mysia, the country ruled by King Telephus, the son of Herakles. In the ensuing battle, Telephus was wounded at the hand of Achilles. When the king's wound had not healed, he sought assistance from the gods by consulting the famed Oracle at Delphi. The cryptic mes-sage from the Oracle came back, "He that wounded shall heal."

Taking this prescription seriously, Telephus stole into Aulis, where the Greek fleet was beached. Disguised as a beggar, he asked Queen Clytem-naestra, the wife of Agamemnon, for her help. Now, Clytemnaestra was displeased with her husband, and because she also happened to be related to Herakles, she advised Telephus to abduct her only son, Orestes, to be held for ransom. He did so and threatened to kill Orestes if Achilles did not attend to his wound.

Achilles had studied healing and medicine with Chiron, the centaur. You may recall from our story in Chapter Four that Asklepios, the Greek God of healing, had also learned his healing arts from Chiron. Nevertheless, Achilles refused to help Telephus, claiming to have no such medical knowledge. This is when Odysseus stepped in to offer a potential solution. He reasoned that if Achilles' spear had wounded Telephus, then it was the spear that should be used to heal him. Odysseus scraped some of the rust from the tip of the spear and applied it to Telephus's wound, which was miraculously cured. In gratitude, King Telephus agreed to guide the Greeks on to Troy.

Although I do not recommend the practice, some will have an alcoholic drink first thing the next morning in order to diminish the effects of a hangover. Likewise, many will successfully soothe an insect sting by applying an acidic substance such as vinegar. Some animals with digestive disturbances instinctively eat grass to induce vomiting for relief. These paradoxical therapeutic tactics run contrary to our typical mode of dealing with illness. They are not unlike that classic cartoon plot where the main character is hit on the head and loses his memory, only to have it return when he is accidentally, or purposely, hit on the head again. It is a version of the "hair of the dog that bit you"—that proverbial prescription, which most of us seldom put into actual practice.

It is known that Hippokrates, the father of conventional medicine, advocated treating an illness with either its opposite *or* its similar. Thus, he believed that some "hot" diseases could be given "cooling" medicines, while others might respond to "warming" treatments. Paracelsus, physician and early contributor to modern chemistry, broke with the predominant Galenic medical thinking of the time, tending instead to side with the notion that most illnesses will best respond to treatment with similars. (See Figure 15.1.) This foreshadowed the system of homeopathic medicine that Samuel Hahnemann was to develop two centuries later. Contemporary alchemist and author Dennis William Hauck points out Paracelsus's belief that treatment with similars could effect both the physical and spiritual dimensions of illness:

*In place of the Galenian slogan of "contrary cures contrary,"
Paracelsus proposed "like cures like." In physical terms, it meant
that a poison in the body could be cured by a similar poison in a
small dose ... In spiritual terms, Paracelsus's dictum "like cures
like" meant that the patient himself was involved in his cure, and
using the proper imagery and suggestion could invoke one's natural healing power ...*[97]

One of the first homeopathic success stories that I witnessed while
studying with Dr. Hotchner in medical school involved a man who had
been stung by a bee. His entire arm had become swollen and in spite of a
full week of therapy with the powerful steroid prednisone, his arm had
shown no sign of improvement. He consulted with Dr. Hotchner, who prescribed a few small doses of a homeopathic medicine called *Apis mellifica*,
a preparation made from the honeybee. To my amazement, most of the
swelling receded within twenty-four hours. This, to me, was powerful confirmation of the effectiveness of treating illness based upon the principle
of similars.

THE MYSTERIOUS SCIENCE

Paracelsus was not only a physician, he was also a master alchemist. Alchemy is one of those disciplines that,
until recently, has been the subject of
much misunderstanding in both lay
and academic circles. Alchemy is popularly depicted as an early and crude precursor to modern chemistry. According
to this interpretation of history, the alchemists were naïve scientists who did
not know what we now know regarding the laws of chemistry and physics
and who therefore believed that they
could discover a method to turn common metals into the most precious

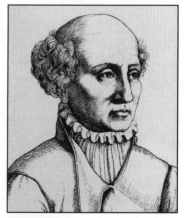

FIGURE 15.1: *Paracelsus, Alchemist
and Chemist*

metal of all, gold. For this reason, alchemy is not usually given credit for the significant contribution it made to early chemistry. But more important, the whole point of alchemy was lost because it was discarded by those who wrongly interpreted it through the lens of scientific materialism.

The Great Work, or *Magnum Opus,* of alchemy was the search for the secret to unlocking the mysteries of physical matter. Alchemists believed that this secret could yield the ability to "transmute" common crude metals into the most perfect form of matter, as represented by gold. The metals could be arranged into a hierarchy from the most impure, lead, to the purest, gold. Because of its rarity and great value, gold epitomized the highest ideals of beauty and perfection. This fundamental precept of the alchemical quest, transmutation from a crude unrefined state into a more refined and balanced state, was a principle that applied to all levels—physical, psychological, spiritual, and cosmic.

The secretive alchemists contributed to misconceptions concerning their work and its purposes by hiding it behind a thick disguise of obscure symbolism, like a spirituo-chemical form of hieroglyphics that most outsiders were incapable of deciphering. In fact, the origins of alchemy can be dated back to the ancient land of Khem, the place that we know today as Egypt. Modern-day alchemist Brian Cotnoir traces the complex lineage of alchemy through the ages:

> *Egyptian technology—both material and spiritual—encountered Greek philosophy, gnosticism, and hermeticism. From this potent mix, alchemy evolved ... Alchemy then flowed from Hellenistic Egypt with the Greeks, via Orthodox monks, throughout such places as Egypt and Syria. These monks were key in the transmission of Greek science and philosophy to Islam, translating texts from Greek into Arabic ... The art and science of alchemy rapidly* ...ced within the Islamic context, nurtured by Islam's embrace *t the natural sciences and gnosis ... Islamic alchemy also* ...*luences from India and China ... From the Islamic realms,* came to Western Europe in February of 1144 ...*[98]*

The medieval European alchemists were under constant threat of persecution by the Christian Church, as were other competing worldviews of the time. As we have seen, Christian authorities considered even the scientific activities of Galileo heretical. Similarly, had the alchemists revealed the true inner spiritual nature of their work, it would surely have led to their demise. Much of alchemy's cryptic symbolism later came to be adopted by other secretive groups, such as the Freemasons and Rosicrucians, who also saw the need to protect themselves from Christian oppression. This secrecy has fed the variety of modern conspiracy theories that have supposedly been decoded from the vast archives of symbolic images and language left behind by the ancient alchemists.

More accurately, the tremendous complexity of alchemy becomes apparent in its multiple purposes and layers of meaning—chemical, psychological, spiritual, and medical. A great deal of Carl Jung's work was based on his investigations of alchemy and what it revealed regarding the nature of the human psyche and the dreams it produces. He was a pioneer who found confirmation of his own experiences and suspicions in the activities and aspirations of the alchemists. In his landmark work *Psychology and Alchemy*, he notes that there is much more to alchemy than meets the eye and, I would add, more than the materialists of science are willing to admit:

> It should now be sufficiently clear that from its earliest days alchemy had a double face: on the one hand the practical chemical work in the laboratory, on the other a psychological process, in part consciously psychic, in part unconsciously projected and seen in the various transformations of matter.[99]

We have benefited immensely from Jung's work, which represents the first true decoding of the alchemical mysteries for consumption by the modern psychological mind. Jung understood that the complex symbology was, in large part, a projection onto matter of the psychic processes taking place within the alchemist—as if the alchemist were working out personal issues of initiation, maturation, individuation, and transformation right there in the laboratory. As such, the thousands of alchemical books, documents, symbols, and art images constitute a vast wealth of material ready to be mined by modern analytical psychology. (See Figure 15.2.)

Taken a step further, alchemy is more than just a mere psychological language of symbols. It actually represents a profound spiritual quest pursued by its original practitioners. It was a quest pursued in secrecy because its implications threatened those who insisted upon the supremacy of their version of the one true male God. As we shall see, this dovetails with our theme of the problem of patriarchal materialism and the oppressive impact it

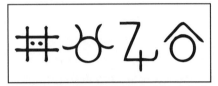

FIGURE 15.2: *Various Alchemical Symbols for the Metal Zinc*

has had upon modern medicine. Contemporary healer, shaman, and alchemist Nicki Scully describes the real intent of the alchemical opus, which reflects the holistic perspective of green healing that we have been delineating thus far:

> For those actually engaged in the Great Work, the transmutation of metals was an allegory veiling their true goal. This goal was a superior and interior achievement—the alchemical gold of enlightenment—through which one transcends duality and illusion and becomes one with the fabric of creation, where creator and creation are one.[100]

The original alchemists were chemists, astrologers, philosophers, spiritualists, and healers all rolled into one. With the rise of materialism the holistic alchemical enterprise became fragmented, as did all other aspects of culture under the influence of mechanistic science. Consequently, at a certain point, alchemy diverged into spiritual alchemy and its material counterpart, conventional pharmacology. Here again we see the divorce between spirit and matter, as "serious" scientists stripped the discipline down to its purely chemical mechanics and discarded all connections to meaning, spirit, and the larger web of life. In a similar vein, the wealth of psychological, cosmic, and spiritual information made available to us through astrology has been reduced to its barest facts and figures as represented by the strictly material science of modern astronomy.

One of the most ancient and important texts of alchemical heritage, *The Emerald Tablet,* or *Tabula Smaragdina,* was purportedly written by Thoth/ Hermes, the ibis-headed Egyptian god of wisdom and writing, and patron of scribes and physicians. Within this brief document the essential precepts of the alchemical worldview are summarized, and from it derives the esoteric axiom, "As above, so below." The microcosm reflects the macrocosm, the interior reflects the exterior, and one's inner spiritual essence is reflected in the attitude toward and the condition of his or her physical body.

Given this underlying doctrine, we can see how the spiritual and psychological dynamics of the person undertaking the Great Work of alchemy are reflected in the physical and chemical aspects of the alchemical laboratory. The alchemical process involves a number of complex steps designed to transmute the original raw material into the refined purity of gold. These are the very same stages that the body-heart-mind-soul undergoes as it grows and changes through cyclical phases of birth, illness, death, reintegration, rebirth, and transformation. Here Dennis William Hauck, in his book *The Emerald Tablet,* confirms the connection between the process involved in turning crude metal into gold and the inner psychic nature of the alchemist's quest:

> *The alchemists attempted to perfect the One Thing of Hermes, what they called the First Matter, by using specific physical, psychological, and spiritual techniques that they described in chemical terms and demonstrated in laboratory experiments. However, while the alchemistic philosophers spoke in terms of chemicals, furnaces, flasks, and beakers, they were really talking about the changes taking place within their own bodies, minds, and souls.*[101]

THE GREEN ELIXIR

Contemporary alchemists are still engaged in the internal alchemical quest long ago disowned by conventional chemistry. They understand that the initial crude energetic substance of the immature psyche can be encouraged to grow in the direction of greater balance, health, and consciousness. The gold, by this standard, becomes an enlightened person who makes use of

her faculties to live in harmony with the surrounding commu-
nvironment. Alchemical healer Nicki Scully, who uses guided
imagery to take people through the various stages of the alchemical process,
is one such pioneer. While orthodox medicine treats the body and ignores
the rest, Scully believes instead that changes on the deeper planes of energy
and spirit eventually precipitate out into changes on the physical level.
Here, she speaks of the significance of bringing body and soul together:

> *It is the goal of the alchemist to bring spirit and matter into align-
> ment and harmony. Within that relationship rests the secret of
> creation, and with it our ability to co-create our own reality and
> to heal ourselves and others.*[102]

The goal of the Great Work, therefore, is to raise the energy of the physical to a higher plane, to bring it more into tune with the vibrations of
spirit. Transmutation involves bringing the spiritual essence locked within
material substance to the fore. The ancient alchemist's endeavor was often
described as the search for the mythical "philosopher's stone" or "lapis
philosophorum," which was the elusive "substance" needed to assist in the
transmutation process—that which could release the inner essence from
the physical vehicle. This inner essence, the Holy Grail of alchemy, was
sometimes called the "Elixir of Life" and it was believed to hold the power
to restore health and vitality. Alchemist Brian Cotnoir describes alchemy
as an approach to spirit through the physical:

> *The alchemical view holds that essence is trapped in matter, our
> inner light imprisoned by matter or obscured by our material fog.
> Alchemy shows a way of ascent, the return to God. It is through
> matter itself that we may find our way. It is an approach to the
> divine through matter.*[103]

The problem that we face, after all is said and done, is that while these
concepts may sound fascinating, they nevertheless remain abstract, antiquated, and rather ethereal. On the one hand, the pharmaceutical industry
has sucked the spiritual life out of the sacred business of creating medicines for healing. On the other, while spiritual alchemy may work on a

deeper level in subtle and imperceptible ways, it lacks a ce:
ness and physical immediacy. This dualistic dilemma seen
some extent, in spite of the attempts of alchemists to br
believe, however, that alchemy is alive and well and that the
tical and reliable methodology for healing that utilizes the energetic essence
of substances to bring body, emotions, mind, and spirit together to resonate as a coordinated whole. But I get ahead of myself. First, allow me to
explain a little bit more.

The alchemists never did seem to find that elusive ingredient that could
transmute physical substance into spiritual essence. At the very least, this
substance is not readily apparent to contemporary man. One would think
that the philosopher's stone would be of such a nature that it would have
a foot in both physical and spiritual worlds. What is it that has the power
to mediate between body, heart, mind, and soul, and how can we use it for
the betterment of health and humankind? All of these efforts of human
intellectual and spiritual activity over centuries of time have led thousands,
perhaps millions, of people to the conclusion that there is "something"
capable of accomplishing the goals of this Great Work. Have we been
deluded or is there something that can actually transmute a state of immaturity, energetic imbalance, and ill health into a golden state of well-being
and higher consciousness? Are we really to believe that from the transformative stone comes the essence, the Elixir of Life, that can be used to heal
the sick? Interestingly, Dennis William Houck equates this intangible elixir
that can restore health with the life force itself and its green quality!

> In physiological alchemy, life and health flow from the Stone in
> the form of the Elixir. It is said this True Medicine could restore
> a man of eighty to the youth of a child in twenty-eight days. In
> the same way that the Stone perfected any substance, the Elixir
> perfected any living tissue. In many ways, the Grand Elixir was
> the principle of life itself, the vital force or the spirit of life, the
> "blessed greenness" contained within the Emerald Tablet.[104]

AN OIL-INDUCED ITCH

Now, let's bring this highly esoteric discussion out of the mysterious ether and back down toward solid ground. Perhaps an example of a patient who consulted me and my wife, who is a registered nurse, will suffice to bring this otherworldly philosophy into focus. Susan, a young woman in her thirties, sought our assistance for a skin condition that developed after she had spent two years teaching in the country of Kuwait. A few months after returning home she began to develop symptoms that she had never before experienced. Her face became very dry and flaky, and started to itch and peel repeatedly. For three years she had consulted dermatologists, and tried antibiotics, assorted creams, and skin peels, but nothing had helped. By the time she consulted us she was distraught over her appearance, especially because her wedding date was rapidly approaching.

Further investigation revealed that Susan had experienced two episodes of severe vertigo over the past year, keeping her virtually bedridden for nearly four weeks. My wife, thinking quickly, reminded me that one of our homeopathic medicines is well known for its ability to *cause* dry skin and vertigo. By virtue of the homeopathic principle of similars, we considered that perhaps this medicine could be used to *treat* Susan's dry skin and vertigo. With this in mind, we began to question her about her time spent in Kuwait. She confirmed what we had suspected. We knew that Kuwait is an oil-rich land and she acknowledged that there were oil fires burning continuously while she was there, "twenty-four hours a day." Although she did not actually see them, she could often smell them in the air. Curiously, a friend who had spent time in Kuwait with her had also developed a similar skin problem.

Surmising that Susan's problem could be related to prolonged exposure to these fumes, we prescribed a few small doses of homeopathic *Petroleum*, a preparation made from purified and refined crude oil. Three weeks later, she returned to our office to report, "My skin is doing so well. It's about 80 percent better. This is the best my skin has been in years." By the time her wedding arrived, two months later, her skin was completely clear. Thereafter, she had one minor flare-up of skin symptoms, which quickly resolved after another dose of the *Petroleum* remedy. She also had no

further vertigo after treatment began, and her skin has
time since. It is interesting to note that allergy symptom
previously experienced, began to emerge as her skin pr
Susan made clear that the allergy symptoms were prefer
condition, and this is in keeping with our concept of the di
as previously discussed.

THE SCIENCE OF SIMILARS

Part of the controversy that has swirled around homeopathy since its incep-
tion two hundred years ago has to do with the scientific establishment's
inability to accept its use of miniscule doses of medicines. Dr. Samuel Hahnemann discovered a process of "serial dilution and succussion," which
enabled him to eliminate the gross toxicity of any given substance while
maintaining its therapeutic effectiveness. He devised a method by which
a substance is diluted in a solvent like water or alcohol, shaken vigorously,
then further diluted in more solvent, and shaken again. This homeopathic
pharmacological process of dilution and succussion, also called potentization, can be repeated for a specified number of times until a designated
potency is reached. This method allows a highly toxic substance such as
snake venom to be used safely in its homeopathic form as a medicine. Paradoxically, the more the process is repeated, the stronger the effect of the
resulting homeopathic medication can be when prescribed to a person
who needs it.

Some proponents of homeopathy, including indefatigable homeopathic
advocate Dana Ullman, MPH, call this system of homeopathic prescribing "nanopharmacology,"[105] an ingenious reference to these minute doses
of healing energies. Conventional medicine, without taking the time to
investigate the actual effects of homeopathic medicines, tends to dismiss
the entire enterprise as nothing more than the use of placebos. Ironically,
all homeopathics that I use in my practice are FDA approved and regu-
lated, but this is apparently not enough to convince nonbelievers. Take the
Petroleum that was prescribed to Susan, for example. If we were to submit
this preparation to a pharmaceutical lab for inspection, any knowledgeable

scientist would have to conclude that it has been diluted to such an extreme that it no longer contains any traces of petroleum. Understandably, a materialistic perspective holds that the preparation can have no medicinal effect since there is "nothing" left in it to produce such an effect. And I would concur, that is, *if* we were to examine this phenomenon from a strictly chemical perspective.

So how can homeopathic *Petroleum* possibly have any effect on Susan's skin condition? Remember now that biology cannot function without chemistry, but it is also true that chemistry cannot function without physics. Although I cannot provide a satisfactory scientific explanation that details exactly how a homeopathic preparation works, I can state with absolute certainty from personal experience that it *does* work. Physicists have studied the issue and have come up with a variety of complex theories. Most are in agreement that although the final solution obtained from the potentization process no longer contains any of the original substance dissolved into solution, it also no longer has the same energetic properties as the original solvent that the process started with. Therefore, the answer lies somewhere in the realm of physics and can be explained as an energetic phenomenon. The true test of any worthwhile treatment, after all, is the final effect that it has upon the suffering individual and his or her illness. Medical historian Harris L. Coulter explains why an understanding of the mechanism of action of a therapeutic substance should not be the determinant of its value:

> Homeopathy rejects the allopathic belief that the mechanisms of medicinal substances can be ultimately explained. The "real action" of a drug will always retreat beyond the investigator's means of discovery if it is sought at the cellular, molecular, or submolecular level, since mechanisms at all of these levels are determined by the behavior of the organism as a whole.[106]

Furthermore, any true skeptic willing to suspend judgment would find that a simple experiment might be capable of challenging his or her materialistic beliefs regarding homeopathic medicines. Hahnemann knew very well that, due to their toxicities, he could not test the crude undiluted substances used in homeopathy on patients. Alternatively, he used the diluted preparations to test their usefulness. If we were to do the same by administering repeated doses of homeopathically prepared *Petroleum* to a group of one hundred individuals without revealing to any of them what they were receiving, a certain percentage of sensitive individuals would begin to complain of symptoms documented as having an association with petroleum—such as dry, cracking, peeling skin and vertigo. Likewise, if we administered homeopathic *Apis* made from the honeybee to the same group, a certain percentage would develop hot, itchy, swollen, hive-like skin symptoms. And yet, pharmacological investigation would conclude that neither the *Apis* nor the *Petroleum* has any trace of the original substances that went into their creation. I have long since ceased trying to "prove" this reality to medical skeptics, who are unwilling to keep an open mind, and have focused instead upon the good that it can do for my clients.

Ecological sustainability is one of the greatest benefits derived from the homeopathic pharmaceutical process. The production of homeopathic medicines never involves animal testing in any form. In addition, the quantity of the original substance chosen to create each given homeopathic remedy is so small as to be negligible in terms of its environmental impact. One small preparation produced by dilution and succussion translates into treatment for thousands of people. What's more, no synthetic chemicals are ever created or employed in the process. As such, homeopathy represents one of the greenest of all medical therapies available to humankind.

Compare this to the devastation the conventional pharmaceutical industry wreaks upon our bodies and the environment. Basic common sense tells us that we must approach with skepticism any therapy that requires the creation of synthetic chemicals that are essentially toxins and that, if handled improperly, taken in the wrong dosages, or even taken according to directions, can cause serious harm to life or limb. The current configuration of the pharmaceutical industry is unsustainable, and if allowed to continue will surely destroy human health and the ecosystem upon which it depends.

Hahnemann was a tenacious and tireless pioneer and proponent of his new method of healing, in spite of resistance from the old school physicians. He endured a great deal of ostracism during most of his professional career and enjoyed popular success only in his later years, before he died at the ripe old age of eighty-eight. The name of this historic physician finds an interesting parallel in the monkey god, Hanuman, one of the most popular deities in the Hindu pantheon. Hanuman, who some consider to be an incarnated manifestation of the deity, Lord Shiva, is worshipped the world over as a symbol of courage, perseverance, devotion, and selfless service.

LIBERATING ESSENCE FROM MATTER

Let us return now to Paracelsus, who said that the goal of alchemy was to transmute crude matter into its "final substance and ultimate essence." Is it possible that Hahnemann discovered a method that could distill the essence from physical substances to be used for therapeutic purposes? Jungian psychotherapist Peter O'Connor speaks of the alchemist's search for such an "agent" or method that can aid in the transmutation process and what the end result of this process could be:

> All that was required was a suitable agent for bringing about this transmutation and redeeming the perfect matter, 'gold,' from the base metal. This redeeming or transmuting agent became known under a wide range of terms, and one can see constant reference to it in Jung, from such terms as the lapis ... or the philosopher's gold. In searching for this stone, the alchemist was endeavoring to liberate the spirit he believed to be concealed in matter; that is, to redeem the divine spirit, the perfect form, from the vessel of matter in which it was held captive.[107]

If conventional pharmacology can determine that a homeopathic preparation contains no physical substance and physicists have measured changes in the energetic properties of the solvent after potentization, then what is it that homeopaths have been using to heal thousands of persons over the past two centuries? Perhaps the best answer to this question is that the solution remaining after the potentization process contains the "essence" or "spirit" of the original substance. Alternatively, we can refer to it as the "energy" of the substance, to make it more acceptable to our modern sensibilities. In any event, the bottom line is that every substance has an energetic imprint or signature that can be employed in its homeopathic form to heal the sick. It is not a question of having faith or believing in the energetic imprint, and it may not satisfy the need of mechanists for a rational explanation, but it is a method of making effective medicines that has been verified over and over again.

Therefore, I would like to state with unequivocal certainty that homeopathic medicine is the literal modern-day embodiment of the alchemical ideal. There is no need to search any further. The transmutation process that converts matter into its pure essence has been found—in fact, it was found over two hundred years ago. The process of serial dilution and succussion can transform any physical substance into its pure gold-like energetic or spiritual essence. Once this Elixir of Life has been produced, it can then be used to restore balance to the vital force of the person who needs it, by bringing matter and spirit back together into alignment once again.

Hahnemann not only discovered this remarkable potentization process, but revealed his true genius in his application of these medicines. He understood deeply, like no other person had before him, the primacy of the principle of similars. Thus, it became a simple matter for him to study the symptoms that could be *caused* by any given animal, mineral, or plant substance in order to understand its indications for *treating* similar symptoms. Like with the scrapings from the tip of Achilles' spear, the use of a substance in healing is determined by the illnesses that it can cause. As the Oracle of Delphi declared, it is the wounder that shall heal.

A genuine appreciation for the profound simplicity of this fundamental law of green healing may require some reflection but, once you understand it, you can see how all substances then become potential agents of healing. The search for the Grail is then transformed into the quest to find the one substance, or sequence of substances, capable of healing each individual's illness. Once we understand that each unique human affliction is characterized by a life force stuck in an energetic vortex vibrating at a certain frequency, we can then seek the substance that is vibrating at a similar frequency out there in the world. Finding a substance that resonates with an illness becomes a matter of matching the symptom patterns of the two. Matching the energetic signature of a medicine with an illness of similar energetic nature assists the life force to "throw off" the illness and find its equilibrium again. The homeopathic methodology is simple in concept, but it can be quite complex in actual practice. When it is done properly, the results can be comprehensive and life changing. In a nutshell, homeopathy brings together the principle of similars and the alchemical transmutation of matter into its energetic essence to form an art and science of healing.

A PERSONAL CONNECTION

Years ago, within weeks of opening my private homeopathic practice, an eccentric fellow named Christopher walked into my office seeking medical care for his ailing father. He brought with him gifts, including old photos and postcards of homeopathic hospitals that had once existed in New York State at the turn of the century. Over the ensuing years we became good friends, as he educated me about the long and rich history of homeopathy in the United States and abroad. Did you know that there were over one hundred homeopathic hospitals in the United States in the

late 1800s? And that some of our current allopathic medical schools were originally founded as homeopathic schools? Did you know that a monument dedicated to Samuel Hahnemann, the founder of homeopathy, was erected in 1900 and still stands just a few blocks from the White House in Washington, DC? (See Figure 15.3.) Well, I didn't either, until Chris taught me all that and much more.

A number of years later, Chris called me one day with a curious tone to his voice, asking if my grandfather had been a doctor. I told him yes, I knew that my grandfather, who had been deceased for

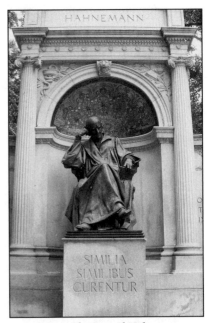

FIGURE 15.3: *The Samuel Hahnemann Monument, Scott Circle, Washington, DC*

over fifteen years, was a family practitioner and had donated much of his time and medical services to the poor. Chris asked if he had practiced in Astoria on Long Island. As I responded that yes this was true, I began to wonder what he was driving at. To my utter astonishment he said that he had found Vincent P. Malerba's name in a Directory of Homeopathic Physicians published in 1936. It listed him as having graduated from New York Homeopathic Medical College and Flower hospital in 1928!

Further research revealed that the college had dropped "Homeopathic" from its title in 1936 as it became a conventional allopathic institution,[108] and that it continues to operate today as New York Medical College. How truly strange this felt to me, since I had been appointed several years earlier by the very same college as an adjunct faculty member because of my experience in homeopathic medicine. My grandfather had apparently graduated from a medical school that was on the historical cusp and was therefore homeopathic in name only. No doubt he must have studied some homeopathy, but I know for a fact that he had gone on to practice mostly conventional medicine. Nevertheless, it had impressed upon my soul a synchronistic congruity that confirmed the life path that I had chosen, or that perhaps had chosen me.

NANOPHARMACOLOGICAL BIOMIMICRY

Homeopathy is pharmacological physics. It is the art and science of matching an illness with an energy dose that resonates at a similar frequency. It is an alchemical healing science that pairs the symptom patterns produced by substances in nature with the patterns of human illness. We can credit homeopathic advocate Dana Ullman, mentioned earlier, for applying the term "biomimicry" to the manner by which the pathological potential of the healing substance mimics the pathology of the suffering individual. Taking Ullman's two terms together, we come to understand homeopathy as "nanopharmacological biomimicry." When the essence of an illness, as expressed through the symptoms produced by the vital force, is brought together with an energy of a substance of similar essence, the result is the liberation of the defense mechanism from the vortex of dysfunction that had, until then, been holding it rigidly in place.

Thus far I have used examples that I have purposely chosen for their ability to clearly portray the connection between the "wounder" and the "healer." The *identical* relationships between the "wounding" substances, burning oil in Kuwait and a bee sting, and their corresponding "healing" energies, homeopathic *Petroleum* and *Apis,* are readily apparent. In both cases we have clear-cut "causes," although it must be recalled from our previous discussions that causation is a tricky concept. We can call the bee sting the "cause" of the swollen arm but there are many who, after being stung in the exact same location, will not develop a swollen arm. In the end, it always comes down to the status of the vital force and its response to the external stressor. This homeopathic concept becomes a little more challenging to comprehend when we recognize that it is based on *similars* and that most illnesses do not offer an *identical* etiology for our diagnostic convenience.

By virtue of our knowledge of the principle of similars, we can tentatively begin to predict the applicability of various substances to certain illnesses, based upon our awareness of the pathology that these substances are known to cause. Poison ivy, for example, as we all know, has a strong tendency to generate itching and blistering. By extension, illnesses that manifest similar symptoms, and that are not necessarily caused by poison ivy, may be amenable to treatment with homeopathic poison ivy. And this is exactly what Hahnemann found. *Rhus toxicodendron,* homeopathic poison ivy, has been effectively used by thousands of practitioners to treat conditions that are similar to poison ivy, such as herpes, shingles, and even chicken pox, especially when these illnesses are characterized by strong itching and blistering.

Mercury is a metal used in making thermometers because of its exquisite sensitivity to temperature changes. Although the list of possible symptoms that mercury can cause is extensive, its temperature characteristics alone provide valuable clues as to the applicability of homeopathic *Mercurius.* And so, *Mercurius* is high on my list of possible homeopathic prescriptions when a client with an illness that involves fever and chills, such as the flu, an ear infection, or a throat infection, reports feeling hot, then cold, then hot, then cold.

THE CASE OF THE POWERFUL WOLVERINE

The following case provides another example of the extraordinary effect that a well-chosen homeopathic prescription can have upon a significant disturbance in the vital energy.

Nora was a remarkable woman with a robust appearance and a powerful presence. It turned out that she was a Wolverine, an alumnus of the University of Michigan, the archenemy of my alma mater, Michigan State, home of the Spartans. I joked that in spite of this shortcoming of hers, I would still pledge to help her as best as I could. Although she was fifty-seven years old, she looked to be closer to forty-seven, and she acted as if she were thirty-seven. She wore a short skirt and her legs were very muscular, like those of an athlete. The symptom pattern that she described reflected her powerful appearance. Well past the average age of menopause, she nevertheless was continuing to have regular menstrual periods, which were characterized by a very heavy blood flow. She described the flow as "very bright red, hot blood. I can feel my heart pumping it out of me."

In addition, Nora had recently developed intense headaches that forced her to lie in bed. "I can't stand the light. They go boom, boom, boom," she said. If someone accidentally bumped into the bed it could cause a severe wave of head pain. Not surprisingly, she also had been diagnosed with high blood pressure four years earlier and, it too, was of a particularly intense nature. Before starting conventional medication, her lower number, the diastolic blood pressure, could reach as high as 110 to 115. "When it's high, it's like my head is exploding." Even at the subconscious level, this power was exhibited in the fact that Nora had had many dreams of "being caught in huge tidal waves."

Fortunately, in this particular case I did not have to think too hard, as I was aware of a homeopathic remedy that matched her symptom pattern well. Homeopathic *Belladonna* is made from a highly toxic plant, the deadly nightshade, and is well known to cause symptoms that can be attributed to the sudden rushing of blood to various specific locations in the body—an effect that resonated with the quality of Nora's menses, headaches, blood pressure, and dreams. In even small amounts, this poisonous plant can kill a person, but in its homeopathic form, it is completely benign.

Given the nature of Nora's symptoms, I proceeded cautiously, prescribing small doses of homeopathic *Belladonna* at long intervals. Her immediate response was to develop a bad headache that lasted for hours. To her delight, she did not have another one until three months later, after she drank a cup of coffee, which I had previously advised her not to do. After one month, she reported that her blood pressure was the lowest it had been in three years, and that her menstrual flow had slowed down significantly. After three months, she said that her blood pressure was even lower. She said that her last period was "normal," and she compared it to periods she used to have thirty years prior. At the five-month mark, Nora had had no further headaches, her blood pressure was stable on less medication, and she had completely ceased to have menstrual periods. Eight months from the start of treatment she said, "On the whole, I feel better than I've felt in years." She later moved out of town but I was happy to receive a letter from Nora updating her status. In it she wrote, "Three cheers for Belladonna! Any more of these good feelings and you will get this Wolverine cheering for MSU!"

PARADOXICAL PARALLELS

Evidence of this paradoxical phenomenon of similars abounds, even in allopathic medical practice. The conventional drug used to treat gout, colchicine, is a synthetic version of an alkaloid derived from the plant meadow saffron. Homeopaths have studied the effects of this plant, which include the distinct ability to generate gout-like symptoms. It is therefore used to great effect as homeopathic *Colchicum* to treat gout. Most people know that Ritalin and other drugs like it are central nervous system stimulants used to treat children and, more recently, adults with symptoms of hyperactivity. I remember being taught in medical school that although the effect of these drugs was a poorly understood paradox, they were nevertheless effective. Even immunizations are an extremely crude application of the principle of similars.

It is not surprising that similars are used in conventional medical practice without awareness as to why the method can produce positive results.

The problem with this use of similars in orthodox medicine occurs when the homeopathic requirement of individualizing each and every case is neglected, and the substances used are toxic and administered in doses too large. Allopathic medicine gives all children the same vaccines, and gives virtually all hyperactive children Ritalin-like drugs. In homeopathy, a variety of different medicines may be prescribed, and the choice is completely dependent upon matching the symptom pattern of the child with the symptom profile of the remedy.

We can see that at the most fundamental level, any genuinely effective psychotherapeutic intervention is also based upon the principle of similars. I am sorry to say it, but people don't overcome the emotional baggage of their past by running away from it. If they attempt to do so, it usually follows behind and haunts them until it eventually catches up to them. When clients tell me that they have put their problems in the past and nevertheless still have a variety of physical health problems, I suspect that the underlying emotional issues have not been dealt with. The only way to adequately and successfully deal with difficult emotional and psychological issues is to turn around and face them squarely and honestly.

Jungian analyst Arnold Mindell describes a particularly remarkable application of the principle of similars in his book *Working with the Dreaming Body*. He refers to the mind-body-spirit unity as the "dreambody" and his work with patients as "process work." The book tells how he came upon the idea of the "amplification" of a person's symptoms and the way in which they are expressed. According to this method, if a man with a headache, for example, says that his head feels worse when pressure is applied and it feels like it will explode, then he is encouraged to apply as much pressure as he can tolerate and to let himself explode. Mindell found that people can have profound, productive, and illuminating experiences when they reach the limit of their tolerance for suffering. Some break down into cathartic emotion, some experience paradoxical relief from pain, and some gain new insights into the roots of their pain and illnesses.

Having read his book, I was amazed that he made no mention of the homeopathic use of similars, since this is exactly the nature of his method. Not surprisingly, his explorations with his patients have yielded some valuable observations regarding the nature of illness and healing. Here he recognizes the value of empirical observation and the uniqueness of each individual and his or her illness:

> *I don't believe in therapy because I don't know any more what is right for other people. I have seen so many strange cases that I have decided to go back to my original idea as a scientist. I simply look to see what exactly is happening in the other person and what happens to me while he is reacting. I let the dreambody processes tell me what wants to happen and what to do next. That is the only pattern I follow.*[109]

Here Mindell acknowledges that people usually do not will themselves to be sick, and he touches upon the meaning behind illness:

> *A chronic disease is often a lifelong problem, a part of someone's individuation process. I don't believe that a person actually creates disease, but that his soul is expressing an important message to him through the disease.*[110]

And here, he quite clearly expresses the homeopathic theme of the wounded healer:

> *Here is quite a paradox. Diseases can be self-healing; the dreambody is its own solution ... Discover the process, amplify its channel, and a symptom can turn into a medicine.... Thus, a body symptom, regardless of how seemingly insignificant, can become the most difficult and exciting challenge in your life! A terrifying symptom is usually your greatest dream trying to come true.*[111]

As mentioned in an earlier chapter, we even have biblical confirmation of the successful application of the principle of similars for healing purposes. And it was none other than Yahweh himself that proposed the remedy to Moses. The *Book of Numbers* from the *Old Testament* recounts one of the stories of the Israelites' wanderings through the desert. When Moses sent messengers to the King of Edom to ask if his people could pass through on the way to Canaan, the King refused and threatened to send an army out against them. The Israelites were obliged to back away and travel around Edom, thus prolonging their journey. The people were unhappy about this turn of events and about life in the desert in general, so they began to complain. They voiced their discontentment to Moses and blamed him and even blamed God. When God heard this, He sent a plague of "fiery serpents" among them to punish them for their lack of faith. Many died from the bites of these poisonous snakes and others became gravely ill. Fearing for their lives, the people repented for their lapse into doubt and mistrust. They beseeched Moses to pray for God's intervention and Moses complied:

> And the Lord said unto Moses, 'Make thee a fiery serpent, and set it upon a pole: and it shall come to pass, that every one that is bitten, when he looketh upon it, shall live.' And Moses made a serpent of brass, and put it upon a pole, and it came to pass, that if a serpent had bitten any man, when he beheld the serpent of brass, he lived.[112]

Now if God had proposed that Moses instruct the people to place tourniquets on bitten limbs and to extract the venom from their wounds, then we could see how the people would be eager to comply. But the prescription offered by God ran contrary to conventional wisdom, further trying the patience and testing the faith of an already weary band of believers. The affliction brought about by Yahweh was designed to teach perseverance in the midst of hardship, and the cure was provided by the same One who had done the wounding. This theme of the wounded healer, the principle of treatment with similars, is also clearly indicated by the fact that the Israelites were cured of their snakebites when they looked up at the "brazen serpent" upon the pole.

Of course, the Christian version of this dynamic is Christ, the ultimate wounded healer, crucified on the "pole" so that humankind would no longer need to suffer. Through his wounds his followers may be healed. The *Gospel of John* in the *New Testament* confirms this connection when Jesus says:

And as Moses lifted up the serpent in the wilderness, even so must
the Son of man be lifted up. That whosoever believeth in him
should not perish, but have eternal life.[113]

A CASE OF COLLEGIATE COLD FEET

The principle of similars can work just as effectively for emotional issues
as it can for physical health problems. Lindsey was a high school senior
who had struggled with a good deal of anxiety over the previous year. She
told me that the anxiety had been particularly difficult since she had begun
the college application process. She felt fatigued, was having trouble falling
asleep, and had even fainted several times. She had consulted a regular doctor, who had ruled out the possibility of mononucleosis and a variety of
other physical illnesses. In addition, she was having some cramping with
her menses and would become very emotional and weepy during that time.
In response to further questioning she said that her legs were also tending
to cramp.

When I asked her about her fears, Lindsey responded, "Going to college. Leaving my mom and dad." After a little more questioning she revealed
that her soccer coach had suddenly died in her junior year of high school.
To compound matters, her grandfather had also passed away a few months
later, during the following summer. My questioning her about the time-
line of events helped Lindsey to realize that the anxiety had started around
the same time that her coach had passed away.

The facts of this case clearly pointed to the likelihood that the deaths
of Lindsey's coach and grandfather had triggered her anxiety, and that her
physical symptoms were simply a by-product of the larger issue. It is not
that she didn't want to go to college. To the contrary, she had very clear
plans and ambitions for her future career, but she was being held back by
the newly developed anxiety. It was reasonable to conclude that Lindsey
had become fearful that, in going off to college, she could also lose her
parents.

Anyone who has studied a little bit of homeopathy may recognize that
stories like Lindsey's are described in many introductory textbooks. The
unique combination of anxiety, grief, fear of loss, and muscle cramps is

well represented by the remedy *Ignatia*, a homeopathic preparation made from the St. Ignatius's bean. Priests found the plant in the Philippines, brought it back to Europe in the seventeenth century and, presumably, named it after the founder of the Jesuit order, Saint Ignatius of Loyola. It is an invaluable medicine, which can release a person from the grips of "spasms" of grief and loss. I gave Lindsey one moderately strong dose of *Ignatia* and instructed her to return in a few weeks.

One month later, she reported that she had had a "meltdown" several days after taking the remedy, during which she did a lot of crying. This had "felt good emotionally" to her and coincided with a distinct reduction in feelings of anxiety. Amazingly, she had also settled on the college of her choice. Several months and a few doses of *Ignatia* later, Lindsey had another cathartic release of grief the night before her high school graduation. "I was sad that my grandfather couldn't be there," she said.

To everyone's delight, she went off to college the following autumn and did very well, until, sadly, her grandmother passed away. It "reopened old wounds" and caused a little anxiety, but I prescribed a booster dose of *Ignatia*, which settled her down, and she returned to successfully complete her first year of college. Lindsey's sadness had become locked up inside, and instead of expressing grief in a healthy way, her body had generated cramps and anxiety. Proper treatment had allowed the life force to be released from this energetic vortex of suffering.

WOUNDED HEALERS

You may recall that Chiron, the centaur, was mentor to both Achilles and Asklepios. Chiron had been abandoned by his parents and later, as an innocent bystander, was accidentally wounded by Herakles. Since he was immortal, he could not die and lived in great pain. Because of this he is the Greek exemplar of the Wounded Healer, who, through the experience of his own suffering, passed his healing knowledge on to others who had suffered a similar fate.

In 1977, astronomer Charles Kowal discovered an object in space that was later named after the mythic Chiron. Orbiting between Saturn and Uranus, it was first thought to be an asteroid, and later a comet. Some believe the discovery of this celestial body to be the fulfillment of a Native American prophecy that foretold of the coming of a planet of healing in the sky. Contemporary astrologers believe that it represents the ushering in of the New Age, and is therefore associated with holistic healing. The placement of Chiron, the Wounded Healer, in one's astrological birth chart is thought on the one hand, to identify the nature of one's woundedness, and on the other to represent the key to overcoming our greatest suffering.

Astrologers who have studied Chiron believe that it signifies the new paradigm of the Wounded Healer. Because it is a comet and not a planet, Chiron has no home in astrological terms, and is therefore considered a wanderer. It is the wounded wanderer in search of healing. Proponents of the emerging green consciousness intuitively understand that the old methods of suppression are no longer viable. Chiron is commonly represented in astrological charts by the image of a key. The very "key" to our healing lies in the source of our woundedness. We cannot have the light without the dark, the male without the female, the medicine without the wound. Martin Lass, musician, astrologer, and healer, captures the message of the new Chiron in the phrase, "The gift is in the wound." The potential of all that we can become is already there within us, waiting to be embraced and developed. The wound is the gift that teaches us about our limitations and shortcomings. The wound nags at us, spurring us on to seek healing.

We may not be aware of what that healing ultimately entails, but if we are successful in our search we realize that it involves bringing to consciousness that which was previously unconscious, thereby restoring balance in the process. Recognition of the process and acceptance of the challenge then provide meaning where previously none was to be found. As healing takes place, polarities are transcended, and a new unity is born. The darkness is brought into the light and integrated into the whole. Lass sums up the lessons that Chiron teaches us:

> When we deny, disown, fail to acknowledge, ignore, try to escape from, condemn and/or try to banish certain parts of ourselves, we are Wounded; we are in denial of the larger Plan and Purpose of the cosmos. Such are the Wounds that Chiron mirrors. However, when we walk willingly into our Darkness, shining a light, so to

speak, we gradually recover the lost pieces of our lives. Gradually, we become whole once more, reconnect with our higher celestial nature and take our rightful place as co-Creators of this magnificent universe.[114]

The principle of similars is the most important and fundamental characteristic that all genuine and effective methods of healing have in common. In the Latin, Hahnemann dubbed it *"Similia Similibus Curantur,"* or "Likes are used to cure likes." While treatment with opposites is an effective tool for stopping or suppressing symptoms under appropriate circumstances, it is usually ineffective as a method of healing the whole. Given the healing capacity of the homeopathic method and the fact that it is the polar opposite methodology to the allopathic use of contraries, it is easy to understand why homeopathy has been historically met with tenacious opposition by the conventional medical establishment. Viewing homeopathy as a competitor, orthodoxy fails to understand that the complementary use of both methodologies is in the best interests of our patients.

The alchemical technique of transmutation exists today as a scientific method of potentization through dilution and succussion, which enables the energetic spirit to be distilled from any material substance. In this form, it can be applied to the art of healing as long as the energy signature of the substance resonates sufficiently with the energetic wound of the suffering individual. Thus, within the nature of our own wounds lies the ultimate source of our self-healing. This approach to healing overlaps and transcends all categories of mind, body, emotion, purpose, meaning, spirit, and soul. In the process, we reclaim the wound as our own. The wound of the wanderer in the desert thus finds a home and a place of balance as it is set once again in its rightful place within the awe-inspiring and magnificent complexity of the energetic whole.

Renewable Healing Resources

Much that passes for illness is a message that should lead into a world that is exciting and filled with lights, colors, sounds, pleasures, tingling, unconstricted breathing, personal growth, and startling vision, to which the world of sterile chemicals and operating tables is a cruel reversal and wasteful joke.

—Richard Grossinger, *Planet Medicine*

The Thunder-beings bring us the raw energy we need to change and renew our lives. We humans are Catalyzers who have electromagnetic, giving and receiving, bodies. We are the bridge that connects Earth and Sky when we are in harmony. Like Mother Earth and Father Sky we are male and female in nature. The command of usable energy comes when male and female are in balance within us.

—Jamie Sams, *Sacred Path Cards*

THE ELECTROMAGNETIC UNIVERSE

The universe is a vast sea of interweaving energy waves, with each ostensibly discrete entity vibrating at its own unique frequency. It is not enough to say that all *living* things are energetic organisms. By virtue of Einstein's equation we know that all physical matter, organic and inorganic, is equivalent to its energetic essence. Matter is just energy vibrating at a much lower frequency. It is moving at such a slow pace that it appears to our limited senses to form the world of solid objects.

Basic conventional science teaches us that the universe is an infinite electromagnetic field composed of a spectrum of waves moving at different amplitudes and frequencies. Way down at the low end of the spectrum are the radio waves by means of which we receive television, radio, and wireless transmissions. A bit higher up, with waves traveling at slightly higher velocities, are microwaves. (Although I do not recommend this method of meal preparation, microwaves can generate enough heat to cook our food.) Next comes a relatively unexplored range of frequencies called terahertz. Above them we find the infrared spectrum, a range of light frequencies just outside the lower end of the visible spectrum, which can be detected as heat and can be seen with special devices that can be used, for example, by firefighters to detect hotspots and by photographers to take pictures in the dark.

As the frequency of a wave becomes faster, its corresponding energy increases, while its wavelength shortens. Therefore, if an infrared ("below red") wave were to become shorter, moving more quickly and with greater energy, it would move into the visible spectrum of light and color. Red, the color of visible light with the lowest frequency, comes just above infrared. The rainbow spectrum of colors, ROYGBIV (red, orange, yellow, green, blue, indigo, violet), which is capable of being detected and interpreted by the human eye, optic nerve, and brain, comprises only a tiny sliver of the greater electromagnetic spectrum.

Moving out of the visible spectrum, just above the highest color frequency, violet, we reach ultraviolet ("extreme violet"). Among other things, ultraviolet light, or UV radiation, assists in the production of vitamin D and can cause skin tanning and burning. Beyond UV frequencies we find X-rays and, ultimately, gamma rays. Both are used in medical radiography for therapeutic purposes and to penetrate the physical body in order to visualize internal structures.

The standard five human senses cannot detect the greater part of the electromagnetic spectrum. This is easily illustrated with the use of a dog whistle, which creates mechanical sound waves that can be detected by some animals but that are generated at frequencies too high to be heard by the human ear. Most of us lose the ability to detect frequencies at the far ends of the sound spectrum as we grow older. My children once found a Web site that accessed various frequencies of sound waves. They played certain higher frequencies that were clearly audible to them, and fell to the floor laughing hysterically when they realized that my wife and I could not hear these sounds.

The theoretical origin of the universe has always generated much speculation and controversy. Some conceptualize it as a vast primordial soup of particles that began to coalesce into the forms that we are familiar with. The Big Bang supposes the manifest universe emanated from some sort of physical or energetic explosion. There are a variety of creation stories. The Bible tells us in one place that "... God said, Let there be light: and there was light."[115] In another place, we are told, "In the beginning was the Word, and the Word was with God, and the Word was God."[116] Regardless of your preferred theory and taking into consideration that even the particles of the primordial soup are, at bottom, energy, the origin comes down to some form of energetic phenomenon, whether explosion, light wave, or sound wave in the form of the voice of God.

SECRET KNOWLEDGE

The conventional exoteric conception of the electromagnetic spectrum takes into account only that which science is capable of perceiving from its materialistic perspective. Esoteric knowledge, on the other hand, indicates that there is much more to the human body and its environment than can be detected by the physical senses or science's instruments of measurement. Exoteric knowledge means the body of publicly accepted information, such as is imparted to us through the conventional sciences and even traditional religious beliefs. Esoteric knowledge encompasses a very broad, unconventional range of information that most would claim to be unscientific, illusory, or even heretical. By this standard, even though I personally understand homeopathic medicine to be based in a rigorous scientific methodology, it nevertheless would get lumped into the esoteric category of the foreign and unfamiliar. The histories of many esoteric disciplines reach back thousands of years. Homeopathy is in its relative infancy compared to such fields as astrology, alchemy, Gnosticism, Kabbalism, and Hermeticism. Esoteric endeavors have often focused upon an understanding of the "inner" nature of human beings, a topic that has become virtually extinct in our externally oriented times.

During the Middle Ages, and further back in time, esoteric studies were standard fare in the curriculum of the well-educated person. Much of this knowledge, primarily due to religious persecution, was kept concealed from the "common" person. There is much evidence confirming the existence of "Mystery schools" as far back as ancient Greece, Egypt and, some would say, Atlantis. Mystery schools were places where "initiates" would go to train to become physicians, priests, scientists, and community leaders. Here the esoteric sciences such as astrology, numerology, and alchemy, and spiritual disciplines such as chant, yoga, and meditation, as well as the exoteric sciences, were taught. Our modern notion of a school is a place where training of the *mind* takes place. But there is an alternate type of training, as Grace Knoche, author of *The Mystery Schools,* explains:

> *A Mystery school is a university of the soul, a school for the study of the mysteries of the inner nature of man and of surrounding nature. By understanding these mysteries, the student perceives his intimate relationship with divinity, and strives through self-discipline and devotion to become at one with his inner god.*[117]

This keeping of the "secret" knowledge was a privilege that at times came to be abused, thus paralleling the behavior of some elite religious hierarchies, the keepers of church dogma. Church fathers made it clear that they alone were the conduits to God. Common men and women had no place in such business other than to obey Church law as ordained by the clergy. As such, God became something that could only be experienced second-hand, vicariously through the privileged few. Likewise, those in possession of the secret esoteric knowledge became more than a little presumptuous in assuming that only the well educated could handle this information.

The inner explorations of the sixties generation opened to our awareness the reality that we do not have to hand personal responsibility for spiritual experience over to authority figures. We learned that, to the contrary, spiritual experience is a deeply personal endeavor that loses much of its meaning if it is sought from an external source. There is an enormous untapped trove of inner knowledge and experience that has been kept from our reach, but the veil of secrecy is being gradually lifted, and the neglected knowledge of the Mystery traditions is now becoming available, as it rightfully should, to all modern seekers. This long forgotten body of knowledge is that which the patriarchs and materialists would deny us.

Some of us are so thoroughly programmed and out of touch with our inner selves that we have come to equate personal spirituality with perfunctory attendance at services once per week. In order to open ourselves to the mysterious and spiritually edifying world of esoteric knowledge we need only to overcome our fears, which come from our lack of familiarity with the subject matter.

According to esoteric understanding, the exoteric electromagnetic spectrum can be expanded to incorporate other energies that have hitherto gone unrecognized by mainstream authorities. Most of these energies can tentatively be placed at either end of the "known" spectrum. Below the lower end of the range of radio waves, as the frequency slows down even further, we can identify the realm of physical matter. The form of matter that vibrates most rapidly is a gas. As a gas slows down and decreases in energy it becomes a liquid. The slowest phase of all, which generates the least amount of energy, is the solid phase of matter. Thus, solid matter is the densest form of energy, is the least energetic, and vibrates at the slowest frequencies.

At the upper end of the spectrum, beyond where the instruments of science can detect, the energies become more speculative and mysterious, at least to many. Here the vibration rates are very fast, and imperceptible to the five senses. This is the frequency range that may account for a wide variety of phenomena that many dismiss, mainly out of fear and ignorance, as the perceptions of eccentrics or psychotics. The visualization of auras, communication with spirit guides and angels, energy healings, psychic abilities, clairaudience, clairvoyance, telepathy, dream premonition, and even intuition and synchronicity are experiences that fall into this vibratory range. The funny thing is that most individuals rarely take these phenomena very seriously, until they experience them firsthand. Because there is little cultural acknowledgment or acceptance of such phenomena, the person who has had such an experience is often placed in the lonely position of having to seek out other persons who have made similar observations.

Various esoteric schools of thought have developed a number of classification systems that define this higher range of frequencies, and, with minor variations, they are all similar. This esoteric "anatomy" derives primarily from the Eastern yogic traditions of India, China, Tibet, and Japan.

Various individuals and groups, especially those representing the Theosophical movement, founded by Helena Petrovna Blavatsky and Henry Steel Olcott, brought many of these occult and mystical teachings to the West in the late 1800s. At that time the Theosophical Society formulated three main objectives: 1) to promote a universal nondiscriminatory brotherhood of humanity, 2) to advocate for the study of comparative religion, philosophy, and science, and 3) to investigate the unexplained laws of nature and the powers latent in man. Many consider Blavatsky, along with Annie Besant, Alice Bailey, founder of anthroposophy and Waldorf education Rudolf Steiner, and others, to be the primary figures that inspired the modern New Age movement.

Esoteric anatomy postulates not only a gross physical dimension but also a series of psycho-spiritual "subtle" bodies and planes of increasing metaphysical significance. One distillation of this knowledge divides all existence beyond the physical plane into *subtle* and *spiritual* planes. Another differentiates the *etheric* from the *emotional* and *mental* planes. A similar classification includes the *etheric, astral, mental,* and *spiritual* planes.

The lower end of this upper range of frequencies begins with the etheric body, which many describe as a subtle energetic extension of the physical body. It is a type of energetic body double that bridges the physical body to the finer electromagnetic forces of the universe. We can reasonably assume that the approximate "location" of the vital force that we have been discussing is in the etheric body, on the etheric plane. The astral body of the astral plane conveys human emotion and desire. It is the channel of love, hate, hope, and fear. The mental plane is the container of mind, thought, and intellectual activity. And the spiritual plane contains the highest and most refined form of energy in the universe. In this golden age of materialism, theses higher energetic planes remain underappreciated, misunderstood, and poorly utilized by most individuals.

The universe, therefore, is a vast keyboard of frequencies ranging from the densest solid to the most high of spiritual energies, which some would call God or the One. Scientists tell us that the energies of the electromagnetic spectrum can travel across space and time in the form of waves. Light can be conceptualized as waves or as energy particles, called photons. By extension, a thought is a form of energy that can travel across the mental plane, often having an imperceptible though significant impact upon its environment. Like light waves, thought waves can also cover enormous distances in split seconds. Similarly, emotions are energies that can traverse the astral dimension, thus having an effect upon many people and many aspects of life, even at a distance.

PATTERN AND PURPOSE

Thought and emotion are so powerful that they can have a direct effect upon the world of physical matter. I once knew a person who dreamt that she was very angry with her mother, but was previously completely unable to express this anger in her waking life. The following morning, as she stood in the kitchen recounting this dream, the Corelle cereal bowl that she was holding spontaneously exploded into a thousand little pieces before her very eyes. Anyone familiar with Corelle knows how difficult it can be to shatter one of its products. If the intensity of this unexpressed emotion could do such damage to an external object, imagine what effects our thoughts and emotions can have upon our physical bodies and our mental and emotional health. Conversely, just imagine the positive things that could be accomplished if the majority of humanity took the very real power of thought and emotion seriously. We can deny or suppress such thoughts and emotions at our own risk, or we can acknowledge their existence before they build in power until they can no longer be contained.

Myriad phenomena that make up the physical and non-physical dimensions exist within this vast electromagnetic field that we call the universe. A holistic glance at this world reveals many repeating patterns and correspondences that we have become accustomed to ignoring out of our materialistic and mechanistic biases. We tend to dismiss these patterns as simple coincidences of little significance, which, as such, do not warrant our attention. For example, what are we to make of the fact that there are, among many other sevens, seven colors of the visible spectrum, seven notes on the Western musical scale, seven original astrological planets visible to the naked eye (the Sun, the Moon, and five planets: Mars, Mercury, Jupiter,

Venus, and Saturn), seven days of the week, seven continents and seven seas, the seven directions of the Native American medicine wheel, the seven days of biblical creation, and the seven heavens of Islamic tradition? Are we to accept all this as mere coincidence, an arbitrary product of the human psyche, or a reflection of patterns and correspondences that replicate themselves throughout the created universe?

For many years I have practiced a form of medical treatment that relies upon the correspondences between the patterns of human illness and similar patterns reflected in the animal, plant, and mineral kingdoms. Such correlations should lead any thoughtful person to consider the possibility of a profound order to a universe that to the rational scientific mind seems random and chaotic. We know that the moon affects the tides and women's menstrual cycles, among other things, and astrologers know that moon cycles affect human emotion and behavior. Is it so far-fetched to believe that the movements of other celestial bodies can also have an impact on the earth and its inhabitants? Conventional medicine completely overlooks the obvious reality of human body and personality types, and yet the significance of these patterns is often recognized by many psychological and alternative healing modalities.

Such patterns are to be found all throughout the natural world and are reflective of the "As above, so below" principle. Acupuncture uses points on the ear that correspond to other parts of the body. Similarly, reflexology, acupressure, and shiatsu points on the hands and feet correlate to other body locations, including the internal organs. Stramonium, which is a nightshade plant similar to Belladonna and is routinely and effectively used to treat persons who have a fear of the dark and a tendency to wake with night terrors, is an example of correspondence in homeopathic medicine. The remarkable parallel here is that the flower of this plant, also known as Jimsonweed, only blooms at night.

Thirteenth-century Italian mathematician Leonardo Fibonacci uncovered a number pattern that remains associated with his name to this day. The Fibonacci sequence begins with zero and one, and each subsequent number is obtained by adding the two preceding numbers. The resulting series begins with the following:

0, 1, 1, 2, 3, 5, 8, 13, 21, 34, 55, 89, 144, 233 . . .

When we tune in, we begin to recognize the many cycles and patterns of nature. Therefore, it should come as no surprise that the number of petals on nearly all flowers conforms to one of the Fibonacci numbers. Lilies, for example, have three petals, buttercups have five, marigolds have thirteen, and asters have twenty-one. (An unusual exception to the rule is the fuchsia, which has four petals.) Botanists have found Fibonacci number arrangements in the branches, leaves, seeds, and pine cones of many plants and trees.

One of the most fascinating correspondences that I have ever encountered is the similarity between the ancient Chinese *Book of Changes,* the *I Ching,* and the crowning discovery of modern science, the structure of DNA. The rungs of the ladder of the DNA double helix are composed of nucleotide base pairs. Each base pair is derived from four possible nucleotides: adenine (A), cytosine (C), guanine (G), or thymine (T). A sequence of three base pair rungs on the spiral staircase of DNA creates the genetic code for an amino acid. Amino acids are the building blocks of the proteins that form the structural basis of all life on our planet. All possible three-letter combinations of the DNA coding units, T, C, A, and G, are used to encode one of these amino acids or one of the three stop codons at the end of a sequence of amino acids. Therefore, the number of potential three-letter combinations derived from A, C, G, and T can be mathematically represented by the following:

$$4^3 = (2 \times 2) \times (2 \times 2) \times (2 \times 2) = 64 \text{ possible nucleotide combinations}$$

The *I Ching* was divined and constructed by the ancients to respond to the petitioner with advice corresponding to all possible life situations and their outcomes. The head and tail pattern obtained from a series of coin tosses indicates a specific reading in response to a question asked. Each reading from the oracle is composed of a hexagram of six lines. A hexagram is further divided into two sets of three lines, or trigrams. Each individual line has two possible configurations—a solid line representing the yang, or a broken line denoting the yin qualities of the universe. The mathematical representation of all possible combinations of six broken or solid lines is expressed by the following equation:

$$2 \times 2 \times 2 \times 2 \times 2 \times 2 = 64 \; possible \; \text{I Ching} \; readings$$

The composition of the *I Ching* and the structure of DNA, therefore, are both based in a binary code consisting of yin/yang and nucleotide base pairs, respectively. Each then translates into triplets, represented by trigrams and the three base pairs of an amino acid sequence. And each system has sixty-four total possible combinations, which form the foundation of all of life's situations and all of life's physical forms. Marie-Louise von Franz, eminent Jungian psychologist, contemporary of Carl Jung, and founder of the C.G. Jung Institute in Zurich, comments on this *I Ching*/DNA correspondence in her book *Number and Time*, which explores evidence supporting the existence of numerical archetypes:

> One cannot escape the impression that these numerical combinations are introspective representations of fundamental processes in our psychophysical nature ... In these genetic findings we are confronted with an exchange of "information" in living cells that corresponds exactly to the structure of the I Ching hexagrams.
>
> This astonishing correspondence seems, more than any other evidence, to substantiate Jung's hypothesis that number regulates both psyche and matter.[118]

Is it possible that this is an accident, a freaky fluke of correspondence between the human psyche and the structure of nature? Or is it powerful confirmation of a patterned universe from which we can derive purpose, meaning, direction, and guidance? There are many who take these numerical motifs and natural patterns as indication of a divine ordering principle. Greek mathematician and scholar Pythagoras was allegedly an initiate of several Mystery schools in the sixth century BCE. Today known as the father of numbers, his namesake is the Pythagorean theorem, the formula that constitutes the foundation of modern geometry. He is also the first to have called himself a philosopher. What we know of his body of work comes primarily from secondhand sources. Manly P. Hall notes that Iamblichus documented thirty-nine aphorisms attributable to Pythagoras. One such aphorism reflects our topic:

> 'Speak not about Pythagoric concerns without light.' The world is herein warned that it should not attempt to interpret the mysteries of God and the states of the sciences without spiritual and intellectual illumination.[119]

Pythagoras viewed life as a religious and scientific synthesis informed by number, form, and pattern as evinced by the natural world and the cycles of the cosmos. He established an educational institution and secret society in southern Italy to promote his beliefs, and is credited with having investigated the use of music and color in the treatment of disease. It should come as no surprise that the Hippocratic oath of modern medicine has its roots in the oath of the Pythagorean Brotherhood. Vera Stanley Alder, author of a number of books that make esoteric thought accessible to neophytes, describes a quote that some attribute to Pythagoras, and others credit to Plato, who was strongly influenced by Pythagoras:

> Pythagoras said: 'God geometrises.' He and other giant intellects have realised that the world is created upon a system of exact vibrations, patterns, symbols and dimensions, and that through a study of these numbered vibrations and rays, the symbols of the way in which they intersect to form certain shapes, and the different grades of matter which their varied frequencies participate, an understanding of the created world, its trend, purpose and the great Consciousness behind it can be acquired and utilised.[120]

My point here is not to feed the reductionistic delusion that we will someday be able to plug all of life's potentialities into some mathematical equation. What I *am* saying is that if we trust our instincts and follow the signs and patterns, they will lead us to a vision of humanity and its relationship to the universe that is deeply satisfying and congruent with a holistic vision of green health care.

THE ENTROPIC ILLUSION

Physical medicine's care for the outer person is predicated upon a denial and neglect of the reality of the all-important inner person. The physical body is but a temporary shell for the soul. Attention paid to the inner spirit and soul will naturally accrue to the benefit of the physical body. The reverse is not necessarily always the case.

I recall that even back in high school, I instinctively rejected the notion of "entropy" as taught by conventional science. Although I could not put it into words, it did not quite sit right with me, as I felt it to be a false assessment of the nature of our universe. Science used the term to denote the randomness of the physical world and its natural tendency toward gradual decay and disorder. This "you are born, gradually decay, and ultimately die" perspective on life is indicative of the nihilistic potential of science.

A life lived with the certainty of entropic decay can cause one to cling onto this physical existence, to grab for all that one can get before it is too late, to resent that one did not get one's share. Its fundamental selfishness fails to comprehend the connection between all things physical and immaterial. It causes one to strain against the natural order of things and against the ebb and flow of energetic influences. It engenders a fear of our own body, its processes, and its symptoms and their meanings. Death, according to this perspective, is to be forestalled at all costs because it represents the entropic conclusion as "proven" to us by science. Consequently, we exhaust most of our resources in this pursuit, rather than exploring a multitude of life-enriching activities and practices that could contribute to health here in this lifetime and also spiritually prepare us for the next.

Even much of contemporary scientific thinking now refutes this simplistic notion. Taken from a strictly materialistic standpoint, there is some limited truth in the notion of entropy, but it only accounts for half of the equation. Any green thumb knows that plants go to seed, sprout and bloom, decline and decay, return to the soil, and contribute nutrients to ensure the initiation and continuation of the next cycle, which contributes to the next cycle, which contributes to the next cycle. The renewable rise and fall, yang and yin interplay of inorganic and organic matter, must always be taken together as a whole to form a true picture of the "Way," as described in Taoist thought. The flip side of the entropic coin, the counterbalance to the meaningless reduction of this life to the decay of the physical body, is an evolutionary vision of the Earth, even the universe, as one giant cosmic organism growing and maturing in the direction of increasing complexity, higher consciousness, greater respect for individuality, and awareness of an unbreakable unity.

Beyond the limited world of drugs and surgeries propelled by economic forces whose bottom line is profit lies a vast cornucopia of healing energies, principles, and methodologies that even the alternative health care community has barely begun to comprehend. Western society has yet to acknowledge the reality of many of these forces and energies that play such vital roles in health and illness, let alone begin to tap into and utilize them to our benefit. But the truth is that there is an overall pattern, in addition to an individual pattern and purpose for each one of us, if we would only find the time to slow down, tune in, learn about these energies, and align ourselves with them. So much ill health and unhappiness arises from struggling against the flow, from a personal will that equates the ego with the center of the universe. A will that is not aligned with one's higher self or one's place and purpose can, in limited ways, through sheer force, achieve fleeting moments of success. But in the end, if not heeded, the higher energetic and spiritual forces will have their final say in these matters.

TUNING IN

We can employ a number of effective methods and health-promoting habits to help us tune in to these energies. The philosophy and science of yoga, which is increasingly popular, is one such method. Some creation stories speak of a god, like the Egyptian Khnum, who breathes life into inert matter. Each life in this world begins with the very first breath, inspiration, and ends with expiration, when the breath finally leaves and the soul begins to depart. Yoga is built upon the science of breath. Unfortunately, most Westerners take breath for granted and are too busy, frantic, and fractured to stop and breathe fully and effectively.

Science teaches that breathing is an autonomic function that, to a certain extent, can be voluntarily overridden. Beyond these simple facts, we tend not to give breathing much thought. But consider for a moment what happens during a frightening experience. Adrenalin pumps, the heart beats faster, and the breath is suddenly drawn in for a moment, sometimes longer. When we are gripped with fear, we have a strong tendency to gasp and then temporarily forget to breathe. I have seen a good number of clients over the years whose problems have originated long ago in a moment of shock. Years later, they sit before me complaining of an inability to breathe properly, even though a conventional medical workup has given them a clean bill of health. It is as if the vital force retains the memory of the shocking moment and is now stuck, thus causing the person to breathe in a shallow or inefficient manner.

In more subtle ways, the normal mechanisms controlling respiratory function can be altered by a stress-filled life, resulting in an insidious decrease in the ability to breathe freely. Slowly, over time, we grow accustomed to improper, shallow, and ultimately restricted breathing. Poor oxygenation of the blood through insufficient inhalation, and inadequate removal of carbon dioxide and other wastes due to improper exhalation, then take their toll on the cardiovascular system. I am convinced that the fast pace and dysfunctional nature of the average person's daily routine, coupled with a lack of compensatory focus upon proper breathing to counteract these negative pressures, are significant factors in the prevalence of heart disease in contemporary cultures. The best solution, short of dropping out of mainstream society, is for people to take up yoga and the breathing disciplines that it has developed over thousands of years.

We all understand on an intuitive level that within this universe of abundant energies and waveforms, some frequencies are going to attract and some will repel each other. Some are in harmony and resonate together, while others can clash, causing dissonance. Some are in sync and others are out of sync with each other. If an E string on one guitar is struck, its vibration can cause the corresponding E string on another guitar across the room to vibrate. Rudimentary physics teaches us that when out-of-phase or out-of-synch waveforms combine, they disrupt each other and lose energy. This is called destructive interference. If two waves and their frequencies are in phase, or in sync, their combination will cause constructive interference, and the overall energy and strength of the resulting wave will increase. The extent of destructive or constructive effect depends upon the degree of synchronization or resonance of two energies.

Some devices, such as radio transmitters, are designed to send energy, while others, such as cell phones, act as receivers. FM and AM radios receive certain energy wavelengths from the radio wave portion of the electro-magnetic spectrum, depending upon the frequency to which they are tuned. These devices then "interpret" this "information" and convert, or trans-duce, it into another form of energy, such as the sounds produced by a radio or cell phone. Likewise, all of the various frequencies of the cosmic spectrum are energies capable of being produced, transmitted, received, and interpreted by something or someone out there in the universe. What physicists refer to as "energy," techies call "information," mystics know as "spirit," and New Agers call "consciousness." The human being is the most exquisitely designed receiver and transmitter of energies in the created world. We are conduits for energy, and it is potentially unhealthy to get our frequency channels jammed. We need to take concerns regarding the health impact from cell phones, microwaves, and other devices that emit energies very seriously.

Yoga understands this reality and provides methods for keeping the channels open and energy flowing. Yogic theory recognizes an etheric anatomy consisting of seven (there's that magic number again) major chakras that align with the spine and correspond to branches of the auto-nomic nervous system and the organs of the endocrine system. A chakra is a bioenergetic vortex of activity that receives, processes, and expresses vital life energy. Each chakra has a name, is associated with a color of the spectrum, and corresponds to certain aspects of human behavior. In fact, the heart chakra is the central chakra or point of balance, and is repre-sented by green, which is also the color that stands at the midpoint in the color spectrum, ROYGBIV. According to yogic discipline, the life force, prana, also known as the kundalini or serpent goddess, rests coiled up at the lowest chakra, at the base of the spine. When this life force is "awak-ened" through regular practice, it flows up the spinal column through the chakras and out the top of the head. Along the way, it invigorates, renews, cleanses, and contributes to health through the proper flow of the life force. With the help of yoga, we can tune in to certain frequencies, resist other potentially detrimental energies, and keep the overall energy of our systems fine-tuned and balanced. Douglas De Long, author of *Ancient Teachings for Beginners*, a nifty little beginner's manual based upon the teachings of the ancient Mystery schools, points out that this mechanism has more than just a physiological effect upon the human body:

> *The extremely high vibratory rates of chakra energy will work in harmony or 'sympathy' with the sympathetic system. This special nervous system or division is attuned to the cosmic vibrations, universal energy, the human aura, and virtually all spiritual energies that originate from the Creator and the heavenly fields above. (It is unfortunate that medical science does not recognize the true potential of this harmonious system, but in time they will.)*[121]

Furthermore, the subtle anatomy of this system consists of three main energy channels, or *Nadis*, that course their way up the spine. According to their Hindu names, the *Sushumna*, which runs from the base of the spine to the top of the head, is the central channel around which winds the *Ida*, the feminine left channel, and the *Pingala*, the masculine right channel. This image evokes obvious structural parallels and is also cosmically analogous to several topics that we have covered thus far. It represents yet another example of how yin and yang, female and male, can work together in balance and harmony for the benefit of health. The modern symbol for this, ironically, is the medical caduceus with its two snakes winding up the winged staff. The awakening of kundalini serpent energy also evokes the biblical image of Moses's people looking up to the fiery serpent on the pole in order that they may be healed. Similarly, the serpent of wisdom is associated with the *axis mundi*, the Tree of Knowledge in the Garden of Eden. And finally, the structural lattice that encodes all life forms derives from the double helix of DNA, like two serpents interwoven to embody the dance of polarities in the mystery of life. These powerful correspondences represent several of those synchronistic patterns that cannot be ignored and, clearly, are not just coincidences.

HONORING THE ANCESTORS

In addition to becoming attuned to the energies, vibrations, frequencies, patterns, and synchronicities of the universe, if we are willing we can open our minds to other powerful sources of information available to us. Perhaps one of the sadder aspects of contemporary culture is its attitude toward the elderly. Here in the information age, we are constantly bombarded with images and messages that essentially equate our elders with illness, infirmity, dullness, and senility. A culture that fears death also fears growing old, and naturally, by extension, avoids and neglects its own elders. Hollywood, often under the guise of comedy, portrays the average "old" person as smelly, unhip, crotchety, and boring. Because thoughts and ideas are forms of energy that do have power, these images contribute to our collective disrespect toward those who brought our parents, their parents, and their parents into the world.

By the grace of God, I was lucky enough to have a special relationship with my maternal grandparents. At the young age of ten, I was privileged to travel with them to their homeland, Ireland. My grandparents, a grand uncle, a grand aunt, and I spent a full month visiting relatives and seeing the sights all across that magical green island. I felt like an honored guest, an emissary of the younger generation, and it gave me a profound appreciation for my ancestral roots, the stories that my elders told, the values that they transmitted, and the wisdom that they imparted. By virtue of this ancestry, I am truly proud of my status today as a dual citizen of both Ireland and the United States.

Ancient Irish culture was not dissimilar from early Native American life. The Celts lived in tribal units, had a deep respect for the land, practiced an earth-centered form of spirituality, and had deep reverence for their spiritual ancestors. In these cultures, the role of the ancestors cannot be overestimated. Matthew Wood, in his book on the roots of vitalistic medicine, *The Magical Staff,* eloquently pays tribute to the role that the ancestors should play in all of our lives:

> *In the life of the Native American, a deep feeling of meaning,*
> *human relationship, and love is derived from the interface with*
> *'the Ancestors' or 'Grandfathers.' This is an element which is super-*
> *natural in the highest degree. . . . By being good, kind, spiritual*
> *people, the Ancestors earned the respect of the Creator, so that after*
> *their death they were allowed to continue as sentient beings. And*
> *now, from the other side, they still look over us, guiding, protect-*
> *ing, teaching, loving us. . . . Through knowing and respecting them,*
> *we are able to become more effective channels for a dispensation*
> *of spiritual healing energy.*[122]

Orthodox medicine is increasingly detached from its own roots, its forebears, and the spiritual realities of life. Conducting scientific studies to determine whether prayer can help cure cancer just won't cut it. The ridiculousness of subjecting "God" to a placebo-controlled, double-blinded study represents the height of materialistic arrogance. It is time for the mechanistic paradigm to stop and acknowledge what millions of people already know deep in their hearts. No "proof" is necessary. And respect is long overdue.

DREAMS AND DREAMERS

One of the most effective ways we can honor the ancestors, besides the obvious marking of anniversaries of their births, deaths, and other important dates, is through our dreams. The ancestors often speak to us in our dreams and, more often than not, we dismiss these events as "just" dreams. However, if we are willing to listen, the messages that they bring can heal us and change our lives. Dreams can also play a powerful role in illness and disease. They can foretell the onset of an illness, provide the key to recovery, and mark the return to health. A dream can be the source of the greater awareness that accompanies genuine healing. Most dreams can offer a new perspective that, prior to dreaming, was only an unconscious potentiality. Once assimilated into consciousness, dreams carry greater power and can act as catalysts to create movement and flow once again after periods of inertia and stagnancy.

In order to harness the true power of dreams we must first overcome the biases that we have assimilated through living in our modern times. The universal historical and cross-cultural belief in dreams as messages from the Other Side, from the spirit world, or from God, is striking and undeniable. It is not surprising that contemporary culture's prevailing mode renders us unable to receive most dream material, which, from our rational perspective, becomes virtually impossible to comprehend. Echoing the role that orthodox medicine has played in the development of this deficiency, John Sanford, Jungian analyst and Episcopal priest, offers some insight into the religious origins of our dream illiteracy:

> For the church, as it became increasingly institutionalized, devalued and denied the reality of the individual soul and its dreams in favor of collectivized creeds, rituals and traditions. In putting the life of the institution above that of the soul, it lost the dream; instead of ministering and listening to the soul, the church sought to mold the individual to the life of the institution. This left the church devoid of its spiritual basis, and open to the same materialism and rationalism that gripped the rest of the world.[123]

Ironically, Christian history and biblical stories abound with accounts of dreams and dreamers that have had significant impact upon their circumstances and cultures.

The story of Joseph, son of Jacob, is one such account. Nobel Prize laureate Thomas Mann turned it into a literary masterpiece, his four-part epic, *Joseph and His Brothers*. Joseph, because of his ability to understand dreams, was thrown into a well and left to die by his brothers after his dream foretold that they would someday bow down to him. Joseph was rescued, sold into slavery, and eventually earned his way out of prison by virtue of his reading, writing, and language skills. In spite of being a non-Egyptian, he rose to the post of Vizier of Egypt, Pharaoh's right hand man, after he had done what no other person could do.

Pharaoh had two dreams. In the first, he saw seven (there it is again) magnificent and healthy cows rise from the Nile, one after the other, followed by seven lean and sickly cows. Later the same night, in a second dream, he witnessed seven fat and healthy ears of corn burst forth from a stalk on the banks of the Nile. The stalk then put forth seven more ears, one after another, but these were all blighted and blackened. Pharaoh had heard of Joseph's facility with dreams, so he summoned him to his side. Mann's accounting of this fateful encounter begins with Pharaoh's query:

> 'And what say you to my dreams?'
>
> 'To your dreams?' Joseph answered. 'To your dream, you mean. To dream twice is not to dream two dreams. You dreamed but one dream. That you dreamed it twice, first in one form and then in the other, has only the meaning of emphasis: it means that your dream will certainly be fulfilled and that speedily.' . . .
>
> 'What means my dream, what would it show to me?'
>
> 'Pharaoh errs,' Joseph responded, 'if he thinks he does not know. His servant can do no more than to prophecy to him what he already knows.'[124]

With great agility, Joseph helps Pharaoh to conclude that seven years of bountiful harvests in the land of Khem will be followed by seven years of famine, and that preparations to stockpile foodstuffs in advance should be made immediately. Pharaoh places Joseph in charge of the project and thus disaster is averted. The brothers, forced to seek assistance during the famine, are ultimately aided and treated with kindness by Joseph, the Vizier of Egypt. Some have speculated that Imhotep, the world's first physician, and Vizier to King Djoser of Egypt's third dynasty, was none other than Joseph himself.

Once we suspend our disbelief, we can take the next step, to welcome dreams with earnest intent. We can prepare ourselves, keeping pen and paper at the bedside, by asking to receive a dream. At the moment of first consciousness on emerging from the dream state, I try to remain motionless with eyes closed, carefully going over all the details of the dream several times until I have it clear in my mind. Only then do I rise to record it on paper. My wife and I regularly tell our dreams to each other over breakfast, and we sometimes retell them later in the day, especially if a dream strikes us as particularly significant.

Dream imagery is a product of the unconscious and its comprehension is not necessarily dependent upon left-brain thinking. Dreams are to be understood in symbolic terms and speak in images that precede language and conceptualization. Some dreams are best when directly experienced rather than interpreted. Some of the life of a dream can be lost when it is subjected to analysis. It is sometimes preferable, when possible, for the dreamer to act out his or her dream. The dreamer should never accept another person's interpretation unless it clearly resonates with the dreamer's own intuitive sense of the dream.

With a little practice, we can learn again to tune in to these messages from the Other Side, which were once a profound source of guidance for our ancestors. Dream explorer and trailblazer Robert Moss envisions a future when dreams are accepted once again as commonplace and are believed to carry with them the power to transform lives:

> I must confess that I have a burning agenda: I want to do everything possible to help rebirth a dreaming culture, a society in which dreams are shared and celebrated everywhere, every when—in the workplace, in our families and schools, in our health care facilities … In our dreaming culture, dream groups will be a vital part of every clinic, hospital, and treatment center, and doctors will begin their patient interviews by asking about dreams as well as physical symptoms.[125]

Well aware of my father's denial of death and his tendency to cling to this material existence, I was concerned about his ability to make a smooth transition after his death from this life over to the Other Side. Although I had no personal experience in such matters, I had heard stories and read about the issue in a few books. I resolved to pray regularly for the quick and uneventful passage of his soul to its intended destination in the afterlife.

My three children were quite fond of my father and had many positive memories of visiting him at his home on Long Island. I was concerned about how they had taken his passing but they seemed to be handling it without too much trouble. Several months after his death, my youngest, who was ten years old at the time, awoke one morning to report that he'd had a dream. He said that "faeries were all over the place, popping out of the furniture." They had granted him a wish but he hesitated. As they were leaving, my son called back to them and said he had one question that he would like answered. He then asked the faeries if they could bring someone back to life. They responded that, regretfully, they did not have the power to grant such a wish. At that moment, he woke from sleep.

Although my son was quite familiar with our Irish heritage, neither he nor I knew very much about faeries other than the "little people" stereotypes that many of us carry regarding these supposedly fictional entities. A little research helped to illuminate the fact that faeries are essentially the Celtic version of spirits. They can take many forms, as some believe them to be angels, nature spirits, or the companions of the departed. Thankfully, Tom Cowan, author of a book about Celtic shamanism, can enlighten us on the subject:

> One of the more intriguing insights into the spirit world, an insight that reappears throughout Celtic faery lore, is the apparent need for human contact on the part of spiritual entities. For reasons not always clear, the faery folk ... actively want to share their secrets, wisdom, and power with us. Seeking human companionship, they either enter our world of ordinary reality or take us into theirs. It is almost as if they recognize in us companion spirits, temporarily assigned a mortal reincarnation, and that their involvement in our lives, even when mischievous, is to assist us in some important way.[126]

Almost a full year had elapsed since my father's passing when the same son announced that he'd had another dream. This time he had seen his grandfather, my father, enter into a tunnel and, halfway through, get himself stuck. My son likened this tunnel to the large cement culvert that carries runoff rainwater from the mountains, under the road, and into a stream that adjoins our property. In the dream, our family went over to the other end of the tunnel, where it opened into a lake. We waded into the water to see if we could help. Just then, a black dog-like animal with erect ears ventured into the tunnel and emerged again dragging my father out with its teeth gripping him by his shirt collar. My father appeared to

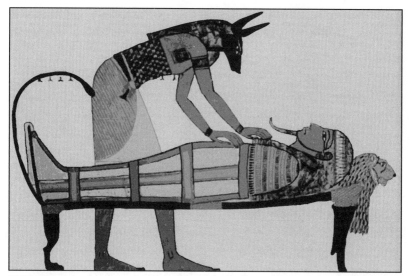

FIGURE 16.1: *Anubis, Egyptian Guardian of the Underworld, Preparing the Body of Sennedjem in Thebes*

be quite well and looked noticeably younger, perhaps forty years old. Then, according to my son, my father stood up, embraced me and thanked me for my help.

This time I did not need to do the research, as I was familiar with the Egyptian Anubis, the black, pointy-eared jackal-headed god who is guardian of the underworld and protector of the deceased. (See Figure 16.1.) Anubis provides safe passage from this life to the next and to those who journey to the other side. I was profoundly touched by this dream, which brought a good degree of closure to one of the more problematic relationships of my life. Since my wife and I took my son seriously and did not dismiss his dreams as silly nonsense, I firmly believe that this left the door open for meaningful communication and provided a formative experience for my son regarding his attitudes toward life, death, and the afterlife. His contact with the faeries and his grandfather brought much-needed healing to my family.

The dream world is a source of healing and higher consciousness accessible to all. It is the place that we all visit when sleeping, and it is the same Otherworld that the shaman visits when seeking assistance from his spirit guides. Freud led the way but gave dreams a materialistic interpretation.

Jung expanded our symbolic understanding of dreams to include the arche-types and the collective unconscious. Organized religion seems to have for-gotten that dreams can be one of God's primary modes of communication. Asklepian priests once conducted healings through dream incubation, nature-based cultures communicate with their departed ancestors, and contemporary society desperately needs to overcome its materialistic bias to be able to once again tap into this powerful source of healing. A dream can often provide the awareness, the spark, the confidence, or the guid-ance necessary to manage in times of ill health.

A patient named Debbie once shared a dream with me that subse-quently turned out to have a clear impact upon her sister's struggle with illness. Debbie's mother had called one day to report that her sister had been diagnosed with breast cancer. Debbie was saddened and concerned, and went to bed that night asking for spiritual guidance and a dream that might assist her sister in this difficult time. When she awoke the following morning, she had brought back a clear image from her sleep. Debbie was walking with her sister along a beach where a large sand dune rose up next to them. Suddenly, Debbie spotted an enormous wave heading toward shore. She quickly instructed her sister to climb the dune. They both started up the dune but her sister turned back and ran toward the wave, where she was swept up and tumbled about. As the wave crashed to shore, her sister was deposited on top of the dune alongside Debbie, battered from the expe-rience but alive and breathing.

Although Debbie's instincts told her that she had received a positive message from the Other Side, she felt apprehensive about reporting the dream to her sister, fearing that it might scare her at a very vulnerable time. Nevertheless, she felt compelled to share the dream, and contrary to expec-tation, her sister seemed to be uplifted by the message. In the difficult months ahead, she was battered by the regimen of radiation and chemotherapy but she held on to the prognosis of the dream. More than once she reported back to Debbie how the image of the dream was like a life preserver that had kept her afloat and breathing with a renewed will to persevere.

A universe of indestructible energies lies waiting to be explored. The patterns have always been there, imploring us to connect the dots. We can transcend the dead-end emptiness of entropy if we strive upward toward better health and higher consciousness. We must begin with the fundamentals. First we learn to breathe, and then we receive the gifts of our dreams and the wisdom that our ancestors have offered us. We can seek to raise our vibrational frequencies so that we may tune in to the energies that science would have us believe do not exist.

We have merely touched upon the tip of the iceberg of that which is potentially available to those who wish to be healers and those who are in need of healing. The esoteric knowledge and spiritual wisdom of the Western Mystery traditions, Eastern spiritual disciplines, Christian mysticism, Hermeticism, Gnosticism, Paganism, numerology, astrology, Theosophy, and anthroposophy, to name just a few, are available to all with open and inquisitive minds. The re-emergence of this holistic knowledge and green wisdom is beginning to fill the void that has been created by the left-brained emphasis upon physical science and the rational mind.

Practical techniques that take advantage of this wisdom for healing, growth, and the raising of consciousness, such as yoga, nutrition, meditation, chakra work, dream work, and energy balancing are making inroads into popular culture. Therapeutic and medical modalities—such as acupuncture, Reiki, color therapy, aromatherapy, homeopathy, chiropractic, osteopathy, shiatsu, healing touch, and Ayurveda—which acknowledge and make use of the multitude of energetic forces that impinge upon health, form the cutting edge of a new green medicine that respects the diversity of the human situation and the unity of all things. It remains for us to simply embrace the tide of change as it ushers us into a deeper respect for ourselves and our connection to creation.

17

Greener Medical Pastures

We are emerging from a long period of such materialism at present, and that is why doctor, priest and public are confronted with the task of learning a great deal all over again, and revising the knowledge of their ancestors before they can carry things a step further.

—Vera Stanley Alder, *The Finding of the Third Eye*

... a master is not merely one who learns and repeats authoritative forms of words passed on from the time of the ancients; he is one who has been born to his wisdom by the mysterious all-embracing and merciful love which is the mother of all being. He is one who knows the unknown not by intellectual penetration, or by a science that wrests for itself the secrets of heaven, but by the wisdom of "littleness" and silence which knows how to receive in secret a word that cannot be uttered except in an enigma.

—Thomas Merton, *Mystics and Zen Masters*

Small wheel turn by the fire and rod
Big wheel turn by the grace of God
Every time that wheel turn round
Bound to cover just a little more ground

—Robert Hunter, "The Wheel"

OLD SCHOOL

Professionalism, once designed to ensure the quality and integrity of a vocation, has instead become contemporary code for territorialism. It delineates boundaries that define the scope of one's functions and serves to prevent others from having an influence in those circumscribed matters. It creates an atmosphere of competition for turf rather than coop-eration for the greater good. The definition of a given field of science as a distinct and separate discipline fulfills a similar territorial imperative. Under the guise of rigorous principles and ethics, medical science sets the stage for the protection of its own self-interest. It, in essence, announces to all that "We are the experts here. Mind your own business." Factionalism of this nature will always fail in the end, and suffering patients will reap the spoiled fruits of such dysfunctional divisions.

A true green revolution in medicine will not be possible until ortho-doxy redefines professionalism to mean the practice of one's science and art to the best of one's ability with honesty, unselfishness, and integrity. Professionalism should not mean that medicine is to be practiced to the exclusion of outside influences. It should not become a prison that stifles originality and creativity. It should mean that medicine will always seek, and remain open to, better ways of serving humanity.

As it stands, the closest thing that we have to a holistic medical pro-fession is the field of naturopathy. The training of naturopathic physicians covers a wide range of alternative and natural therapies, but there is one significant restricting condition placed upon their licensure—they cannot prescribe pharmaceutical drugs or perform conventional surgeries. On the other side of the fence, orthodox medicine grudgingly allows the rare token of holism into its domain, as when recently it accepted glucosamine and chondroitin as viable anti-arthritic therapies. Conventional medicine must dispense with the pretense of giving fair consideration to alternative thera-pies while judging them according to impossible standards. Licorice, for example, should not be judged based upon its applicability to treating cancer patients. Whether or not licorice is a useful measure in dealing with indigestion should be sufficient standard to judge its therapeutic value. Making alternative therapies jump over such unrealistic hurdles creates a neat and convenient divide that separates conventional from holistic doctors.

While, admittedly, there is a smattering of daring individuals deter-mined to overcome this false dichotomy, the wide gulf between orthodoxy and holism remains the normative reality. As long as there are two separate systems, health care will remain inadequate and will tend to fall short of the ideal. If conventional medicine is ever to heal itself of its fragmented state, it must first acknowledge its brokenness and admit that it needs to transcend its rigid and limited conception of what constitutes desirable and viable therapies. "Treatment of the whole person" must become more than just a corporate slogan or marketing gimmick.

Likewise, the mavericks of alternative medicine can also, at times, be a little narrow-minded, sometimes eschewing all pharmaceutical options. "Natural" does not necessarily equate to "superior," and not infrequently, a conventional drug or surgery is the best plan of action. On the other hand, practitioners of the healing arts must resist allowing their arts to be made over into sciences out of the overwhelming desire to seek "respectability." We already see this trend, as some holistic practitioners promote their therapies with questionable scientific rationales. Some areas of knowledge are well suited to scientific investigation, while others are not. Some things, especially in the realm of healing, will always retain a sense of mystery, and are best appreciated in their natural state. Spiritual and energetic forces, when subjected to the parameters of clinicians and their mechanistic bias, often lose their power to heal. The standard should not be whether a therapy can be dissected and understood by the rational mind, but whether it is of true benefit to the sick and the suffering. Scientific "proof" should be of secondary concern, especially when a therapy demonstrates efficacy in clinical practice.

Professionalism also engenders and legitimizes the dominance of medical specialization. Specialists are legally protected by the well-defined parameters of their scopes of practice, which virtually guarantees that they do not attempt to connect the dots in any manner of holistic thinking. The primary difference between a generalist and specialist is that one is supposedly trained to be mindful of the bigger picture while the other maintains a narrow focus. The few generalists that remain today are, in reality, specialists narrowly defined by their mechanistic orientation toward the physical body. More important, contemporary internists and general practitioners are the only ones who demonstrate even a semblance of philosophical consideration for the way in which symptoms and events are connected, whereas, a true green generalist should be defined by his or her profound understanding of the inextricable interconnections between body, mind, soul, family, community, culture, and environment.

No consciously chosen discernable philosophy that unifies conventional medicine in its pursuit of health and healing exists, and therein lies its greatest weakness. Without guiding principles, medicine has become a dangerous and haphazard smattering of toxic drugs, redundant tests, fleeting fads, and invasive procedures administered and performed by technocrats who have little reason to communicate or cooperate with each other and whose livelihood is largely determined by insurance bureaucrats whose bottom line is profit. The patient's welfare barely factors into the equation. While most medical professionals have the best of intentions, the U.S. health care system as a whole does not constitute a vocation of service to the sick. It is a market-based economy that places profit before patients. The most accurate way to describe the ideology of modern medical practice is as a corporate industry that markets goods and services to medically uneducated consumers. These consumers are deliberately kept in the dark and naively accept the grossly simplistic notion that all symptoms are bad and must therefore be stopped, without regard for the fallout and long-term consequences. As long as the profit motive takes precedence over patients, the results will be mediocre at best. And those who would equate socialized medicine with communism are just poorly informed. We seem to forget that public schools, public parks, libraries, Medicare, and highway repair, to name just a few, are government funded socialized services that we capitalists have come to cherish.

A medicalized culture depends upon the docility, compliance, and ignorance of the masses. The culture, rather than seeing symptoms as the messengers of disharmony that they are, elevates them to the status of foes to be vanquished. Our current overemphasis upon diagnosis serves as a form of medical trickery, designed with the unconscious ulterior motive of distracting and appeasing the public. Technological medicine focuses on diagnosis precisely because its therapeutic options are lacking in imagination and limited to the standard drugs and surgeries. Contemporary medicine is bereft of any coherent philosophical orientation, let alone holistic understanding. The inherently shortsighted nature of medical interventions that generate more illness than they are designed to alleviate creates a revolving door of sick individuals in constant need of medical services. The medical economy thrives on the iatrogenic disease that it generates. While this works especially well for the perpetuation of established medicine, it is oftentimes harmful to the suffering individual.

The dynamic of suppression that pervades virtually all orthodox medical interventions must be acknowledged and understood for what it is. If the profession is unwilling to do so, it is incumbent upon patients to educate themselves as to the dangers of suppression, and this is one of the primary purposes of this book. The strict physicality of our illnesses is mostly an illusion. Regardless of what the proponents of the mechanistic paradigm would have us believe, most chronic physical ailments run much deeper than the physical plane. This is why treatment on the physical level yields such superficial, temporary results. If such means do happen to force a disease into remission, it is usually because the treatment has suppressed it, in which case we can expect more problematic health issues somewhere down the road. Effective treatment for most chronic illness requires a more sophisticated approach, which includes consideration of the mental, emotional, spiritual, and energetic planes.

We must come to differentiate occasions when suppressive measures are unavoidable from instances where they are just a matter of convenience, because each dose of medication taken can harm the psyche and deaden the spirit just a little further. Most physical symptoms, especially those indicative of chronic illness, are merely a reflection of an internal state. If the symptoms are treated superficially, the illness will proceed unchecked, thus leading to deeper pathology. Medicine's materialistic cookie-cutter approach, which in and of itself is conducive to the generation of further illness and disease, reflects a homogeneous culture that is losing its creative capacity to appreciate the diversity of human life and the uniqueness of individuals. Preserving the body at the expense of the soul and to the neglect of the spiritual dimension is a hazardous dead-end strategy. Only at the point of crisis will Western medicine begin to more closely examine its mechanistic and materialistic bias, its false claim to objectivity, its exclusion of intuition, creativity, and common sense, and its lack of underlying philosophy and begin to connect the various fragments of its frequently inappropriate methods of treatment.

We are blinded to realities that are all around us by the scientific method that dominates our times. We simply need to expand our conceptual framework in order to see them. If I do not believe in the existence of woodchucks, then when I finally do see one I will mistakenly assume that it is just a really big squirrel. We must recognize the serious limitations the randomized, double-blinded, placebo-controlled, scientific "gold standard" of modern medicine imposes upon our perceptions. While the value of this approach is occasionally relevant, its elevated status as the highest standard of proof deserves a significant demotion in the overall hierarchy of health priorities. A more complete understanding of modern medical science makes it evident that economic medical reform only scratches the surface of the real underlying issues. Rather, it is the substance of medicine that must undergo serious revision from the ground up, and it must start by incorporating a cohesive philosophy that begins to make some sense out of its chaotic and often harmful practices.

Health is not a commodity that can be purchased. The medical system must cease taking advantage of the weakest members of society—the elderly, the poor, and the infirm. For physicians to continue to routinely prescribe, and patients to continue to take, medications that pose distinct risks of serious illness and death is, to me, an unacceptable standard of care. The notion of better living through pharmaceuticals is a failed experiment, the repercussions of which are likely to reverberate for generations to come. Faith-based vaccinations that continue to maim our children are the tragic result of stubborn adherence to a failed philosophy not borne out by fact. Those who choose such medical lifestyle options as cosmetic facelifts, boltulinum toxin injections, and erectile dysfunction drugs should be forewarned that this is not medicine designed to heal, and it involves the risk of placing your life in the hands of those who may not be motivated by the best of intentions.

NEW SCHOOL

The hypertrophy of the masculine principle, which divides, dissects, and differentiates, grows at the expense of the feminine principle, which connects, encompasses, and unifies. An unholistic approach that obsesses over lab values and physical symptoms becomes unholy when it disregards the roles of meaning, purpose, and the spiritual dimension. We must educate ourselves and come to understand the issues in order to determine when we want technical experts to repair the physical body and when we need well-rounded physicians to heal the whole. The reality, of course, is that we need both, but we must not delude ourselves that one is the other or that physical repair is an acceptable substitute for whole-person healing.

A new tradition of medical dissent must be established if true change is ever to take hold. In order to accomplish this we must resist the disproportionate and intimidating power wielded by medical authorities and institutions. For it is fear that keeps the voices of patients and professionals alike from being heard. It is fear that paralyzes and prevents change. Orthodox medical church dogma must be questioned and challenged, and the irrational rigidity of its rationalism must be made clear. Proper education of the populace will enable it to resist exploitation. We must learn to cut through the layers of propaganda in order to perceive the unfiltered empirical facts. Education, clarification, and demystification will lead to enlightenment and empowerment.

While the medical profession deserves our respect, it should not command our subservience. There should be no medical authority that supersedes the patient's own personal authority without the patient's explicit consent, and he or she should always retain the right of refusal regardless of all prior agreements. Another issue that goes hand in hand with personal autonomy is privacy, which, in turn, is of prime importance to a person's experience of health and well-being. Third-party access, the current trend that allows someone other than patient and physician to access medical records, is unconscionable. A just and compassionate society must provide the right to health care for all, regardless of ability to afford or pay for it. And, above all, citizens should retain the right to choose or refuse health care options and modalities as they see fit.

The guiding principles of green medicine are founded on the truth that all things are connected. All is one. As above, so below. Everything is energy. From this follows the need for a medical system of inclusivity. In actuality, one person's poison can be another person's cure. We cannot dismiss individual human experiences just because statistical probabilities say such events are unlikely. Respect for the diversity of approaches to health and healing, and for the uniqueness of individuals, their illnesses, and solutions, is of paramount importance. Differences of medical philosophy and practice do not have to create divisions. They simply provide additional options for discerning patients and practitioners. A non-denominational medical culture of unity within diversity will ensure the best possible outcome for the greatest number.

Treatment of the whole person is not just a slogan, as there are a variety of methodologies that come very close to this ideal. Correspondingly, when we use the whole of our human capacities, we accomplish this goal best. A left-brain, cause-and-effect approach will achieve superior results when it is wedded to a right-brain, intuitive perspective. We must not give the rational function the role of final arbiter in all medical situations. What the rational mind judges to be coincidence is often perceived by the holistic mind as a meaning-filled synchronicity. Information that may contain the key to cure according to one perspective runs the risk of being discarded by the other. An empirical, experiential acceptance of the way things are as per first-hand observation is the perfect complement to the analytical thought process that weighs and measures. Employing one without the other is akin to attempting to swim with one arm and one leg.

The green principle of wholeness also entails an understanding of biology, chemistry, and physics as one cohesive phenomenon based in energy, spirit, information, or cosmic consciousness—whichever you prefer. By this standard, it defies all logic to assume that any symptom can be separated from the whole. The life force, its patterns, and dynamics must be respected if the healing process is to be successful. Symptoms are not the enemy—lack of understanding is the true enemy. Symptoms are the vital force's attempt to heal the whole. If it fails in its mission, a symptom tends to get stuck, persisting or recurring in a negative feedback loop. The aim of the healer should be to restore freedom of flow to the bioenergetic life force by penetrating to the source, to the center of gravity of the disturbance, whether it be on the physical, emotional, mental, or spiritual plane— or on more than one plane. Once balance is restored, symptoms are no longer necessary, as the life force will have no further need to complain.

The human body is an energetic relay station, a vehicle designed to receive and transmit a wide array of waveforms, vibrations, electromagnetic phenomena, and psychic and spiritual energies. To restrict our understanding to the crudest of these energies grounded in physical matter is a colossal waste of human potential. We can keep our channels tuned to the equivalent of AM stations with spotty reception, occasionally picking up a signal here and there—or we can learn to tune in to, to detect, to process, to understand, and to transform and transmit these varied energies for the betterment of our individual, collective, and planetary health. The techniques available to do so have been around for thousands of years, but our materialistic high-tech bias prevents us from perceiving and developing them.

Health is not a black-and-white phenomenon. It is all gray area. To deny this is to lend credence to the dangerous war-against-disease mentality. Disease will not, cannot, and should not ever be eradicated. This would entail eradication of parts of ourselves, both literally and figuratively. One's state of health is an ongoing ebbing and flowing process of balance and imbalance, and the absolutism of right or wrong and good or bad only contributes to the imbalance. Yin and yang, feminine and masculine, dark and light, and the spiritual and the physical are all part of the cosmic plan, and all yearn to be expressed within the oneness of creation.

Illness is the beacon that points us in the direction of harmony with the forces of the universe within us and around us. It is purposeful and contains potential meaning to those willing to tune in to its messages. The direction toward cure is the same as the path toward greater awareness, higher consciousness, and personal fulfillment. The easiest way to achieve this is to go with the flow. It is the path of least resistance. Our illness is our model for healing. While treatment with opposites can temporarily put out the fire, and this may sometimes be necessary, it nevertheless goes against the flow and, hence, the embers are likely to continue to smolder. Repair of the physical body should not be equated with healing of the whole. Treatment with similars, which seeks to mimic the healing mechanism of the vital energy, works with the forces of nature, and is the most likely method to encourage the direction of cure. Disease contains within it the potentiality of cure. The deepest, most problematic wound provides the best opportunity for meaningful healing. It is the wounder that shall heal. And finally, no healing philosophy or methodology is viable if it is not based in the most important principle of all—that of love.

The principles that inform green medicine are the very same ones that the evolutionary impulse of mankind is already beginning to manifest on a global scale. The information age is rapidly transforming the world into a smaller, more interdependent place, thus forcing its inhabitants to come to terms with cultural and philosophical differences. The only way forward that promises a successful outcome lies in respect for differences and the uniqueness of individuals within a cooperative framework of unity. The old and inherently destructive ways of patriarchal competition for resources, dominance of one group over another, and war, is rapidly approaching obsolescence. We will either destroy our planet and ourselves or we will begin to accept the changes of perspective necessary for adaptation. Freedom of expression in lieu of suppression, and a masculine rapprochement with the feminine are the guiding principles that will ensure global, ecological, societal, local, and individual health for a long time to come.

The highly celebrated and sophisticated Mayan calendar has garnered much attention in recent years largely because the end of a 26,000 year cycle approaches. The Mayans were expert astronomers and astrologers, and their calendar, which reflects this fact, has been found to be more accurate than our own Gregorian calendar (which is of Christian origin). According to Mayan belief, on December 21, 2012, at the winter solstice, our current cycle will come to a close and a new age of spiritual transformation will begin. This 26,000-year cycle corresponds to the precession of the equinoxes. Many predict this date indicates a crucial turning point for the evolutionary consciousness of humankind. They say a period of significant upheaval will precede this transformation. The outcome may depend upon the choices that we make and the strategies that we employ to bridge our differences. Mechanists and skeptics will be tempted to dismiss this as foolishness, but those who perceive the connectedness of things may want to give it some serious consideration. Will we choose aggression and competition or will we opt for cooperation and compromise?

My wife once had the privilege of attending and participating in a ceremony performed by two Yachak shamans from the Andean mountains of Ecuador. In this re-enactment of the Ceremony of the Eagle and the Condor, which originally took place in 2001, the Eagle symbolizes the Mind of the Northern Hemisphere and the Condor represents the Heart of the Southern Hemisphere. She found this to be a moving experience that has shaped her beliefs and our intentions in the time since. As prophesized by the Yachak ancestors, a bridge needs to be created between the ancient wisdom and our modern ways, in order to ensure a successful transition to the new age when the eagle and condor will once again fly together. As the world enters a new phase of unity and peace, the heart and mind, and the feminine and masculine, shall join together to work as one.

There is nothing inherently wrong with orthodox medical science when it is promoted and practiced with a genuine awareness of its boundaries and limitations. Unfortunately, in its present state, it lacks all sense of proportion and appropriate boundary. Like a profit-driven corporation, it seeks constant expansion, and frequently presumes to impose its perspective upon disciplines and cultures that, until then, had been doing just fine without it. While scientific and medical knowledge will and should always continue to expand, it will never and can never come to encompass all. Many aspects of life, illness, and death will always rightfully remain a mystery.

Orthodox medicine must begin to acknowledge the one-sidedness of its perspective. It must begin to recognize the harm that mere symptomatic treatment can cause. It must come to terms with whether it is sufficient to be technically proficient at repairing the physical body, or if it is willing to expand its horizons toward the goal of healing the body-heart-mind-soul. Preserving the body while deadening the spirit is not a viable option. The medical patriarchy must free itself from authoritarian dogma, overcome its material bias by acknowledging the reality of the non-material, and become actively inclusive of new ideas and methods. One size does not fit all, and each personal health situation requires an individualized solution aided by well-rounded and enlightened healers. No medical philosophy or practice is acceptable unless it is based in respect for the whole patient and the healing process.

The green physician of the future must shed the pretense of privilege and false professionalism and reclaim the role of doctor/priest/healer/ teacher. The physician who embraces the emerging holistic paradigm must reclaim responsibility as educator and find the courage to speak firmly on important contemporary issues that impact our individual and collective health, such as war, poverty, inequality, education, the food chain, and the environment. The green physician must check his or her ego, stop shilling for corporate interests, cease defending mechanistic medical dogma, and turn full attention to issues that directly concern the patient's well-being. The physician should stop hiding behind scientifically contrived words that are designed to keep patients at a distance, but that add not a whit to the physician's healing abilities. When the patient's illness has its roots in societal dysfunction, the physician must have the courage to name it for what it is. Patient autonomy and empowerment should take precedence over pharmaceutical crutches that enable someone to be fitted into, and to perform for, the sick culture of materialism that has contributed to the illness in the first place. Green medicine is personalized and humanized, not sanitized and corporatized.

True healers must welcome dissent and entertain the value of new modalities of healing, which, in many cases, are simply old methods that have been prejudicially discredited and discarded by the mainstream. Old and low-tech need not be equated with inferior. A vast wealth of alternative therapeutic resources, indigenous healing methods, spiritual traditions, and esoteric knowledge stands waiting to be deployed. New/old methods should be evaluated based upon the benefit they can provide for suffering individuals, not whether they can be proven or invalidated by abstract statistical studies. In the end, the patient's voice and own assessment of his or her progress (or lack thereof) should be the most important gauges of success.

GREEN SCHOOL

I have long wished for a proper venue in which to express the ideas articulated in this book. I have been blessed with numerous opportunities to speak to the general public and to medical professionals over the years, but usually under very specific and circumscribed conditions. In most cases, I was either preaching to the choir, addressing a group of holistic practitioners or health-conscious citizens who were familiar with these ideas, or I was given an hour or so to explain some of the basics to a room full of conventional doctors, nurses, or students. These have hardly been the circumstances to describe such concepts in any kind of meaningful depth. Hence, I have felt the compelling desire to put these words into print in the hope that they will be welcomed by receptive minds.

As the final piece to this work, I would like to share my vision for the future of medical education—how it can be and how it should be. Admittedly, I will be painting an idealistic image, made up of lofty aspirations. I am not naïve enough to believe that it can be achieved overnight, but someday, maybe the Academy of Green Medicine and Healing (AGMH) will become a reality. The alternative is to continue with a system that is increasingly out of touch with real people, out of financial reach for the average American, and becoming so dysfunctional that it is likely to eventually collapse upon itself.

I envision a health care system in which the most gifted healers are wise, kind, well educated, and disciplined. If we are to take our health care seriously we must begin to nurture and train our healers more seriously. Because it is crucial that we remove the profit motive from the field of healing and medicine, we must eliminate the deceptive practice of direct-to-consumer advertising by the pharmaceutical industry. We must minimize opportunities to corrupt the intentions of health practitioners. Medical training should be highly selective as to its applicants and should be relatively inexpensive, because in the end, the astronomical debt of the average medical graduate only gets passed on to patients, in the form of higher prices and less time spent with them.

Entrants into the Academy of Green Medicine and Healing should not be chosen primarily for their test-taking abilities, but according to their temperament and aptitude for their calling in life. Medical school should not be filled with students who have chosen their path for the prestige and financial rewards that the profession can bring. The Academy should admit applicants based on whether it is the most appropriate place for them to pursue a vocation, the way a seminary or a monastery does. Some individuals may show signs of having such a calling at an early age, and teachers and elders who have the individual's best interests at heart should recognize and nurture the calling in appropriate settings. Some may come to their calling later in life and this, too, should be acknowledged as a legitimate avenue into the Academy. The Academy will expect most, if not all, applicants to be well-versed in methods of physical and spiritual self-care, such as regular exercise, good nutrition, meditation, yoga, and tai chi, and, if they are not, will expect them to develop these practices during their time at the AGMH.

Candidates will have completed prerequisite coursework in astronomy, comparative religions, psychology, mythology, and linguistics, in addition to the usual mathematics, biology, chemistry, and physics. The future AGMH will combine the attributes of an allopathic school with those of a naturopathic school and an ancient Mystery school—conventional medicine, natural and alternative medicine, and esoteric thought and healing all rolled into one. Biochemistry, physiology, cell biology, and hematology will be taught alongside Ayurveda, homeopathy, acupuncture, and herbology. Psychoanalysis, anatomy, astrology, cardiology, yoga, gynecology, osteopathy, pharmacology, and reflexology, to name just a few, will all have a place in the curriculum. The study of the inner person will be just as important as the study of the outer physical being. Experiential learning will be emphasized just as much as book learning. The history and philosophy of spiritual healing, psychic healing, and medical healing will round out the syllabus of a program that will nurture and develop each individual student's unique gifts and talents.

The Academy of Green Medicine and Healing will produce well-rounded generalists and will also recognize those that have a particular gift for a specific area of medicine or healing. Some may have psychic abilities, while others may be exceptional diagnosticians. Some will be well suited to work with children in pediatrics, and others may have a talent for working with dreams. Some will be excellent spiritual counselors, while others will have a knack for casting limbs and mending broken bones. There will be no more assembly line cookie-cutter medicine, and no more standard-issue white coats and stethoscopes.

The Academy will not be modeled after allopathic education. It will not be a closed system, an impenetrable fortress impervious to all new ideas and innovations with the exception of the latest products developed by Big Pharma. It will instead be a thriving environment of organic learning open to ideas from all sides. Its philosophy and methods will not be set in stone, but will change and evolve just as humanity changes and evolves. It will encourage medical dissent and differences of opinion. The AGMH will use the scientific method as a form of genuine inquiry rather than a weapon to defend the status quo.

The principles and dynamics of healing presented in this book are the result of many years of observation and clinical trial and error conducted by thousands of unconventional physicians and healers. As such, these principles are every bit as scientific, if not more so, than the standards of the defenders of conventional medical science who would seek to discredit them. Furthermore, these principles should not be discarded because they are scientific, paradoxical, and enigmatic all at the same time.

The Academy's environment will promote the health of its trainees so that graduates will exhibit the very same characteristics that they hope to achieve for their patients. It will produce no more stressed-out doctors telling us that we need to reduce our stress levels. Physician/healers will be mature individuals, with good interpersonal skills, who seek to understand health issues in a kind, humble, patient, and non-judgmental manner. The physician's demeanor should have a contagious and beneficial effect upon the client's state of mind. In similar fashion, professors and educators at the Academy will be well balanced, experienced individuals who love to teach and who exhibit similarly desirable qualities. They will not be chosen based upon power, prestige, and the number of scientific papers that they have authored.

The current cut-throat, boot camp, military model of medical education produces overworked, cynical, burnt-out, bleary-eyed warriors against disease. It is understandable that only the exceptional individual is capable of surviving such grueling indoctrination while maintaining the aforementioned characteristics and virtues. A high-stress environment that neglects the emotional and spiritual needs of its trainees only produces highly stressed graduates poorly suited to tending to suffering individuals and their needs.

The principles of healing put into practice by AGMH graduates will begin to significantly reduce iatrogenic disease produced by the practice of mechanistic medicine. The vicious cycle of treatment needed for the side effects of treatment will be broken. Academy graduates will advocate for early education programs that promote the understanding of methods of physical, emotional, and spiritual self-help. They will raise the bar from the current woefully underwhelming standards of hand washing and the food pyramid. By promulgating the values of mutual respect for race, culture, and religious traditions, graduates will create an atmosphere conducive to mental, emotional, and spiritual health. Greater emphasis upon ecological values will increase the odds that changes will be made in time to save Mother Earth and the many forms of life that she supports. These projected changes are idealistic, yes, but even if only partially achieved, they will have an extraordinary effect upon our collective personal, societal, and environmental health.

At some point in the not too distant future, the medical establishment must consciously decide whether it wishes to remain a purely technical science of physical-body repair or if it wishes to embrace holism and the greater quest for healing. It must not be allowed to put forth its beliefs and practices as equivalent to, or an acceptable alternative to, genuine healing that leads to greater overall health. Reality will demand a clear differentiation of the two, and the two will be necessary and complementary components of a comprehensive and unified green health care system that can accommodate the needs of its clients. The role of technician and the role of healer must not be confused. Sometimes physical repair is required and sometimes healing the whole takes precedence.

I hope that I have provided a solid foundation and a compelling rationale that will prompt you to begin questioning the medical status quo and seeking solutions through unconventional and alternative channels. If we make wise and educated decisions regarding our own health care basing them in greater awareness of the issues and stakes involved, we will begin to exert pressure upon the medical establishment to change. Resistance, I believe, will be futile, as the principles described and the forces at play are part of the evolutionary trajectory of our planet and its inhabitants. The green physician/priest/healer/teacher of the future will be knowledgeable in matters of the heart, the mind, the spirit, *and* the physical body. The health care system must open its arms to the unique variety of historical and cross-cultural healing practices and modalities, which can, in turn, then be made available to us all. If not, our only reasonable alternative will be to create a parallel system that focuses its energy upon genuine health and healing. This sort of schism would be less than the ideal, but it is the likely precursor to a more profoundly integrated arrangement of green physicians, healers, technicians, and support staff of the future.

May God/dess bless you on your journey toward greater awareness, wholeness, personal health, and healing. Aho/Amen/Namaste.

Epigraph Credits and Permissions

INTRODUCTION
Richard Grossinger, *Planet Medicine* (Revised edition published by North Atlantic Books, Berkeley, California, 2003), Shambhala Publications, Inc., Boulder, Colorado, 1980, pp. 348–49.

CHAPTER 1
Teilhard de Chardin, *Hymn of the Universe*, William Collins Sons & Co. Ltd., London, Fourth Impression, 1969, p. 83.

CHAPTER 2
Linn J. Boyd, MD, *A Study of the Simile in Medicine*, Boericke and Tafel, Philadelphia, 1936, p. 371.

CHAPTER 3
Vera Stanley Alder, *The Initiation of the World*, Samuel Weiser, Inc., York Beach, Maine, 2000 (first published 1939), p. 21.
Matthew Wood, *The Magical Staff: The Vitalist Tradition in Western Medicine*, North Atlantic Books, Berkeley, California, 1992, pp. xiv–xv.
Thomas Ashley-Farrand, *Healing Mantras: Using Sound Affirmations for Personal Power, Creativity, and Healing*, Ballantine Wellspring, Random House Publishing, New York, 1999, p. 113.

CHAPTER 4
Man and His Symbols, Edited with an Introduction by Carl G. Jung, Dell Publishing Co., Inc., New York, 1964, p. 84.
Richard Grossinger, *Planet Medicine* (Revised edition published by North Atlantic Books, Berkeley, California), Shambhala Publications, Inc., Boulder, Colorado, 1980, p. 371.

CHAPTER 5
George Vithoulkas, *A New Model for Health and Disease*, North Atlantic Books, Berkeley, California, 1991, p. 62.

CHAPTER 6
Teilhard de Chardin, *Hymn of the Universe*, William Collins Sons & Co. Ltd., London, Fourth Impression, 1969, p. 78.
Werner Heisenberg, *Physics and Philosophy: The Revolution in Modern Science*, Harper & Row, New York, 1958, p. 58.

CHAPTER 7
Christian de Quincey, *Radical Knowing: Understanding Consciousness through Relationship*, Park Street Press, Rochester, Vermont, 2005, p. 91.
Teilhard de Chardin, *Hymn of the Universe*, William Collins Sons & Co. Ltd., London, Fourth Impression, 1969, pp. 68–69.

CHAPTER 8

The Wizard of Oz, Noel Langley, Florence Ryerson, Edgar Allen Woolf, from the book by L. Frank Baum, Edited screenplay copyright 1989 by Michael Patrick Hearn, Faber and Faber Limited, 2001, p. 97.

Harris L. Coulter, *Divided Legacy: The Conflict Between Homeopathy and the American Medical Association,* North Atlantic Books, 2nd Edition, 1982, p. xii.

CHAPTER 9

Franz Kafka, *The Metamorphosis,* 1915, from *Franz Kafka: Collected Stories,* Alfred A. Knopf, Inc, New York, 1993, pp. 75, 121, 122, 123.

CHAPTER 10

"I Want a New Drug (Called Love)," By Chris Hayes and Huey Lewis, © 1983 WB Music Corp., Huey Lewis Music and Kinda Blue Music, All Rights Administered by WB Music Corp., All Rights Reserved, used by Permission.

Bumper sticker message.

Ivan Illich, *Limits to Medicine: Medical Nemesis, The Expropriation of Health,* Marion Boyars Publisher, London & New York, 2002 (originally published 1975), p. 166.

CHAPTER 11

Bob Frissell, *You Are a Spiritual Being Having a Human Experience,* Frog, Ltd., Berkeley, California, 2001, p. 86.

Richard Grossinger, *Planet Medicine* (Revised edition published by North Atlantic Books, Berkeley, California), Shambhala Publications, Inc., Boulder, Colorado, 1980, p. 14.

CHAPTER 12

Bobby Petersen, "Unbroken Chain," Grateful Dead lyrics, © Ice Nine Publishing Company. Used with permission.

Olivier Clerc, *Modern Medicine: The New World Religion,* Personhood Press, Fawnskin, CA, 2004, p. xviii .

Linn J. Boyd, MD, *A Study of the Simile in Medicine,* Boericke and Tafel, Philadelphia, 1936, p. 203

CHAPTER 13

Lao Tzu, *Tao Te Ching,* Translation by Stephen Mitchell, Harper Collins, New York, 1988, Chapter 28.

Jocelyn Almond and Keith Seddon, *Egyptian Paganism for beginners,* Llewellyn Publications, St. Paul, Minnesota, 2004, p. 189.

Marvin Meyer, *The Gnostic Gospels of Jesus,* HarperSanFrancisco, 2005, p. 12.

CHAPTER 14

David Spangler, *Explorations: Emerging Aspects of the New Culture,* Findhorn Publications, Lecture Series, Scotland, 1981, p. 30.

Ivan Illich, *Limits to Medicine: Medical Nemesis, The Expropriation of Health,* Marion Boyars Publisher, London & New York, 2002 (originally published 1975), p. 147.

The Gospel of Thomas: Annotated & Explained, Translation and annotation by Stevan Davies, SkyLight Paths Publishing, Woodstock, Vermont, 2002, verse 70.

CHAPTER 15

Manly P. Hall, *The Secret Teachings of All Ages,* Reader's edition, Tarcher/Penguin Books, New York, 2003 (originally published 1928), p. 494.

Nicki Scully, *Alchemical Healing: A Guide to Spiritual, Physical, and Transformational Medicine,* Bear & Company, Rochester, Vermont, 2003, p. 14.

CHAPTER 16

Richard Grossinger, *Planet Medicine* (Revised edition published by North Atlantic Books, Berkeley, California), Shambhala Publications, Inc., Boulder, Colorado, 1980, p. 26.

Jamie Sams, *Sacred Path Cards: The Discovery of Self Through Native Teachings,* HarperSanFrancisco, 1990, p. 271.

CHAPTER 17

Vera Stanley Alder, *The Finding of the Third Eye,* Weiser Books, Boston, 1970, p. 46.

Thomas Merton, *Mystics and Zen Masters,* Farrar, Straus and Giroux, New York, 1967, pp. 72–73.

Robert Hunter, "The Wheel," Grateful Dead lyrics, © Ice Nine Publishing Company. Used with permission.

Notes

INTRODUCTION

1. Thomas Merton, *The Seven Storey Mountain,* Harcourt Brace Jovanovich, Inc., New York and London, 1948.

2. Richard Grossinger, *Planet Medicine* (revised edition currently published by North Atlantic Books, Berkeley, CA), Shambhala Publications, Inc., Boulder, CO, 1980.

3. Alvin Toffler, *Future Shock,* Random House, Inc., New York, 1970.

CHAPTER 1

4. Ted J. Kaptchuk, OMD, *The Web That Has No Weaver: Understanding Chinese Medicine,* Congdon & Weed, New York, 1983, p. 35.

CHAPTER 2

5. Portions of this case history were originally published in *Homeopathy Today,* November 1997, and are reprinted with permission of the National Center for Homeopathy.

CHAPTER 3

6. First lines of the Hippocratic Oath, attributed to Hippocrates, fourth century BCE.

7. Manly P. Hall, *The Secret Teachings of All Ages,* reader's edition, Tarcher/Penguin Books, New York, 2003 (originally published 1928), p. 96.

8. William Sherwood Fox, PhD, *The Mythology of All Races, Volume 1, Greek and Roman,* Marshall Jones Company, Boston, 1916, p. 280.

9. Edward Tick, PhD, *The Practice of Dream Healing,* Quest Books, Theosophical Publishing House, Wheaton, IL, 2001, p. 22.

10. William Sherwood Fox, PhD, *The Mythology of All Races, Volume 1, Greek and Roman,* p. 301.

11. *The Bible, King James* translation, Matthew 10:16.

CHAPTER 4

12. Bill Plotkin, *Soulcraft,* New World Library, Novato, CA, 2003, p. 91.

13. Michael Harner, *The Way of the Shaman,* Harper & Row, Publishers, Inc., 1980.

14. Tom Cowan, *Shamanism as a Spiritual Practice for Daily Life,* Crossing Press, Berkeley, CA, 1996, p. iv.

15. Michael Harner, *The Way of the Shaman,* p. 57.

16. Philip Gardiner and Gary Osborn, *The Serpent Grail,* Watkins Publishing, London, 2005, p. 43.

17. Bill Plotkin, *Soulcraft,* p. 25

18. Bill Plotkin, *Soulcraft,* p. 29

19. *The I Ching,* translated by Hellmut Wilhelm and Cary F. Baynes, Bollingen Series XIX, Princeton University Press, Princeton, NJ, third edition, 1967, p. 10.

20. Mickey Hart, *Drumming at the Edge of Magic,* HarperCollins, New York, 1990, p. 174.

21. Sandra Ingerman, *Soul Retrieval,* HarperSanFrancisco, 1991, pp. 11–12.

CHAPTER 5
22. Rajan Sankaran, *The Spirit of Homeopathy*, Homeopathic Medical Publishers, Bombay, 1994, p. 12.

CHAPTER 6
23. Thomas S. Kuhn, *The Structure of Scientific Revolutions*, The University of Chicago Press, Chicago, second edition, enlarged, 1970, p. 46.

24. Thomas S. Kuhn, *The Structure of Scientific Revolutions*, p. 24.

25. Edward C. Whitmont, MD, *The Alchemy of Healing: Psyche and Soma*, North Atlantic Books, Berkeley, California, 1993, p. 39.

26. Richard Grossinger, *Planet Medicine* (revised edition currently published by North Atlantic Books, Berkeley, California), Shambhala Publications, Inc., Boulder, Colorado, 1980, pp. 23–24.

27. Michael Polanyi, *Personal Knowledge: Towards a Post-Critical Philosophy*, Routledge, London, 1958.

28. Thomas S. Kuhn, *The Structure of Scientific Revolutions*, University of Chicago Press, 1996, pp. 84–85.

29. Thomas S. Kuhn, *The Structure of Scientific Revolutions*, University of Chicago Press, 1996 pp. 150–151.

30. F. David Peat, *Synchronicity: The Bridge Between Matter and Mind*, Bantam Books, 1987, p. 114.

31. Vera Stanley Alder, *The Finding of the Third Eye*, Weiser Books, Boston, first published 1938, this edition 1970, pp. 14–15.

32. Ivan Illich, *Limits to Medicine: Medical Nemesis, The Expropriation of Health*, Marion Boyars Publisher, London & New York, 2002 (originally published 1975), pp. 47, 48.

CHAPTER 7
33. Jean Shinoda Bolen, MD, *The Tao of Psychology: Synchronicity and the Self*, Harper & Row, San Francisco, 1982, p. 9.

34. *The I Ching*, translated by Hellmut Wilhelm and Cary F. Baynes, Bollingen Series XIX, Princeton University Press, Princeton, New Jersey, third edition, 1967, p. xxiv.

35. Jean Shinoda Bolen, MD, *The Tao of Psychology*, pp. 6–7.

36. Christian de Quincey, *Radical Knowing: Understanding Consciousness through Relationship*, Park Street Press, Rochester, Vermont, 2005, pp. 91, 122.

37. Robert Moss, *Dreamways of the Iroquois: Honoring the Secret Wishes of the Soul*, Destiny Books, Rochester, Vermont, 2005, p. 178.

38. Fritjof Capra, *The Tao of Physics: An Exploration of the Parallels between Modern Physics and Eastern Mysticism*, Shambhala, Boston, fourth edition, 2000, p. 56.

39. Ibid, p. 203.

40. Christian de Quincey, *Radical Knowing*, p. 118.

41. Ibid., pp. 119–120.

42. Jean Shinoda Bolen, MD, *The Tao of Psychology*, p. 55.

43. Ervin Laszlo, *Science and the Akashic Field: An Integral Theory of Everything*, Inner Traditions, Rochester, Vermont, second edition, 2007, p. 80.

44. Jean Shinoda Bolen, MD, *The Tao of Psychology*, p. 63.

45. F. David Peat, *Synchronicity: The Bridge Between Matter and Mind*, Bantam Books, 1987, pp. 35, 114.

46. Fritjof Capra, *The Tao of Physics*, p. 327.

47. *The I Ching*, translated by Hellmut Wilhelm and Cary F. Baynes, p. 208.

CHAPTER 8

48. www.fda.gov/bbs/topics/NEWS/2006/NEW01385.html

49. www.fda.gov/bbs/topics/NEWS/2006/NEW01385.html

50. www.909shot.com/Diseases/HPV/HPVrpt.htm

51. www.reuters.com/article/pressRelease/idUS123707+09-Feb-2009+BW20090209, NVIC Vaccine Risk Report Reveals More Serious Reaction Reports After Gardasil, Mon Feb 9, 2009.

52. www.cdc.gov/vaccinesafety/vaers/gardasil.htm, Reports of Health Concerns Following HPV Vaccination.

53. *Direct-to-consumer advertising and expenditures on prescription drugs: a comparison of experiences in the United States and Canada*, Steven G Morgan, Open Medicine, Vol. 1, No 1 (2007), www.openmedicine.ca/article/view/23/26.

54. Kaiser Family Foundation report, *Prescription Drug Trends*, May 2007.

55. Ivan Illich, *Limits to Medicine: Medical Nemesis, The Expropriation of Health*, Marion Boyars Publisher, London & New York, 2002 (originally published 1975), pp. 152, 154.

56. Robert S. Mendelsohn, MD, *Confessions of a Medical Heretic*, Contemporary Books, Chicago, 1979, p. xii.

57. Samuel Hahnemann, MD, *Organon of the Medical Art*, edited and annotated by Wenda Brewster O'Reilly, adapted from the sixth edition of the *Organon*, 1842, Birdcage Books, Redmond, WA, 1996, p. 60.

58. Ivan Illich, *Limits to Medicine: Medical Nemesis, The Expropriation of Health*, p. 170.

59. Robert S. Mendelsohn, MD, *Confessions of a Medical Heretic*, Contemporary Books, Chicago, 1979, pp. 74–75.

60. Ivan Illich, *Limits to Medicine: Medical Nemesis, The Expropriation of Health*, pp. 114–115.

CHAPTER 9

61. *The I Ching*, translated by Hellmut Wilhelm and Cary F. Baynes, Bollingen Series XIX, Princeton University Press, Princeton, NJ, third edition, 1967, p. 217.

62. Ivan Illich, *Limits to Medicine: Medical Nemesis, The Expropriation of Health*, Marion Boyars Publisher, London & New York, 2002 (originally published 1975), pp. 160–161.

63. René Dubos, *Mirage of Health: Utopias, Progress, and Biological Change*, Rutgers University Press, New Brunswick, NJ, 1996 (first published 1959), pp. 71–72.

64. René Dubos, *Mirage of Health: Utopias, Progress, and Biological Change*, pp. 75, 76.

65. René Dubos, *Mirage of Health: Utopias, Progress, and Biological Change*, pp. 67, 72, 74.

66. This translation of the *Emerald Tablet* is taken from Dennis William Hauck's *The Emerald Tablet*, Penguin Compass, New York, 1999, p. 45.

67. Edward C. Whitmont, *Return of the Goddess*, Crossroad Publishing Company, New York, 1982, pp. 57–58.

68. Carol K. Anthony, *The Philosophy of the I Ching*, Anthony Publishing Company, Stow, MA, 1981, p. 8.

CHAPTER 10

69. Robert S. Mendelsohn, MD, *Confessions of a Medical Heretic*, Contemporary Books, Chicago, 1979, pp. x-xi.

70. Ibid, p. xi.

71. Lewis Mumford, *Technics and Civilization*, Harcourt Brace Jovanovich, New York and London, 1963 (originally 1934), p. 4.

72. Ivan Illich, *Limits to Medicine: Medical Nemesis, The Expropriation of Health*, Marion Boyars Publisher, London & New York, 2002 (originally published 1975), pp. 78, 79.

73. Robert S. Mendelsohn, MD, *Confessions of a Medical Heretic*, p. 118.

74. Ivan Illich, *Limits to Medicine: Medical Nemesis, The Expropriation of Health*, pp. 62, 76.

75. Ibid., p. 135.

76. *Is US Health Really the Best in the World?* Barbara Starfield, MD, MPH, Journal of the American Medical Association, Vol. 284, No 4, July 26, 2000.

CHAPTER 11

77. George Vithoulkas, *A New Model of Health and Disease*, North Atlantic Books, Berkeley, CA, 1991, pp. 151–52.

78. George Vithoulkas, *The Science of Homeopathy*, Grove Press, New York, 1980, p. 112.

CHAPTER 12

79. Ivan Illich, *Limits to Medicine: Medical Nemesis, The Expropriation of Health*, Marion Boyars Publisher, London & New York, 2002 (originally published 1975), p. 106

80. Ibid., p. 116

81. René Dubos, *Mirage of Health: Utopias, Progress, and Biological Change*, Rutgers University Press, New Brunswick, NJ, 1996 (first published 1959), p. 157.

82. René Dubos, *Mirage of Health: Utopias, Progress, and Biological Change*, pp. 73–74.

83. Jamie Murphy, *What Every Parent Should Know About Childhood Immunization*, Earth Healing Products, Boston, 1993.

84. Patricia Savage, "A Mother's Research on Immunization," in *Vaccinations: The Rest of the Story*, Mothering Press, Santa Fe, NM, 1992.

85. Neil Miller, *Vaccines*, New Atlantean Press, Santa Fe, NM, 1992.

86. Harris Coulter and Barbara Loe Fisher, *A Shot in the Dark*. First published in 1985, this is one of the first and most historic books on this controversial topic.

87. www.nvic.org, also: www.909shot.com.

88. "First Do No Harm," An interview by Neenyah Ostrom of the Chronic Illness Research Foundation with Barbara Loe Fisher of the National Vaccine Information Center, www.chronicillnet.org/online/Fisher.html.

CHAPTER 13

89. Gareth Knight, *Magic and the Western Mind*, Llewellyn Publications, St. Paul, MN., 1991, p. 59.

90. Edward C. Whitmont, *Return of the Goddess*, Crossroad Publishing Company, New York, 1982, p. vii.

91. Erich Neumann, *The Great Mother: An Analysis of the Archetype*, Bollingen Series XLVII, Princeton University Press, Princeton, NJ, second edition, 1963, p. 212.

92. Jocelyn Almond and Keith Seddon, *Egyptian Paganism for Beginners*, Llewellyn Publications, St. Paul, MN, 2004, pp. 200, 201.

93. Linda Johnsen, *The Living Goddess: Reclaiming the Tradition of the Mother of the Universe*, Yes International Publishers, Saint Paul, MN, 1999, pp. 174, 175.

94. Edward C. Whitmont, *Return of the Goddess*, p. 173.

CHAPTER 14

95. Teilhard de Chardin, *Hymn of the Universe*, William Collins Sons & Co. Ltd., London, Fourth Impression, 1969, pp. 93–94.

96. Bill Plotkin, *Soulcraft*, New World Library, Novato, CA, 2003, p. 50.

CHAPTER 15

97. Dennis William Hauck, *The Emerald Tablet: Alchemy for Personal Transformation*, Penguin Compass, New York, 1999, p. 299.

98. Brian Cotnoir, *The Weiser Concise Guide to Alchemy*, Weiser Books, San Francisco, CA, 2006, p. 16.

99. C. G. Jung, *Psychology and Alchemy*, Bollingen Series, Volume 12, Princeton University Press, Princeton, NJ, second edition, 1968, p. 270.

100. Nicki Scully, *Alchemical Healing: A Guide to Spiritual, Physical, and Transformational Medicine*, Bear & Company, Rochester, VT, 2003, p. 7.

101. Dennis William Hauck, *The Emerald Tablet*, p. 151.

102. Nicki Scully, *Alchemical Healing*, p. 9.

103. Brian Cotnoir, *The Weiser Concise Guide to Alchemy*, p. 52.

104. Dennis William Hauck, *The Emerald Tablet*, p. 305.

105. Dana Ullman, MPH, *The Homeopathic Revolution: Why Famous People and Cultural Heroes Choose Homeopathy*, North Atlantic Books, Berkeley, CA, 2007, pp. 24–28.

106. Harris L. Coulter, *Homeopathic Science and Modern Medicine: The Physics of Healing With Microdoses*, North Atlantic Books, Richmond, CA, 1981, p. 102.

107. Peter O'Connor, *Understanding Jung, Understanding Yourself*, Paulist Press, Mahwah, NJ, 1985, p. 83.

108. Leonard Paul Wershub, MD, F.A.C.S., F.I.C.S., *One Hundred Years of Medical Progress*, Charles C. Thomas, Springfield, IL, 1967, p. 31.

109. Arnold Mindell, *Working with the Dreaming Body*, Routledge & Kegan Paul, London and New York, 1986, p. 9.

110. Ibid., p. 13

111. Ibid., pp. 15, 27

112. *King James Bible*, Numbers 21: 8–9.

113. Ibid., John 3: 14–15.

114. Martin Lass, *Musings of a Rogue Comet: The New Chiron Paradigm,* www.martinlass.com/chirpara.htm, 2003.

CHAPTER 16

115. *King James Bible,* Genesis 1.

116. Ibid., John 1:1.

117. Grace F. Knoche, *The Mystery Schools,* Theosophical University Press, online edition, second and revised edition, 1999 (Originally published in 1940 by Theosophical University Press).

118. Marie-Louise von Franz, *Number and Time,* Northwestern University Press, Evanston, IL, 1974, pp. 105–106.

119. Manly P. Hall, *The Secret Teachings of All Ages,* reader's edition, Tarcher/Penguin Books, New York, 2003 (originally published 1928), p. 201.

120. Vera Stanley Alder, *The Initiation of the World,* Samuel Weiser, Inc., York Beach, ME, 2000 (first published 1939), p. 16.

121. Douglas De Long, *Ancient Teachings for Beginners,* Llewellyn Publications, St. Paul, MN, 2003, p. 138.

122. Matthew Wood, *The Magical Staff: The Vitalist Tradition in Western Medicine,* North Atlantic Books, Berkeley, CA, 1992, pp. xiii, xiv, xv.

123. John A. Sanford, *Dreams and Healing,* Paulist Press, New York, 1978, p. 8.

124. Thomas Mann, *Joseph and His Brothers, Volume IV: Joseph the Provider,* Alfred A. Knopf, New York, 1944, pp. 119, 120.

125. Robert Moss, *Dreamways of the Iroquois: Honoring the Secret Wishes of the Soul,* Destiny Books, Rochester, VT, 2005, p. 11.

126. Tom Cowan, *Fire in the Head: Shamanism and the Celtic Spirit,* HarperSanFrancisco, 1993, p. 17.

Bibliography

Alder, Vera Stanley. *The Finding of the Third Eye*. Boston: Weiser Books, 1970 (first published 1938).

———. *The Initiation of the World*. York Beach, ME: Samuel Weiser, Inc., 2000 (first published 1939).

Almond, Jocelyn, and Keith Seddon. *Egyptian Paganism for Beginners*. St. Paul, MN: Llewellyn Publications, 2004.

Anthony, Carol K. *The Philosophy of the I Ching*. Stow, MA: Anthony Publishing Company, 1981.

Ashley-Farrand, Thomas. *Healing Mantras: Using Sound Affirmations for Personal Power, Creativity, and Healing*. New York: Ballantine Wellspring, Random House Publishing, 1999.

The Bible translation. www.Biblos.com.

Bolen, MD, Jean Shinoda. *The Tao of Psychology: Synchronicity and the Self*. San Francisco: Harper & Row, 1982.

Boyd, MD, Linn J. *A Study of the Simile in Medicine*. Philadelphia: Boericke and Tafel, 1936.

Capra, Fritjof. *The Tao of Physics: An Exploration of the Parallels Between Modern Physics and Eastern Mysticism*. Boston: Shambhala, fourth edition, 2000.

Clerc, Olivier. *Modern Medicine: The New World Religion*. Fawnskin, CA: Personhood Press, 2004.

Cotnoir, Brian. *The Weiser Concise Guide to Alchemy*. San Francisco: Weiser Books, 2006.

Coulter, Harris L. *Divided Legacy: The Conflict Between Homeopathy and the American Medical Association*. Berkeley, CA: North Atlantic Books, second edition, 1982.

———. *Homeopathic Science and Modern Medicine: The Physics of Healing with Microdoses*. Berkeley, CA: North Atlantic Books, 1981.

Coulter, Harris L., and Barbara Loe Fisher. *A Shot in the Dark*. Avery Trade, 1991.

Cowan, Tom. *Fire in the Head: Shamanism and the Celtic Spirit*. HarperSanFrancisco, 1993.

———. *Shamanism as a Spiritual Practice for Daily Life*. Berkeley, CA: Crossing Press, 1996.

de Chardin, Teilhard. *Hymn of the Universe*. London: William Collins Sons & Co. Ltd., Fourth Impression, 1969.

De Long, Douglas. *Ancient Teachings for Beginners*. St. Paul, MN: Llewellyn Publications, 2003.

de Quincey, Christian. *Radical Knowing: Understanding Consciousness through Relationship*. Rochester, VT: Park Street Press, 2005.

Dubos, René. *Mirage of Health: Utopias, Progress, and Biological Change*. New Brunswick, NJ: Rutgers University Press, 1996 (first published 1959).

Fisher, Barbara Loe. An interview by Neenyah Ostrom of the Chronic Illness Research Foundation. "First Do No Harm." www.chronicillnet.org/online/Fisher.html.

Fox, PhD, William Sherwood. *The Mythology of All Races, Volume 1, Greek and Roman*. Boston: Marshall Jones Company, 1916.

Frissell, Bob. *You Are a Spiritual Being Having a Human Experience.* Berkeley, CA: Frog, Ltd., 2001.

Gardiner, Philip, and Gary Osborn. *The Serpent Grail.* London: Watkins Publishing, 2005.

The Gospel of Thomas: Annotated & Explained. Translation and annotation by Stevan Davies. Woodstock, VT: SkyLight Paths Publishing, 2002.

Grossinger, Richard. *Planet Medicine.* Boulder, CO: Shambhala Publications, Inc., 1980 (revised edition currently published by North Atlantic Books, Berkeley, CA, 2005).

Hahnemann, MD, Samuel. *Organon of the Medical Art.* Edited and annotated by Wenda Brewster O'Reilly, Adapted from the sixth edition of the *Organon,* 1842. Redmond, Washington: Birdcage Books, 1996.

Hall, Manly P. *The Secret Teachings of All Ages,* reader's edition. New York: Tarcher/Penguin Books, 2003 (originally published 1928).

Harner, Michael. *The Way of the Shaman.* Harper & Row, Publishers, Inc., 1980.

Hart, Mickey. *Drumming at the Edge of Magic.* New York: HarperCollins, 1990.

Hauck, Dennis William. *The Emerald Tablet: Alchemy for Personal Transformation.* New York: Penguin Compass, 1999.

Heisenberg, Werner. *Physics and Philosophy: The Revolution in Modern Science.* New York: Harper & Row, 1958.

Homeopathy Today. Newsletter of the National Center for Homeopathy. Alexandria, VA: November 1997.

The I Ching, or Book of Changes. Translated by Hellmut Wilhelm and Cary F. Baynes. Bollingen Series XIX. Princeton, NJ: Princeton University Press, third edition, 1967.

Illich, Ivan. *Limits to Medicine: Medical Nemesis, The Expropriation of Health.* London & New York: Marion Boyars Publisher, 2002 (originally published 1975).

Ingerman, Sandra. *Soul Retrieval.* HarperSanFrancisco, 1991.

Johnsen, Linda. *The Living Goddess: Reclaiming the Tradition of the Mother of the Universe.* Saint Paul, MN: Yes International Publishers, 1999.

Jung, C.G. "Approaching the Unconscious." In *Man and His Symbols.* Edited by C.G. Jung. New York: Dell Publishing Co., Inc., 1964.

————. *Psychology and Alchemy.* Bollingen Series, Volume 12, Princeton, NJ: Princeton University Press, second edition, 1968.

Kafka, Franz. *The Metamorphosis.* 1915, from *Franz Kafka: Collected Stories.* New York: Alfred A. Knopf, inc., 1993.

Kaptchuk, OMD, Ted J. *The Web That Has No Weaver: Understanding Chinese Medicine.* New York: Congdon & Weed, 1983.

Knight, Gareth. *Magic and the Western Mind.* St. Paul, MN: Llewellyn Publications, 1991.

Knoche, Grace F. *The Mystery Schools.* Theosophical University Press, online edition, second and revised edition, 1999 (Originally published in 1940 by Theosophical University Press).

Kuhn, Thomas S. *The Structure of Scientific Revolutions.* Chicago: The University of Chicago Press, second edition, enlarged, 1970.

Langley, Noel, with Florence Ryerson and Edgar Allen Woolf. *The Wizard of Oz, The Screenplay.* From the book by L. Frank Baum. Edited by Michael Patrick Hearn. London: Faber and Faber Limited, 2001.

Lao Tzu. *Tao Te Ching.* Translation by Stephen Mitchell, New York: Harper Collins, 1988.

Lass, Martin. "Musings of a Rogue Comet: The New Chiron Paradigm." Available from: Chiron Astrology and Healing Pages. www.martinlass.com/chirpara.htm, 2003.

Laszlo, Ervin. *Science and the Akashic Field: An Integral Theory of Everything.* Rochester, VT: Inner Traditions, second edition, 2007.

Mann, Thomas. *Joseph and His Brothers, Volume IV: Joseph the Provider.* New York: Alfred A. Knopf, 1944.

Mendelsohn, MD, Robert S., *Confessions of a Medical Heretic.* Chicago: Contemporary Books, 1979.

Merton, Thomas. *Mystics and Zen Masters.* New York: Farrar, Straus and Giroux, 1967.

———. *The Seven Storey Mountain.* New York and London: Harcourt Brace Jovanovich, inc., 1948.

Meyer, Marvin. *The Gnostic Gospels of Jesus.* HarperSanFrancisco, 2005.

Miller, Neil. *Vaccines.* Santa Fe, NM: New Atlantean Press, 1992.

Mindell, Arnold. *Working with the Dreaming Body.* London and New York: Routledge & Kegan Paul, 1986.

Moss, Robert. *Dreamways of the Iroquois: Honoring the Secret Wishes of the Soul.* Rochester, VT: Destiny Books, 2005.

Mumford, Lewis. *Technics and Civilization.* New York and London: Harcourt Brace Jovanovich, 1963 (originally published 1934).

Murphy, Jamie. *What Every Parent Should Know About Childhood Immunization.* Boston: Earth Healing Products, 1993.

National Vaccine Information Center. www.nvic.org; also, www.909shot.com.

Neumann, Erich. *The Great Mother: An Analysis of the Archetype.* Bollingen Series XLVII, Princeton, NJ: Princeton University Press, second edition, 1963.

"NVIC Vaccine Risk Report Reveals More Serious Reaction Reports After Gardasil." Reuters Web site: www.reuters.com/article/pressRelease/idUS123707+09-Feb-2009+BW20090209. Feb 9, 2009.

O'Connor, Peter. *Understanding Jung, Understanding Yourself.* Mahwah, NJ: Paulist Press, 1985.

Peat, F. David. *Synchronicity: The Bridge Between Matter and Mind.* New York: Bantam Books, 1987.

Plotkin, Bill. *Soulcraft.* Novato, California: New World Library, 2003.

Polanyi, Michael. *Personal Knowledge: Towards a Post-Critical Philosophy.* London: Routledge, 1958.

"Reports of Health Concerns Following HPV Vaccination." Centers for Disease Control and Prevention Web site: www.cdc.gov/vaccinesafety/vaers/gardasil.htm.

Sams, Jamie. *Sacred Path Cards: The Discovery of Self Through Native Teachings.* HarperSanFrancisco, 1990.

Sanford, John A. *Dreams and Healing.* New York: Paulist Press, 1978.

Sankaran, Rajan. *The Spirit of Homeopathy.* Bombay: Homeopathic Medical Publishers, 1994.

Savage, Patricia. "A Mother's Research on Immunization," in *Vaccinations: The Rest of the Story,* Santa Fe, NM: Mothering Press, 1992.

Scully, Nicki. *Alchemical Healing: A Guide to Spiritual, Physical, and Transformational Medicine.* Rochester, VT: Bear & Company, 2003.

Spangler, David. *Explorations: Emerging Aspects of the New Culture.* Scotland: Findhorn Publications, Lecture Series, 1981.

Tick, Edward, PhD *The Practice of Dream Healing.* Quest Books, Wheaton, IL: Theosophical Publishing House, 2001.

Toffler, Alvin. *Future Shock.* New York: Random House, inc., 1970.

Ullman, MPH, Dana. *The Homeopathic Revolution: Why Famous People and Cultural Heroes Choose Homeopathy.* Berkeley, CA: North Atlantic Books, 2007.

U.S. Food and Drug Administration Web site. www.fda.gov/bbs/topics/NEWS/2006/NEW01385.html

Image Credits and Permissions

3.1. Imhotep: Bronze statuette, the Louvre, Paris, Source/Photographer: Hu Totya, Creative Commons Attribution Share Alike 3.0 License.

3.2. Thoth in ibis form: Kunsthistorisches Museum, Vienna, Author: Gryffindor, Creative Commons Attribution ShareAlike 3.0 License (June 2006).

3.3. Asklepios: Epidaurus Museum, Mycenae, Greece, courtesy of Michael F. Mehnert, Creative Commons Attribution ShareAlike 3.0 License (9/11/2008).

4.1. Shaman: modeled after a cup found in the Craig Mound, Le Flore County, Oklahoma, courtesy of Heironymous Rowe, Creative Commons Attribution ShareAlike 3.0 License (2008).

4.2. *I Ching* Hexagram 2: courtesy of Ben Finney.

4.3. Shaman's Drum from Tibet: Source: Vassil, on Wikipedia, public domain (6/04/2007).

7.1. Ouroboros: from Greek alchemical manuscript.

7.2. *I Ching* Hexagram 53: courtesy of Ben Finney.

8.1. Thoth: Photo by Jon Bodsworth, www.egyptarchive.co.uk/html/luxor_temple_15.html (11/12/2006).

9.1. *I Ching* Hexagram 56: courtesy of Ben Finney.

13.1. Egyptian Queen Isis: courtesy of The Yorck Project.

15.1. Paracelsus.

15.2. Various Alchemical Symbols for Zinc.

15.3. Hahnemann Monument: Scott Circle, Washington, DC, courtesy of AgnosticPreachersKid, Creative Commons Attribution ShareAlike 3.0 License (6/27/2008).

16.1. Anubis.

Index

About the Author

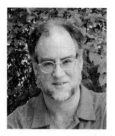

Larry Malerba, D.O., has been a practitioner, educator, and leader in the field of holistic medicine for more than twenty years. He is Clinical Assistant Professor at New York Medical College, is board certified in Homeotherapeutics, and is a frequent lecturer at Albany Medical College, the Albany College of Pharmacy, and the SUNY Utica Nursing Program. He is the author of numerous articles in alternative medical journals—including the *American Journal of Homeopathic Medicine* (where he was assistant editor from 2002–2006) and the *New England Journal of Homeopathy*—and has held positions as president (Homeopathic Medical Society of the State of New York), vice president (American Institute of Homeopathy), and board member of various conventional and homeopathic organizations. In addition, Dr. Malerba has edited journals and newsletters, organized conferences, created educational programs for a variety of organizations, and appeared on TV and radio programs including National Public Radio and Vox Pop. He lives and maintains a private practice in upstate New York.